Guide for the Beginning Researcher

The torch shall be extinguished which hath lit
My midnight lamp—and what is writ, is writ;
Would it were worthier!

> Lord Byron
> Childe Harold's Pilgrimage

Marsha Rowland

Guide for the Beginning Researcher

MABEL A. WANDELT, R.N., PH.D.

Professor of Nursing, College of
Nursing, Wayne State University,
Detroit, Michigan

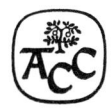

APPLETON-CENTURY-CROFTS
EDUCATIONAL DIVISION / MEREDITH CORPORATION
New York

Copyright © 1970 by MEREDITH CORPORATION

All rights reserved. This book, or parts thereof, must not be used or reproduced in any manner without written permission. For information address the publisher, Appleton-Century-Crofts, Educational Division, Meredith Corporation, 440 Park Avenue South, New York, New York 10016.

7111-2

Library of Congress Catalog Card Number: 74-109163

Second Printing

PRINTED IN THE UNITED STATES OF AMERICA
390-91860-1

To my students:

They made it necessary for me to think.

Acknowledgments

All who endeavor to contribute, in whatever way, to assistance and welfare of fellow humans are aware that no contribution is an individual or solo work. Any endeavor that results in worth to others is supported and enhanced by more persons that the credited individual can even know, let alone name by way of acknowledging the assistance. These writings are no exception.

Primarily, I am indebted to students. By dedicating the writings to them, and by expressing appreciation to the students whose works are cited in references, I express appreciation to individuals and to the many students from whom I have learned and whose works may have served equally well to illustrate various points in the book.

I believe that each faculty colleague has provided some elements of assistance. From some, there has been moral support; from many, accommodations of schedules and assumption of various faculty responsibilities to relieve me for prolonged periods of writing. Dean Margaret L. Shetland and Miss Mildred Gottdank, Professor and Director of the Graduate Program of the College, must be credited with large contributions in the latter areas. Sr. Rosemary McLain, Miss Kathlene Monahan, and Mrs. Dawn Zagornik, Assistant Professors of Nursing, and Dr. Joyce Passos, Associate Professor and Chairman of the Medical-Surgical Nursing Department, read and made valuable criticisms of the writings. I am grateful to them for their guidance to improved presentation and for their encouragement, which gave confidence in the worth of the work.

Miss Maria C. Phaneuf, Associate Professor and Chairman of the Public Health Nursing Department, merits the gratitude of the reader, as well as my own. She read and criticized virtually every draft, beginning with general comments about early drafts and persisting to offer precise criticisms of detailed facets of the final draft. It is to her that I must make acknowledgment of my indebtedness for much of the good in the writings and of my assumption of all responsibility for retained flaws and limitations.

Mrs. Edith Patton Lewis accepted the task of editing the manuscript. All "good" terms used to describe the process and results of editing apply to the work she did—eliminated wordiness, tightened presentation, clarified ideas, preserved my meaning and tone—in short, improved the entire text. The scope and artistry of her contribution, although they cannot be known by others, deserve extensive praise and acknowledgment. There are no words and there is no way adequately to express my appreciation.

My family have long since accepted my nondependability; once more they have put up with my busyness and stood available when I needed them. It is impossible to thank my mother, and the others, for their patience, understanding, and acceptance in respecting my time and freedom to do what I think I must do. They continue to care.

To the many friends who have variously expressed tolerance of my asocial behavior, including not crossing me off their Christmas card lists, I say, "I have not been unaware, and I thank you."

Preface

This book is addressed to nurses seeking an introduction to research and guidelines to problem solving. They may possess various educational backgrounds, and the reasons for their interest may be varied. A major purpose, in addition to providing an introductory text for students, is to encourage all nurses to expand their visions of the meaning of research. It is hoped that many will be prompted to view themselves as participants in, contributors to, and replicators of research, as well as users of research findings. The guides will serve all who are concerned with the study of health related problems: whether they be students or practitioners, and whether their interest be assessment of patient care problems, problem solving, or research.

The outline of 13 steps composing the research process evolved as I planned a short-term course for nurses interested in quickly learning to do fact-finding studies. The approach proved so successful that I adopted it for teaching masters students. The several concepts in each step are delineated in precise terms, rather than with generalizations and abstractions usually selected to describe them. Although the presentation may at times seem overly simplified and too rigidly patterned, my experience with students has been that these devices are useful. The beginner can achieve understanding more expeditiously when he is provided with a framework of concretes, unobscured by the many shadings of qualifying statements about when, and under what conditions, concepts do and do not apply. The discussions of the steps are essentially a blueprint to planning and executing any study where facts are sought to enhance understanding, to reveal new knowledge, or to serve as bases for alleviation or solution of problems.

The 13 steps have been effectively used to introduce the beginner to the total process of scientific inquiry. Individual steps have proved useful, both within and outside of a research context, when concern has been with specific aspects of search for and utilization of facts. For example, Step 3, Definition of Terms, and Step 5, Kinds of Data Needed, are helpful for practitioners and teachers concerned with evaluation processes. Steps 12 and 13, Outcomes, provide supervisors, administrators, and researchers, as well as practitioners and teachers, with guides for identifying meanings of facts and proposing reasonable courses of action. In other words, the book may be used as a guide for developing a plan for a complete study, or it may serve as a reference for planning particular phases of securing and utilizing facts.

Contents

Acknowledgments		vii
Preface		ix
Contents		xi
Foreword	Margaret L. Shetland	xiii
Introduction		xv

STEP

1	Definition of Problem	1
2	Statement of Purpose (Determine the Focus for Study)	63
3	Definitions of Terms	101
4	Assumptions	127
5	Kinds of Data Needed	133
6	Method of Study and Sources of Data	161
7	Techniques	181
8	Tools	201
9	Collection of Data	223
10	Organization of Data (Coding, Tabulation, Classifying)	239
11	Analysis of Data	259
12 & 13	Outcomes	291
Glossary		313
Index		319

Foreword

Nursing is generally agreed that the body of knowledge on which the practice of nursing should be based must be developed and structured. Primarily derivative in nature, at least at this time, nursing depends upon the selection, systematic application, and evaluation of knowledge from basic sciences. It is through the creativity with which this knowledge is utilized in advancing nursing practice and in modifying the systems for providing nursing services that nursing evolves its own significant contribution to the human good. Thus, nursing is developing its own body of knowledge.

There is less agreement, and rightfully so, among nurse educators as to the appropriate methods and the placement of organized content dealing with the process of systematic investigations. Many believe that the approach to teaching and learning of professional nursing should be a process of problem identification, selection of knowledge from the basic and related sciences, formulation of approaches based upon assessment and relative knowledge, application, and evaluation. Unfortunately, in spite of verbal acceptance of investigative approaches to nursing practice, the fact is that much of nursing remains largely imitative and intuitive rather than creative, empirical, or scientific in nature. In order to reverse this emphasis in actual practice, more nurses must be introduced to the methodology of systematic investigations in a formal manner.

Doctor Wandelt's book grew out of her years of experience in introducing graduate students in nursing to research methods. The demand for her to put together the materials that she has developed has come from her former students. Students moving on to doctoral study have shared their class materials with their student colleagues in other disciplines who also find them useful. Some may criticize the approach as simplistic or limiting. This is not the intention of the author who envisions the framework she presents as an orderly plan within which individual creativity can be pursued.

MARGARET L. SHETLAND, R.N., ED.D.
Dean, College of Nursing,
Wayne State University,
Detroit, Michigan

Introduction

Research is a many faceted process. However, the detailed description of the 13 steps into which the process may logically be outlined should help the beginning researcher to understand and use this complex process. Each step will be introduced with definitions of pertinent terms. Although the student will be familiar with most of them, the definitions of these terms, as they are used in research parlance, will be new: if not in basic concept, at least in specific referents. By way of introducing the steps of the research process and the mechanism of defining terms for clarification of concepts, the term, *research*, will be first defined.

There are almost as many definitions of research as there are researchers; certainly, there are as many definitions as there are definers. The definitions vary from the simple: "Research is an organized investigation of a problem," to 10-page chapters in books titled *Introduction to Research*. A succinct, usable definition was proposed in 1956 by the Committee on Research of the American Public Health Association:

Definition of Research

> Research is the studying of a problem in pursuit of a definite objective through employing precise methods, with due consideration to the adequate control of factors other than the variable under investigation and followed by analysis according to acceptable statistical procedures.[1]

This definition, however, leaves many types of bona fide scientific investigations outside the realm of research. A more encompassing, yet still simple, definition uses elements from the APHA definitions and others:

> Research is a quest for new knowledge pertinent to an identified area of interest (a problem), through application of the scientific process. Essential components of the process are:

—definition of the problem, including what others have experienced, learned, and thought about the problem;

—delineation of the focus for study (specification of the particular dimension of the problem on which inquiry will focus);

—determination of the facts pertinent to the focus (selected from among those identified as being germane to the problem);

—employment of appropriate and expedient techniques and precise measurements for collection of facts, with due consideration to adequate control of factors other than the variable under investigation;

—decisions about degrees of breadth and depth sought, which in turn, influence the nature, scope, and sources of facts, as well as the characteristics of subjects, selected for study;

—submission of quantitative or quantifiable data to statistical analysis;

—selection of the data analyses to be done (statistical, theoretical, and descriptive), and use of original, imaginative thinking to reveal previously unrecognized relationships between or among variables;

—proposals of generalizations based on findings and applicable to populations larger than the one studied—included will be hypotheses recommended for testing in future investigations. (Hypotheses, explicit or implicit, are part of all scientific investigations: as focuses to guide the pursuit of a study, hypotheses are sometimes left implicit; as outcomes of analyses of facts collected in a study, they will be made explicit.);

—presentation of findings and results of analyses in communicative and verifiable form.

Identification of specific elements in the scientific process fosters recognition of the broad applicability of the process of research to the search for knowledge and for understanding of phenomena. It underscores the appropriateness of the research process for organizing, planning, and guiding various types of investigations, in addition to those concerned with testing hypotheses. And it encourages inclusion of descriptive, exploratory studies in the realm of scientific inquiry.

Research Versus Problem Solving

Problem solving may be defined in a construction paralleling the definition of research:

Problem solving is a systematic approach to the solution or alleviation of simple, complex, immediate, or long-term problems, characterized by sequential execution of the following observational, thought, and action processes:

—identification and definition of the elements composing the problem and interrelationships among the elements;

—specification of the crux of the problem, along with theorizing about relevance of background facts and theories;
—determination and systematic collection of facts germane to the proposed crux of the problem;
—analysis, interpretation, and synthesis of the collected facts along with previously known facts and theories judged to be relevant to the problem;
—proposal of strategic courses of action calculated to solve or alleviate the problem;
—selection of a course of action;
—action;
—observation and evaluation of outcomes of action, followed as warranted by modifications in the course of action.

Problem solving and research are frequently compared, sometimes to the extent that they are purported to be one and the same thing. Nonetheless, if the researcher and the problem solver keep in mind the fundamental difference between the two, they will avoid many pitfalls along the paths to their different goals.

The fundamental difference is that of purpose. *The purpose of research is to reveal new knowledge; the purpose of problem solving is to solve an immediate problem in a particular setting.* The fact that knowledge obtained through research may contribute to the solution of a problem, or that an exercise in problem solving may reveal new knowledge applicable beyond the immediate problem, does not alter the validity of this fundamental difference. Many process differences between research and problem solving may be noted, but these vary with each situation cited, whereas the fundamental difference is constant and applies in all situations.

Some of the process differences may be identified by considering the elements essential to research and noting the nature and degree of differences of parallel elements in problem solving.

Process Differences

RESEARCH

All elements of a scientific inquiry must be explicitly and precisely described.

Where research data are quantitative or quantifiable, they are analyzed with appropriate statistical procedures.

PROBLEM SOLVING

The same explicitness and precision, though they may be utilized, are not usually demanded of problem solving.

Detailed statistical analyses are seldom done, and quantitative data are usually limited to simple frequency counts.

Elaborate pains are taken to control for factors other than the variable under study.	Such controls are not imposed.
A primary aim is to ensure that findings are generalizable to a population larger than the one subject to study.	The primary aim is the solution of a problem existing in the population being studied; addresses little or no attention to whether findings may be expected to apply to a larger population.
The search for new knowledge through hypothesis testing must be done in a setting and with study subjects different from those which gave rise to the observations that prompted the study and hypotheses (lest there be circularity: from problem, to evidence, to "proof").	The facts for the investigation are always gathered in the same setting and from many of the same subjects that gave rise to the proposal that the study be done.
Entails a plan written in sufficient detail and explicitness that the study may be replicated and the findings verified.	Entails no such requirements.
The researcher has the moral obligation to report his findings in writing that others may share the new knowledge.	The problem solver needs only to provide information, in verbal or tabular form, to those in the immediate setting of the problem and to propose changes that will help them solve the problem that prompted the study.

To be classed as research or scientific inquiry, an investigation must encompass all of the elements delineated in the definition of research. On the other hand, problem solving, while it may encompass many of these elements, need not include all of them; in problem solving, measurement may be less precise, and subject and process identification, less specific. Research *must* utilize the many process steps attributed to it, and problem solving *may* utilize all the steps. But, always, purpose as previously delineated, is the fundamental difference between the two.

Of Equal Value

In discussions about research and problem solving, one sometimes hears expressions of differences in values, with the implication that research is "better," a more worthy endeavor, an exercise providing greater status for the investigator. Such a belief, of course, is ridiculous and reveals a lack of understanding of the two concepts. Since each is undertaken for a specific purpose, the purpose of one being quite different from that of the other, one can not be "better" than the other. It is no more reasonable to say that research is better than problem solving as a method of inquiry than it would be to say that an atomic-powered passenger liner is better than a surfboard as a mode of travel. The surfboarder is apt to be bored to distraction by the inactivity imposed by the passenger liner, whereas, the passenger liner could hardly be replaced by a surfboard for intercontinental travel.

Just as the process of problem solving can not be expected to yield data in the form of new knowledge generalizable to a larger population, so the process of research cannot be expected to produce information necessary to solve an immediate problem. Each of the two processes is invaluable for attaining the outcomes it was designed to produce, for accomplishing its specific purpose.

The process of research may be divided into varying numbers of phases or steps along varying lines of consideration. There may be a simple categorization of phases, such as the 4-phase outline: (1) planning, (2) data collection, (3) data analyzing, and (4) report writing. Some have proposed as many as 20 or more phases. There is a general agreement, however, that there is a meshing of the content and the developmental thinking between various phases. This is equally true for the 13 steps or phases to be outlined here; elements of one step will overlap and mesh with those of other steps, and the student should never be unmindful of this fact. Yet, despite this constant mingling of elements between steps, it is possible to designate particular phases of the process, as identifiable entities—ones which may be placed in a sequential hierarchy of steps. The 13 steps herein identified are suggested as the major steps that must be undertaken, in sequence, both in developing and in executing the plan for an investigation. Each step will be discussed as a separate entity.

Major Steps in the Research Process

Guide for the Beginning Researcher

STEP 1
DEFINITION OF PROBLEM

TERMS DEFINED

Problem: The problem may be thought of simply as an "irritation": the irritation that stimulates interest and prompts investigation.

Problem-defined: The problem-defined must be thought of as a complex entity, and it may be viewed as being made up of seven components:

1. The irritation: portrayed in a real live story
2. Elements in the situation: factors supporting, causing, impinging upon the problem
3. The problem in its largest universe: what others have experienced, learned, and thought about the problem
4. The ideal situation: no problem exists
5. Suggestions for moving toward the ideal
6. Potential results of each suggestion in Component 5
7. Investigator's frame of reference.

Component: A component is any of the simple or compound parts of some complex thing or concept.*

---

* Excerpts and bases for definitions of all terms in this text are from *Webster's New World Dictionary of the American Language, College Edition*. New York, The World Publishing Company, 1962.

Component of a problem-defined: A component of a problem-defined may be thought of as being composed of many elements and possessing many facets.

Element: An element is a basic, irreducible part or principle of anything, concrete or abstract.

Facet: Facet, literally or figuratively, applies to any of the faces of a many-sided object (facets of a diamond, personality, etc.).

Entity: An entity is a being or existence; a thing that has real and individual existence, in reality or in the mind; anything real in itself.

Crux: A crux is a crucial point: the essential or most important point; a critical moment.

Crux of the problem: The crux of the problem is the focal point around which the problem will be defined. It is the "irritation" identified and selected by the researcher as the one about which he thinks something should be done. It is the manifestation of the problem about which he proposes to seek new and extended knowledge, with the view to contributing to alleviation of the problem.

Fact: A fact is an observable phenomenon or entity.

Phenomenon: A phenomenon is any fact, circumstance, or experience that is apparent to the senses and that can be scientifically described or appraised: as bereavement is a psychological phenomenon; the appearance or observed features of something experienced as distinguished from reality of the thing itself.

The concept of phenomenon encompasses the concept of entity. That is, phenomenon is a more encompassing concept than entity. An oversimplification, for the sake of distinguishing the two, is to view an entity (a being or existence) as a "thing," and a phenomenon as a "thing" *or* a "process." From this, all entities may be classed as phenomena, but not all phenomena are limited to the category of "static" entity. For example, the fact or observation of a leaf on a tree may be identified as either an entity or a phenomenon. The fact or observation of a leaf falling from a tree would be classed as a phenomenon; it would not be classed as an entity.

CONCEPTS PERTINENT TO DEFINED TERMS

A clear distinction between "problem" and "purpose" would seem essential to soundly conceived research and accurate interpretation of findings. Yet these terms, with varying definitions and associated concepts, are frequently used interchangeably. The result is confusion—not only for students first learning about the research process, but also for sophisticated scientists trying to communicate with one another about research. Because most researchers use the terms interchangeably, although they also endeavor to define them as individual entities, it is difficult to identify exactly how they usually use these terms. Generally speaking, though, their usage may be summarized as follows:

A problem is a felt difficulty, a condition that needs to be improved. The problem must be defined. The researcher, through a review of the literature, must determine what others have learned about the problem. As a part of the definition of the problem, he will use this information, along with what he knows about it, to develop a theoretical framework to illustrate the interrelationship of the various elements of the problem—to provide a context in which the various elements may be visualized and discussed.

Most researchers propose that the "stated purpose" of the study identifies the solution to be sought for the "problem" and, further, that the "problem for study" derives from the stated purpose. These proposals are followed by instructions about stating the "problem for study" with suggestions that the "statement of the problem for study" takes the form of hypotheses to be tested, or questions to be answered, or specifically identified information to be sought.

Herein lie the difficulties: the problem is first described as the felt difficulty, the something that needs to be solved. The purpose is described as identification of the solution of the problem. Then the term "problem" is again used—but this time to identify the specific element or elements composing the "problem" about which information will be sought. The above sequence involves (1) recognizing a problem (a felt difficulty), (2) defining the problem, (3) deciding on the purpose for the study (the solution of the problem through research), and then (4) delineating the "problem for study." The explanation given for this design is that the problem for study is derived from the purpose for the study. Such planning obviously involves using the term "problem" to denote two distinct concepts and to identify two distinct steps in the research process.

Confusion: Problem Denoting Two Entities

This dual concept of problem used by some researchers to suggest that the problem derives from the purpose can be illustrated and perhaps clarified by an analogy: constructing or setting up a problem in mathematics. The irritation (that which prompts the investigation) presented to the mathematician for solution might be the increase in automobile accidents on a certain highway. The purpose of the study might be to determine the stretches of highway with high and low accident rates. The mathematician would construct "problems" to be solved through calculations of relationships between numbers of vehicles, rates of speed, miles of highway, times of day, and so forth. When these "problems" have been solved—that is, when there are answers to these "problems"—it might be anticipated that

Analogy: "Problem" in Mathematics

there would be new knowledge applicable to planning for actions for the alleviation of the original irritation.

Thus, in this analogy, the problems of study (calculations of relationships among rates of speed, number of vehicles, times of day, and so forth) derived from the desire to learn something about a particular aspect of the larger problem. The aspect of the larger problem to be studied was identified in the stated purpose of the study: to determine stretches of highway with high and low accident rates. Although this reasoning is valid, it makes for confusion in communication. Identification of the elements in the process requires the use of the word "problem" to mean two very distinct entities: (1) the original irritation and all elements and theories appertaining to it, and (2) the constructed pattern (mathematical problem or other ideational construct) that will serve to identify facts and show relationships among them that will lead to new information about the original "problem." Furthermore, the conceptualization—implicitly, if not explicitly—suggests that the purpose of the investigation is to solve the original problem. When the word "purpose" is so used in planning research, the investigator tends to be influenced throughout his planning by concern for solution of a specific problem in a particular setting. This concern blocks him from focusing attention on the acquisition of new knowledge that may be applicable to the problem situation in any setting.

Don't Interchange Problem and Purpose

It is the contention of this book, therefore, that there are multiple reasons for not interchanging the use of these two terms; that it is possible to identify distinct meanings for each of them and to eliminate the need to use them interchangeably; and that each can be used to refer to a single and separate step in the research process.

Before elaboration of the meanings and concepts denoted by the two terms, "problem" and "purpose," however, here is one initial and ready reminder that may be helpful in clarifying the distinct meaning of each term: refer only to *"definition* of the problem" and to *"statement* of purpose," and don't interchange these accompanying words. This is a reasonable rule, if the problem is viewed as the irritation along with all the many elements that compose it, and the purpose is viewed as the single precise statement that identifies the focus of the investigation.

Thus, the definition of problem will identify and describe the many elements and their various facets of which the problem is composed. The statement of purpose will identify one particular set of elements of the problem about which new knowledge will be sought. Distinguishing between the two terms in this way reminds us also that the goal of research is not the solution of particular problems but, rather, the revelation of new knowledge.

The problem should be perceived as an entity too large to be the subject of a single investigation. Any one problem is composed of so many varied elements that no single investigation could possibly be devised to seek information that would provide a complete solution to it. The most that can be planned and hoped for in a single investigation is information related to a single facet of the problem that will serve as a basis for its partial alleviation or, at least, information that will add to prior knowledge and thereby contribute to alleviation of the problem. The purpose, in contrast, is the identification of the particular facet about which information is to be sought in any one scientific investigation. The statement of purpose provides a definitive focus for a single investigation.

Problem Too Large For Single Investigation

The perceptions on which this distinction is based clearly differ from those of most persons who describe the early steps of the research process. The beginning researcher will find it easier to understand and remember the proposed distinct uses of the two terms, the rationale for the uses, and the specific entity of the research process denoted by each, if he keeps in mind the following concepts:

REMINDERS

1. A problem-defined is so multifaceted and complex that no single investigation could possibly yield a solution to it.
2. The reason for doing research is to seek and reveal new knowledge that will be applicable to alleviation of the problem in whatever setting it may be found; it is not to solve a particular problem as it exists in a single setting.
3. A statement of purpose is a single statement that identifies the specific facet of the problem that will be the focus for the investigation—the precise facet of the problem about which new knowledge will be sought.
4. The sequence in the research process is, first, definition of problem (Step 1) and, second, statement of purpose (Step 2).
5. No one step in designing an investigation can be efficiently or precisely planned until the planning for prior steps has been virtually completed.

The concept that the problem is too complex to be solved through a single investigation encourages the student to plan an investigation directed to the search for and study of a limited variety of facts and phenomena. It helps him to understand that he does not have to do everything in a single study and that many investigations can stem from a single problem.

One Problem, Many Studies

One moment of great dismay for the beginning researcher frequently is expressed in: "Someone has already done my study!" This moment may occur after an extensive review of the literature, at the completion of the study design, or even after the investigation has been completed. Of course, there is immediate consolation for the student who has completed his research: someone may have studied one facet of his problem, but no one except himself has done *his* study. For the student who meets the consternation earlier, there is the steadying information that, regardless of the amount of study a particular problem has had, there are facets that have not been studied. For nurses, such assurance is grounded in fact. Replication of studies is good science practice, and there has been almost none in nursing research. No problem of concern to nurses has been exhaustively studied.

Essentially, then, "problem" refers to the initial step in the research process: the recognition of the irritation and the detailed description of all entities thought and observed to appertain to it. The term "purpose" refers to the second step in the research process: the single statement that identifies the specific facet of the problem about which new knowledge will be sought, the focus toward which the investigation will be directed.

DEFINING THE PROBLEM

All who write about the process of research state that defining the problem is perhaps *the* most important step in the total process. According to John Dewey, "A problem well-defined is half solved." But few writers attempt to describe how to define a problem, and none has been found to describe the process in full. Some have said that it is impossible to teach the student how to define the problem because of the complexity and uniqueness of each problem. I shall presume to try, however, by analyzing the process of defining the problem and suggesting some guidelines that may be helpful in this most important step.

Problem-Defined: Components

The problem-defined may be analyzed into seven components. The term "component" is used in contrast to the term "step": for two reasons: (1) to prevent confusion with the 13 steps in the research process which are the theme of the total book, and (2) because, even though both terms refer to individual sections of larger units, the sections to which each refers differ in character. The *steps* of the total research process are complete entities, whereas the *components*, the sections of the problem-defined, although individually identifiable, are not complete entities in themselves.

The components mesh, and no one component can stand alone. To pull one component from the total definition of problem would rob other components of some elements belonging to them. The student may consider the seven components in sequence as he develops the definition of problem. Yet, if he fully developed each one as a single entity, he would have to repeat large portions of details in delineations of two or more components. This aspect of the interrelatedness of the content of the various components (particularly components 3, 5, and 6) will become clear in the following outlines of the seven components of the definition of a problem, along with elaborations of how each one might be developed.

COMPONENT 1

The "irritation"

A real, live episode.
What first aroused your interest?
What was the first observation that started you thinking that "something needs to be done"?
What was the setting?
Who were the persons immediately involved? (usually limited in number: you and one or two others.)
What happened?
What were your thoughts and feelings?

One of the most frequent and perhaps the greatest deterrent to progress for the beginning researcher is difficulty in delimiting a problem to the point where a beginning can be made in its investigation. The difficulty may stem from several interrelated factors. A primary one is the likelihood of the student's identifying a problem through knowledge gained through study, rather than through personal experience and observations in work and life settings. This leads him to identify a problem of such global proportions that it can be identified by categorical title: the shortage of nurses, teaching patients, accidents, or others. In such instances, the student is hard put to compose a single sentence that will place his problem in any kind of organizational or population context. Once he has identified such an encompassing problem and then tries to define it, he finds that, try as he may, it continues to remain *too broad*. He cannot get it to anything he can handle, nor can he identify a direction to be taken to study it. To add to his difficulties, he usually receives the helpful advice that he must delimit his problem, but with no directions for ways to go about the delimiting. The implication of such advice is that the delimiting is a perfectly routine matter and that all that is needed is merely to proceed. The individual offering this advice usually leaves no room for the student to ask "How?"

Essentially, this approach amounts to the student's selecting a general problem (something "everyone talks about, but no one does anything about") and attempting to find within it a specific situation about which

Problem Too Broad

something might be done, thereby delimiting the problem. But always he is plagued by the larger problem and frustrated because no proposal seems adequate to solve the problem. He begins with a broad, general, essentially faceless situation and, with every attempt to describe the problem, the scope seems to enlarge and to acquire new appendages until it seems a veritable giant octopus. There seems no way to segregate and handle an individual part, without other parts interfering.

In contrast, it is suggested here that the student start by identifying a specific, concrete problem: a personally experienced "irritation." From it he can move to describing the broad problem that is illustrated by his specific experience. The description of the broad problem will, in turn, serve to account for his personal "irritating" experiences. He then can move to suggesting ways for coping with the specific irritation and, in turn, with the larger problem. With such a beginning, the student always has a concrete referent from which to work and to take direction. The beginner should be assured that learning about the specific illustrative situation will contribute knowledge relevant to the global problem of his concern.

An Irritating Situation

It is therefore proposed that the student begin by looking to his own experiences and describing a situation that he has experienced and that irritated him: one that led him to think, "Something ought to be done about this." It has been said that "research is to see what everyone else has seen, and to think what no one else has thought." An idea for a scientific inquiry may stem from a single observation but, more likely, it will stem from repeated observations of similar episodes. Nonetheless, it will be helpful for the student to recall the episode that first led to his thinking "something ought to be done." He should then describe in detail exactly what happened: what was the setting, who were the people, what happened? Students often find it difficult to believe that anything so simple and prosaic can possibly be a part of research. They can verbalize an episode and its relation to a researchable problem, but they cannot bring themselves to tell it the same way in writing. When convinced (or coerced) to at least try it, they will present, as a first endeavor, a fictionalized "they" episode, with "the" nurses, "the" doctor, and "the" patient. This remains a personally noninvolved beginning. With continued noninvolvement, as they move on to further definition of the problem, they move too rapidly to broad generalizations without a concretely envisioned base from which to proceed.

To help overcome the self-consciousness, the student is encouraged to think of telling a real, live story and to use first person in the writing. The relating of the actual happening, the recalling of feelings at the time of its occurrence, the thinking through of just what it is that irritates him—all these provide the student with a concrete base from which to start and to which to return in order to maintain relevance. Actually, students do very well in *telling* their stories, but writing them is something else. To many persons, anything put in writing must be formal and "important," not a simple tale about what happened, say, to a patient or to the student himself. But with the second or third try, the student usually manages to make a story live, both for himself and for his reader.

A Real, Live Story: A First-Person Situation

The student might well begin by recalling an "irritating" situation pertinent to the concerns of the course for which study of the problem will be a "learning experience." The beginning researcher who has identified and who now must narrow a "too broad problem," should attempt to recall an episode in which he was involved that is illustrative of the problem. The resort to describing a real, live episode also serves a second, very important purpose. It permits the student, in the very early stages of developing a scientific investigation, to determine his degree of familiarity with the problem and the extent of his feeling of personal involvement. This knowledge helps him to predict his potential for successfully executing the investigation. If he is unable to recall a real, live experience that illustrates the problem, he might consider turning his attention to another problem area, one with which he has had intimate experience. The reason for this suggestion is that research must deal with concretes; the student who has not experienced, directly, a situation illustrative of the area of his concern and who has not felt keenly the irritation caused by it, will find it difficult to identify concrete and specific elements in the problem. Always his perceptions of elements will be abstractions, broad generalizations. He will be unable to delineate observable specific units that compose the broad problem.

The Global Problem and Personal Involvement

Whether the student's problem derives from a personally experienced irritation or is a global problem about which everyone expresses concern, he will proceed in the same way to develop his definition of problem. He will describe the real, live episode: narrate a personal anecdote. In the subsequent components of the definition of problem, he will elaborate the general problem his experience illustrates. The student who began by thinking about a broad problem will have difficulty refraining from thinking about, and including in the writing, generalizations from the larger problem. With discipline, however, and attention to what he is writing, he will be able to do so. As he moves to writing later components of his definition of problem, and particularly when he develops later steps in his design, he will recognize the value of having written the anecdote in a simple, direct, living narrative. He will see the use and value of the specifics about what he witnessed, who was involved, how he was involved, how he felt, and precisely what irritated him—what, in his opinion, needed attention and correction.

EXAMPLE 1A*

In order to illustrate the various elements to be described, a paraphrase of the "real, live story" from three studies done for masters theses will be briefly outlined.[1,2,3] Many of the specifics from the paraphrase, 1A, will be used as illustrations throughout this text.

> It was Mrs. A's first postoperative morning, following a cholecystectomy. I had learned from the morning report that Mrs. A had had a quiet night, with no complaints since having a hypo at midnight. As I entered her room, I heard a low moan. Mrs. A was lying slightly on her side, facing away from the door. I went around the bed and asked if she were in pain. Evincing considerable discomfort, she stated that she ached all over from holding herself still so as not to break her stitches. On inquiry, she told me she had not changed her position nor had she been encouraged or assisted to cough and deep-breathe throughout the night and early morning hours. She went on to say that, of course, she could not cough, since she might tear her stitches. I suggested that I would help her to move and proceeded to remove the many pillows that served to prop her into the position she had been in since midnight. She expressed fear about moving, lest the stitches pull loose; she was also experiencing some incisional pain.
>
> During her early morning care she expressed fear of tearing her stitches whenever it was necessary for her to move. When I proposed to assist her to deep-breathe and cough, she at first refused. I explained the need to do this and assured her that her stitches would not tear and that I would help her so the pain would not be too great. The proposals that she dangle and that later in the day she would get out of bed were met with the same expressions of fear. It took much persuasion, along with extensive time and patience, to assist Mrs. A to perform these necessary activities. After the first two trials, with nothing more untoward than a moderate amount of pain, and with reassurance from her surgeon during his visit, Mrs. A finally was willing to engage in ambulation activities when encouraged to do so.
>
> My concern stems not only from Mrs. A's reluctance to move and cough while I cared for her, but also from the fear she expressed and her

---

* Most examples used are taken directly from student materials or are paraphrasings of the work of two or more students. Essentially, the example, 1A, is a paraphrasing of the work of three students. A few examples are pure fiction. Because the introduction of the many names, sometimes for a single brief reference, could be confusing, each example is ascribed a symbol identity. The digit in the symbol is that of the step in which it is first used; the letter indicates the sequence in which the example appears in the step. For instance, the symbol 1A is ascribed to the first example introduced in Step 1. Examples 2A through 2Q are used in Step 2. An individual example may be used in discussion of more than one step but, wherever one is used, it will be referred to by the symbol first ascribed to it. This labeling device permits tracing an example to various steps in which it is used. In the narrative, the symbol will often be used as though it were the name of an individual.

lack of understanding about the need to move and about the possibility of her stitches tearing. Even more, I was concerned that she had not been performing these activities during the first 20 hours after her abdominal surgery. Mrs. A's is only one story that could be told of patients' not knowing, before their surgery, that they will be expected to perform early ambulation activities, and of their being extremely fearful of doing injury to the operative site.

It is hardly necessary to describe in more detail the real, live episode that first aroused student interest in the problem. It created sufficient irritation to make 1A think that "something must be done about it" or that there ought to be a way to help surgical patients with their early ambulation.

COMPONENT 2

Elements in the situation

Here move toward generalizations about the existence of the problem of which your real, live episode is an illustration.

Limit your focus to concretes: to the institution, organization, community in which the real, live episode occurred.

What elements make up the total situation?

What things (persons, settings, policies, demands, etc.) are part of the problem?

What things possibly cause the problem; support the problem; impinge upon the problem?

What things are part of the problem?

What elements in the physical setting—immediate environment; total institutional environment; community?

What persons are involved? How?

Who are the victims? What is happening to them?

Who are the supporters? How do they contribute to the problem?

Who attempts to alleviate the problem? What do they do?

(Describe direct and indirect influences.)

Following the real, live story of the episode, including description of the irritation felt, the student should move on to describing more about the irritation. The presentation should now be broadened to portray the larger setting; other persons concerned with the problem beyond those directly involved in the episode; the more encompassing problem. 1A observed, for instance, that Mrs. A. expressed fear that her "stitches would break" each time she was urged to ambulate. The second phase of defining the problem was to develop a description of other patients being urged to perform early

Persons
Setting
Actions

ambulation activities. First described were nursing personnel giving direct care to patients, with reference to patients having the same type of surgery and on the same unit as that on which the real, live episode had occurred. Policies about teaching patients and the head nurse's encouragment of the practice were next mentioned; included were the surgeons' wishes about patients' being taught. The description extended to teaching for all patients on the ward unit, without limitation to any type of surgery. Third, the discussion extended to policies and practices in the still larger setting, the entire hospital, and to persons more distant from the single episode: the nurse supervisors, the chief of surgery, the hospital administrator.

Problem in Larger Context

Discussion of the problem in the larger context should describe elements in the situation, both near at hand and remote, that contribute to the problem. It should delineate the elements that possibly cause, impinge upon, or sustain, the problem; elements that are part of the problem, that possibly limit it, that describe the victims of the problem. The discussion of this component of the problem-defined is best limited to actual things that are known to exist in the setting, but not necessarily to factors that the investigator has actually observed or is absolutely certain are elements of the problem. In addition to identifying elements that are likely to be involved, the investigator should speculate about the nature of their involvement in the total problem situation as it exists in the specific institution. He should identify possible interrelationships and interactions among the elements and possible types of influence of the various elements.

For example, one of 1A's speculations was that nursing personnel who were providing direct care for patients had never discussed teaching patients with any of the surgeons and that the nurses did not know what the surgeons thought their patients should be taught. Nor, she speculated, did the surgeons have any idea what instructions nurses were giving or failing to give to their patients. These speculations derived from casual observations of nurse behaviors and lack of any contradicting observations.

Persons Places Processes

Included in the general description of the problem within the particular institution should be counterparts of the narrative description of the real, live episode. Here, the student may find it helpful to convert the concepts of persons, setting, and actions to persons, places, and processes. What is the physical setting? who are the people involved, and how many? what does each one do? why does he do what he does? what is the effect of what each does, on the doer and on others? who are the victims of the problem? who and what supports the problem? As the student moves from describing a single observed episode to describing elements in the larger setting that are related to the episode, so he begins to move toward the generalizations that will compose the problem-defined.

Restricting generalizations to factors that are actually known to exist or very possibly exist in the single setting of an individual hospital, agency, or community may seem to be leading to a plan for problem-solving rather than to a plan for research. Such is not the case. Rather, this restriction in the early stages of defining the problem should help the student think through many of the elements in the problem in a concrete context, before moving on to generalizations that become progressively more abstract. Indeed, the description of the real, live episode as it occurred, was observed, and illustrated a problem in a particular setting may eventually seem to have little import in relation to the investigation as it is finally reported. This type of description, however, serves as a concrete base on which to develop planning. Furthermore, it facilitates visualization of subsequent, more abstract, and generalized elements of the problem.

Concrete Base: Point of Reference

COMPONENT 3

The Problem in Its Largest Universe

> What have others experienced, learned, done, and thought in relation to the problem and to analogous problems?
> Consult the experts:
> Review the literature
> Confer with individuals
> Observe in other settings.
> Think along same patterns as those in Component 2: setting, persons, happenings. But consider all in the largest potential universe.
> Report not only occurrences of problem episodes, but also pertinent thinking about them: theories that suggest reasons for the occurrence of the problem; theories that suggest actions that may contribute to alleviation of the problem.
> Report what others have done about the problem or analogous problems; include results and potential for similar situations.
> Extend your exploration to experiences of disciplines other than your own.

In the previous component, the problem as it exists for potentially known patients in a known setting, involving readily identifiable persons, was described. Essentially, the description was concrete, with specific identification of persons, settings, and actions. But in Component 3, the problem is described in a larger context, with descriptive and generalized statements about varieties of patients, in varieties of settings, and in various interactions with various categories of persons—varieties all introduced by specific representative examples in Components 1 and 2. For example, in Component 1, Mrs. A represented all abdominal and thoracic surgery pa-

Specific to General

tients in one hospital; these were introduced in Component 2. But, in Component 3, all abdominal and thoracic surgery patients in one hospital represent "all" abdominal and thoracic surgery patients in all hospitals, and are introduced and discussed in that context.

It is as we begin to account for elements in the third component of the definition of problem that the boundaries between components start to become blurred. This may even happen during development of the second component, but it is best to resist considering elements of the third component until the second component has been thoroughly explored and definitively written. Speculation, in the delineation of the second component, should be limited to probabilities in the setting or the single institution, agency, or community. For further discussion of this and a shading of grey to the black-and-white proposal, the student is referred to the discussion on selection of the crux of the problem on pages 34–40.

What Others Have Experienced, Learned, Done, Thought

In Component 3, generalizations move to a broader area. By reviewing the literature, the researcher learns about the problem in other settings and what others have learned and done about it.

The general reminders for thinking about and recording elements pertinent to Component 3 can be the same as those used in the first two components: persons, places, and processes. Just as delineations of ideas about each element were more extensive and more general for the second component than for the first, so those for the third will be broader than for the preceding two. It is at this point that the researcher moves to the full conceptualization of the irritation as a researchable problem. He begins to think of it in terms of its application to a large population: to a total universe. He moves from thinking about the problem of Mrs. A, an abdominal surgery patient (Component 1); to all abdominal and thoracic surgery patients in Hospital X (Component 2); to "all" abdominal and thoracic surgery patients in all hospitals (Component 3). As he does this, he relies not only on his own knowledge and speculations, but he also discovers what others have known and learned about the problem. And he moves still a step further and considers what others have learned and proposed about problems analogous to the problem of his concern and to specific elements within his problem. He begins to identify materials to be used in the theoretical framework of his problem: theories that will help to explain the existence and process of his problem and that will provide ideas for suggested solutions to the problem.

The theories will be of two types: (1) tested theories from various sciences, and (2) nonformalized theories, represented by the theorizing and speculations of others and by his own. The theorizing, essentially, will consist of identification of science theories potentially relevant to the problem. It will include speculation of what the relationship of science principles to the problem might be, and how they may contribute to understanding, accounting for, and possible alleviation of the problem.

The speculations will be described by hypothesizing possible relationships among various elements in the problem situation. The hypothetical relationships constitute possible explanations of why the problem is what it is; they suggest actions that may lead to alleviation of the problem; and they identify outcomes that may be anticipated from the actions. Although the student may include some of his own speculations, he is advised to limit the speculations in Component 3 to those proposed by others, and to introduce his own speculations after the completion of Component 4. In so doing, he will limit the number of personal speculations to those closely related to the focus of his own personal interest. This suggestion will become clear in discussion of Components 5 and 6.

Pertinent Observations Plus Pertinent Theories

Just as in the second component, part of the content of the third component will be descriptions of observed elements, and a large part of the content will be proposals about possibly relevant elements. In the first category will be those elements observed by the investigator in settings other than the ones described in the first two components, and those described by others and gleaned by the investigator either through discussions with others or from the literature. The possibly relevant (speculative or theorized) elements will derive from the same sources but, rather than being observations of the investigator and others, they will be identifications of elements (facts and theories) proposed by the investigator and others as being potentially inherent in the problem.

Identifying and suggesting interrelationships of various speculative elements is a form of theorizing. It may be (1) educated guessing (by either the investigator or others), or (2) suggesting pertinence of theories developed by others to various aspects of the problem at hand. The latter kind of theorizing may be thought of as an intellectual "trying on for size." It is the attempt to identify reasons for the *why* of various elements (persons, places, and processes) and for their interrelationships in the problem. As may be seen, Component 3 encompasses several elements that other writers identify as individual steps in the process of research: most notably, the review of the literature and the development of a theoretical framework. But it would seem that viewing these activities as processes and their results as individual entities makes for confusion, requires many interspersed qualifying statements throughout the plan, and is, in many ways, illogical.

Some authors suggest that the process of research proceeds in this order: (1) identification of the problem, (2) review of the literature, (3) definition of the purpose for the study, (4) a second review of the literature, (5) statement of the specific problem for investigation, and (6) a

Review of Literature; Theoretical Framework

third review of the literature. But the authors who propose such a procedure frequently fail to identify the need to search the literature in relation to other steps in the research process. Many don't even mention various steps, let alone discuss the elements composing them. In this, they fail to serve the beginning researcher. The concept of the multifarious and complex nature of the problem-defined makes it logical and consistent to propose that the theoretical framework is an integral part of the definition of problem. This framework is an entity that cannot stand alone, and it alone requires a particular review of the literature. As I see it, neither the theoretical framework nor the review of the literature are entities that can stand whole and alone. Each, like the definition of problem itself, is never completed, and each is pertinent to the development of several individual steps in the research process.

I would therefore propose that both the theoretical framework and review of the literature be viewed as a support for the various individual steps in which they are employed. The review of the literature may be viewed as the accumulation of structural materials. The theoretical framework may be viewed as the structure developed with these materials—a structure that makes explicit the relationship of the various theories and principles to the facts of the problem. All, when reasonably identified and described, compose basic structures in the problem-defined. These concepts will take on clarity and additional meaning as they are applied in the development of later steps.

The Bulk of the Problem-Defined

Identification and description of pertinence of elements in Component 3 make up the bulk of the definition of problem. Because of this, blurring of boundaries between the third and other components is inevitable and extensive. Component 3 identifies the irritation in its largest universe: describes the problem as it has been known to exist, or as it may exist, in various forms and settings. Information that may explain its existence is described. Factors that may alleviate or aggravate the problem are delineated. These many elements are derived from the experiences, knowledge, and thinking of the investigator and of others. Of the latter, many, though not all, of the elements come from the literature. This is also true of the concepts used to construct the theoretical framework. The researcher will use ideas from the literature as he develops Components 5 and 6, where he will propose actions that may be taken and outcomes that may be anticipated from the actions. As part of Component 3, the researcher will describe the experiences, knowledge, thoughts of others; in Components 5 and 6, he will use these elements as the bases for his own proposals and thinking.

Thus, the elements composing the third component are also appropriately elements composing Components 5 and 6; the boundaries between these components are blurred. It is possible, of course, to identify individual components in detail and to develop each one as a complete entity, but to do so would necessitate extensive duplication in the definition of the problem. It is therefore proposed that the components be viewed as integral parts of the single initial step in the process of research: the problem-defined.

By way of example, then, in developing Component 3, the investigator will describe what is known about the problem in its largest context. He will also suggest theories that might explain the various elements and interrelationships that compose it. 1A identified examples of patients being taught about their illness and treatment and about what they could do to help themselves. She reported not only on patients having surgery but on patients with prostheses, paralysis, heart impairment, tuberculosis, diabetes, and many other disease conditions. She described the persons from the various disciplines concerned with and contributing to the care of the sick, with particular attention to individuals teaching patients and helping them to understand their own roles in their treatments. She considered the various settings in which patients are taught, types of teaching programs and tools used for teaching, and reports of studies of effects of teaching practices and programs. She reported some theories of learning and of group organization, as well as theories from psychology, physiology, and other sciences that seemed logically to be related to various elements in her problem. She related many of the identified theories to the problem by elaborating on how they might explain the existence of the problem and how some might serve to guide planning for improving the situation.

Example 1A

This outline of content, which merely suggests some of the elements to be identified and interrelationships to be described, makes it clear that Component 3 contains elements in common with Components 5 and 6. This will be made more explicit when the latter components are discussed, but it is helpful for the planner first to delineate the content of Component 4.

COMPONENT 4

An ideal situation

What would the situation be like, if no problem existed?
Dream: Envision that everything is lovely!
Redescribe your real, live episode; only this time eliminate all signs of problem, all cause for irritation. Tell what the setting would have been, what people would have done, what would have happened to and been responses of the victims in an "ideal" setting, where no problem exists.

By the time the investigator has reached this point in the planning, he has already presented his irritation. He has thought through and identified all elements that possibly cause and relate to his problem. He has consulted with others, in person and through the literature. He has described many facets of his problem and has explored the relationships of many of these facets with the particular irritation that he has identified as the crux of his problem. He has identified relevant theories and described ways in which they help to explain the existence of the problem. Now, in Component 4, he will describe a situation in which the problem does not exist—in other words, an "ideal" situation. Component 4 does not include, however, suggesting solutions to the problem or proposing things that might be done to eliminate or alleviate it. Rather, this phase should portray a situation in which there is no such problem. The planner may think back to the first and second components and now rewrite the real, live episode. This time, however, he should describe the setting, the persons, and the actions in the situation as he thinks they *should* be. He should portray a situation where there is no irritation (at least, none relevant to the problem of concern).

An Ideal— No Fairy Tale

For example, 1A, in developing Component 4, may have described Mrs. A as she received instructions about her anticipated surgery from her surgeon and her nurse. She would have described how the nurse, the afternoon prior to surgery, demonstrated deep-breathing and coughing to Mrs. A and helped her to practice the actions. She may have told of the patient's behavior and progress following the surgery. She would have described the planning by the nursing personnel for teaching each patient according to his own needs. The scheduling of teaching sessions, the identification of the persons responsible for the teaching, and the sharing of planning by persons of various concerned disciplines would have been described. The setting and equipment provided for teaching patients, along with the provisions for helping nursing personnel to learn what and how to teach patients would have been included. This delineation may seem like a fairy tale. But, actually, in any mention of a problem and a proposal to do something about it, there is the implicit suggestion that an "ideal" should be established. Immediately, one thinks of creating a situation in which no problem exists.

The Goal— Not the Process for Attaining It

For the ideal, the planner might very well describe what he has thought might be the goal of "doing something about" his irritation, remembering that the description of the goal (the portrayal of the ideal) does not include description of the means for its attainment. The planner should dream! He should envision and describe the ideal as an idyllic drama: a drama, simple and pleasing, portraying the happiness of heroes and heroines; a drama without villains. To discuss means for attaining this ideal would require identification of the irritation and the introduction of tribulation into the lovely idyll. The goal of "doing something about it" is an envisioned ideal situation, with no elaboration of the intricacies of the path to its attainment.

The goal thus made explicit can serve as a standard against which to measure proposals for solution to the problem. In addition, it will suggest actions that may be taken. Just as Components 1 and 2 focus on a specific problem in a particular setting, suggesting concern for solving the problem in that setting alone, so does Component 4 focus on the portrayal of the ideal. Nonetheless, the student is reminded that these components in the definition of problem are meant to serve only as illustrations of the broad problem of concern.

Elements in each of the components provided concrete materials on which to base visualizations of counterparts in the general problem, which affects many persons in many similar settings. The ultimate plan is to seek information that will be generalizable to a large population in a universe of settings. But in order to make suggestions and planning meaningful, general concepts must be viewed as they pertain to specific persons, in specific settings, involving specific actions.

Specifics for Concrete Base— Not for Problem Solving

No problem can possibly be solved through one single piece of research. By the time the investigator has written down the details of the first three components of the definition of problem, this fact should be obvious to him. Yet it is natural that he would like to make as large a contribution as possible to information needed for alleviation of the problem. With the picture of the ideal situation made explicit, he provides himself with something concrete against which to consider, evaluate, and make decisions about paths likely to yield the most fruitful results. Essentially, then, in Component 4, the student has described an ideal situation in which there is no mention of irritation, no manifestations of the problem: all is as it should be. In Components 5 and 6, he will move to propose actions that might change the conditions described in the first three components to the conditions described in Component 4.

COMPONENT 5

Suggestions for moving toward the ideal

What might help to achieve the situation you describe as ideal?
Suggest all actions that might contribute to development of the ideal situation:
Changes and innovations in setting, in behaviors of people, and in policies, procedures, and routines.

Utilize materials from Component 3 to develop ideas and to provide rationale for your suggestions.

Direct most attention to elements of greatest interest and concern to members of your own discipline.

Address proposals to actions that may be taken, independently or cooperatively, by members of your discipline.

Where there are glaringly obvious suggestions pertinent to members of other disciplines, these should be mentioned but not extensively elaborated.

Identify and describe all potential suggestions *before* describing the one you consider the primary one, thereby avoiding mind-set, which acts to block extended thinking.

COMPONENT 6

Results to be expected as outcomes of suggestions

Describe results to be expected from each action suggested in Component 5.

These will *not* be repetition of Component 4. The ideal describes a situation where no problem exists, where there is no need to suggest changes.

Research cannot attack a total problem, composed as it would be of the many elements identified in Component 3.

A single investigation can deal with but a small segment of a total problem. Many segments will be identified through suggestions for actions and possible outcomes of actions.

Development of Components 5 and 6 leads to ideas for the most effective approaches to alleviation of the problem, for identifying actions that may be expected to make the greatest impact on the problem within the scope of the planned investigation, and for new knowledge that may be pertinent to the problem.

Do Components 5 and 6 together, using materials from Component 3 to provide rationale for proposed results. Proposed results will serve as rationale for suggested actions.

Do not repeat all descriptions from Component 3; rather, refer to them.

The elements in components may be thought of as suggestions for actions that might be taken or situations that might be developed to change the conditions described in the first three components (the problem situation) to the conditions described in Component 4 (the ideal situation). The elements of Component 6, in contradistinction, may be thought of as descriptions of results to be expected from each suggested action in Component 5. Included will be theories and speculations used to rationalize suggested actions and to provide bases for expecting the proposed outcomes. Pertinent theories that have been discussed in developing earlier components need only be referred to as Components 5 and 6 are elaborated. It is in these two components that the investigator will introduce his own speculations about possible elements composing the problem, along with suggestions to explain them. His speculations will include the potential applicability and relevance of the experiences, thinking, and theories of others to his immediate concerns.

Obviously, there will be more than one suggestion for possible attainment of each aspect of the ideal, and many and varied results may be anticipated from each suggested action. A part of the presentation of each suggestion and anticipated result will be ideas and theories delineated in Component 3 which provide bases and rationale for the proposals. From this it may appear that Components 5 and 6 will be repetitious of Component 4, but this is not the case. The ideal is described with no suggestion of the elements that will compose it and with no rationale for believing that things would work as described. Furthermore, the ideal will portray only one set of circumstances, whereas, in Component 5, many alternative suggestions for actions will be delineated, as well as many situations and programs to be instituted and developed. Component 6 will describe many possible resulting situations, each being an example of an ideal or an approach to an ideal; each will be an example of some degree of alleviation of the problem. In Components 5 and 6, the logic for making the suggestions and the bases for proposing the anticipated results will be made explicit.

Supporting Rationale

Components 5 and 6 are distinct entities within the definition of problem, and each will be described individually. They are listed together, however, because it is expedient to develop them concomitantly, both in describing them and in their development. As the researcher pursues the process of defining his problem, he will want to think through and describe the results to be expected (Component 6) from each suggested action immediately following identification of the action or element (Component 5).

Develop Components 5 and 6 as a Unit

Combined planning for these two components has two advantages: (1) it avoids repetition in identifying suggested changes and innovations; (2) it allows the investigator to carry thinking and planning about any one suggestion to a reasonable conclusion as the ideas about it occur to him, rather than having to make notes of these ideas as they accompany development of Component 5, to be used later for development of Component 6.

Step 1: Definition of Problem

Long before the investigator has reached this phase in defining his problem, he will have thought about actions that might alleviate the problem. These thoughts may have come even before he has fully recognized that certain observed situations provoked an irritation or constituted a problem. Most persons confronted with an irritation are likely to offer suggestions for corrective action before considering all aspects of a problem; they have confidence in the worth of the hastily identified "solution." But the prompt suggestion and hasty solution can establish a mind-set that will preclude thinking of other ideas.

Avoid Mind-Set

To avoid the limiting influence of a mind-set, the investigator, before he writes his primary suggestion, should write down all the suggestions he can think of that could conceivably contribute to establishing the ideal. He should also delineate many of the outcomes that may be anticipated from each suggestion. Not until he has exhausted all possible suggestions should he identify his primary suggestion and its expected influence, along with ideas that explain and support his proposal.

This process requires considerable self-discipline, but it will get the investigator past the inhibiting mind-set of the primary suggestion. It also ensures that the investigator will not rush on with further planning before he has thoroughly explored and delineated the many elements and facets of his problem. If he has included considerable detail in his third component, he will have already written many of the ideas and concepts pertinent to the fifth and sixth components. He need not repeat them in full, but may merely allude to them. Furthermore, if details were fully outlined in Component 3, he will not have difficulty in resisting the rush to the primary suggestion, since these details will remind him of many suggestions that may be made and various results that may be anticipated.

Definition of Problem: Never Completed, Just Stopped

Early in his thinking about Components 5 and 6, the investigator will ask himself whether there will ever be an end to defining the problem. What with consideration of the many elements that compose a problem; the many elements that impinge upon it; the many theories that may possibly explain why things are as they are and that provide rationales for proposing changes; and the need to describe the interrelationships of all these elements and theories—surely, it seems to him, there can be no end. Indeed, this is true: *no problem is ever completely defined*. So the researcher must make a decision about when the problem has been *thoroughly* defined and then direct his attention to the next steps in planning the investigation.

Planning the Stopping Place

Beginning to plan for closure of definition of problem occurs rather early in the development of Components 5 and 6. The approximate place will depend on the competence of the investigator and the scope of the investigation to be undertaken. Since most problems likely to be investigated by nurses will involve persons from several disciplines and knowledge and theories from many sciences, there is the potential for including in Components 5 and 6 suggestions for actions from persons from other disciplines; possibly applicable theories from many sciences may also be included here. If the study is likely to involve persons from many disciplines, then there will be many, many suggestions needing to be identified and described in full. If the study is of a more limited scope—one that a nurse might accomplish alone or with only limited consultation with or involvement of persons from other disciplines—then proposals in Component 5 should be limited to those that a nurse or nurses might effect. Should there be definite and conspicuous proposals for actions by members of other disciplines, they, of course, should be recorded.

The nurse researcher, however, can begin to limit the scope of the definition of the problem by thinking of things nurses might do to make the situation as she thinks it should be. If the scope of the study is to be markedly limited, she may want to limit her suggestions to actions the nurse performs independently and for which she assumes full responsibility. This may mean that many actions with considerable potential for alleviation of the problem will not be elaborated. But there is little point in delving into facets of the problem which the investigator cannot carry beyond the planning stage. The final and definitive move toward closure of the definition of the problem is delineated in Component 7.

COMPONENT 7

Investigator's frame of reference

> How do you view the interrelatedness of the many elements composing the problem?
>
> What, explicitly, is your frame of reference? To which theories do you subscribe as having pertinence for the problem?
>
> Identify, precisely and succinctly, the crux of the problem, as you see it, and the specific theories you believe hold most promise for explaining the problem and for providing direction for search for new knowledge germane to the problem.
>
> This component may be viewed as a summary of the problem-defined, with explicit identification of elements and their interrelationships that are of primary interest and concern to the investigator and to members of his discipline.

As Components 3, 5, and 6 were developed, many elements appropriate for use in constructing a theoretical framework for the problem were identified and, in Components 5 and 6, many large sections of the framework itself were constructed. Now, in Component 7, the investigator will identify the elements of most direct concern to him and describe his conceptualization of the problem-defined as he chooses to investigate it. He will identify precisely how he envisions theories explaining the existence of the problem. He need not give detailed explanations of why he sees the total as he sees it, nor why he views it one way and not another. He may want to identify more than one way in which he might view it, and then make explicit the particular line of thinking he will pursue as he plans his study and thinks through potential interpretations of anticipated findings. He will draw from the other six components to summarize the many elements that compose the problem as he sees it and as he will study it.

A GEODESIC DOME

It may help the beginning researcher, at this point, to begin thinking of his problem-defined as analogous to a geodesic dome, with its many structural units whose facets are seemingly of various sizes, shapes, and subdivisions (Exhibits 1-5). The analogue of the dome rather than of a geodesic sphere is suggested, since the dome is a portion of a sphere. The sphere is the natural, completed geodesic structure and is a complete, closed entity, whereas a problem-defined is never a complete, closed entity. Thus, the concept of the dome as a whole can provide an analogue to the total problem-defined: a constructed whole, yet without a natural completion. In addition, many analogies may be drawn wherein structural parts and composite units of the dome correspond to the elements, composition, and construction of the problem-defined. Individual units of the dome and relationships among them are shown in Exhibits 2 and 4.

Two Types of Hexagonal Units

In large geodesic structures, such as the United States Pavilion at Canada's Expo '67 (Exhibit 1), construction utilizes two distinct types of hexagonal units. One type of unit is three-dimensional, a hexagonal pyramid, with the vertex pointing outward from the structure and the open base of the pyramid facing the inside of the structure. The second type of unit is two-dimensional, a hexagonal plane.

Pyramids Independent Units

Each three-dimensional pyramid may be envisioned as an independent unit, constructed of its own materials and not sharing structural materials of another unit (Exhibit 2, pyramid A). That is, the spokes that make up the frame and the materials (they may be glass, canvas, wood, or others) of which the sides (triangular faces) are composed are the materials of one pyramid, and not a part of another pyramid. The only material shared by more than one pyramid is the frame bar of the base side of each triangular face of the pyramid. Here, two pyramids share one base structural bar common to one face for each of them, and one pyramid will share six base-bars, each one common to a single base-bar of each of six adjoining pyramids (Exhibit 3).

In contrast to the relative independence of each pyramidal unit, the two-dimensional hexagonal planes are not structurally complete individual units. As Exhibits 1 and 2 show, the hexagonal planes are constructed by the spokes radiating from the vertexes of the pyramids. They are the framework supporting the "walls"; in a geodesic structure, the framework, instead of providing support from within, is in the form of a superstructure that provides support from without. (The structure is similar to the shell of the crustacean, which supports the muscle and organ units of the animal, instead of the internal skeleton that supports the body structures of most animals.) The spokes of the planes may be thought of as connecting the individual pyramids to adjoining pyramids. A single hexagonal plane may be identified by focusing on the vertex of one pyramid and moving to the ends of the six spokes radiating from it to the vertexes of the six surrounding and adjoining pyramids. Exhibit 3 shows that the spokes attached to the vertex of pyramid A and radiating to the vertexes of pyramids B, C, A', G, H, and I provide the sides for the triangular units of the plane, while one of the spokes connecting the vertexes of any two of the pyramids adjacent to pyramid A, e.g., C and A', provides the structure for the base of one of the triangular units of the hexagonal plane. Obviously, the hexagonal planes are not independent structures with individual, self-contained structural materials. Rather, from one to three units of any one plane may be units of one or more other planes. To ascribe a particular triangular unit to one hexagonal plane is, in effect, to deprive another plane of one of its triangular units. Thus, triangle AA'C is common to both the X and Y hexagonal planes. Triangle AA'G is also common to X and Y; in addition, it is common to a third plane, Z.

Planes Share Common Structures and Faces

Among other features of the structural relationships of the dome is the fact that there are 12 spokes that meet at the vertex of each pyramid (Exhibits 1 and 2). Six of these spokes compose the supporting structures of the sides of the triangles of the hexagonal pyramid; they slope to the base of the pyramid and there meet base-ends of the spokes from adjoining pyramids. The other six spokes composing the hexagonal planes are those that extend outward from the vertex of the pyramid and are horizontally parallel to the bases of the pyramids. The spokes of the pyramid enclose and support the materials of which the faces of the pyramid are made. For the purposes of the analogies to be drawn among elements of the problem-defined and the units of the geodesic structure, varicolored glass is envisioned as the material composing the faces of the pyramidal units. The spokes of the hexagonal planes connect the vertexes of the pyramids and

Twelve Facets Radiate From One Pyramidal Vertex

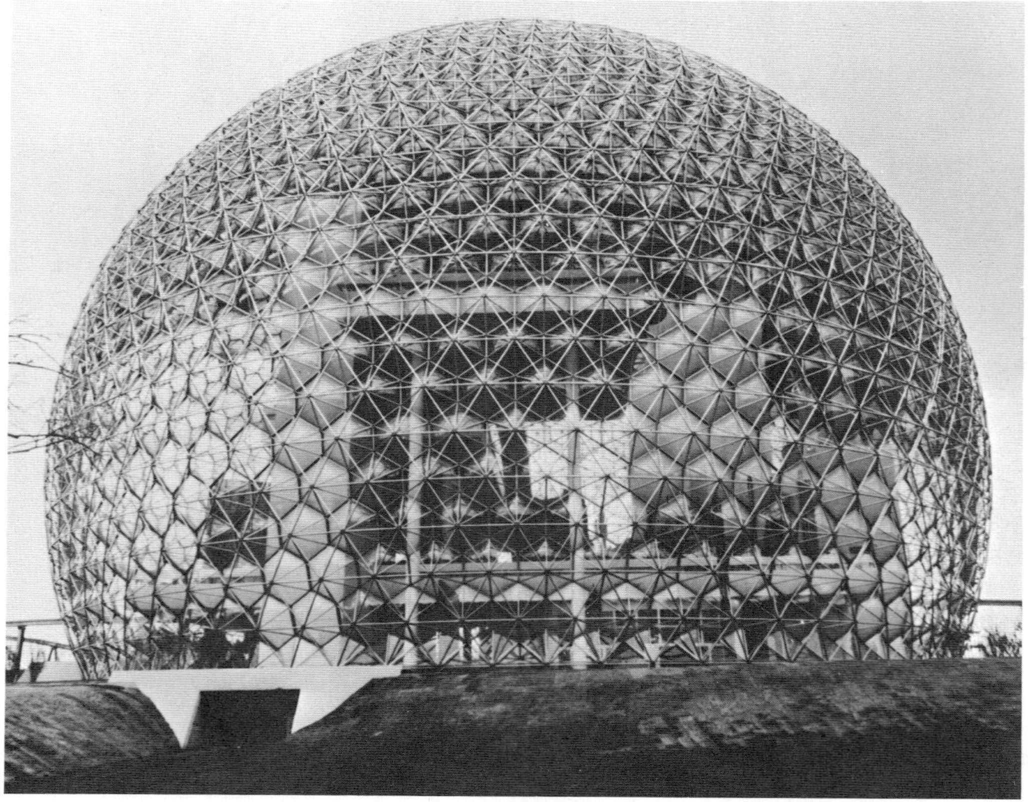

Exhibit 1. Photograph of a geodesic dome. Individual features, isolated and described in Exhibits 2 through 5, may be identified, and their relationships to each other and to the total dome are portrayed.

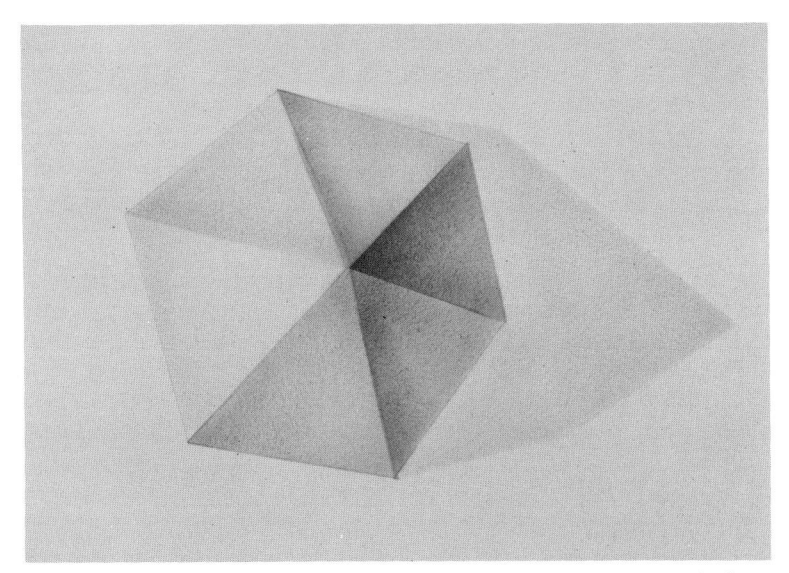

Exhibit 2. Pyramid A. Schematic portrayal of a single hexagonal pyramid, showing six sides framed by base bars that form a hexagon and spokes that extend from base-bar intersections to vertex.

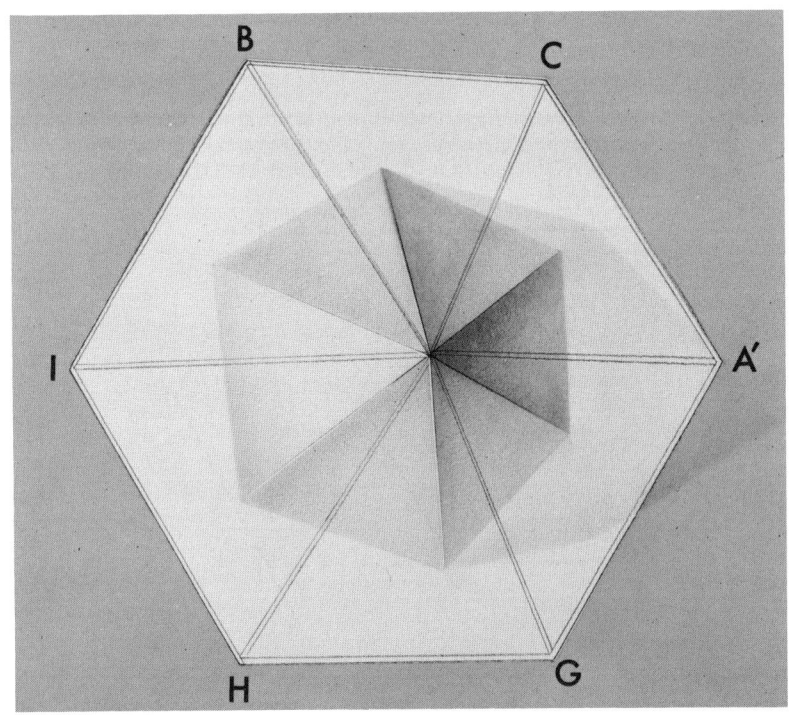

Exhibit 2. Plane X. Schematic portrayal of a single hexagonal plane formed by superstructure spokes that radiate from the vertex of an underlying pyramid to vertexes of six adjoining pyramids. Underlying pyramids correspond to pyramid A and those adjoining it in Exhibit 3. Only pyramid A is portrayed; those adjoining it are identified by labels at the points of their vertexes.

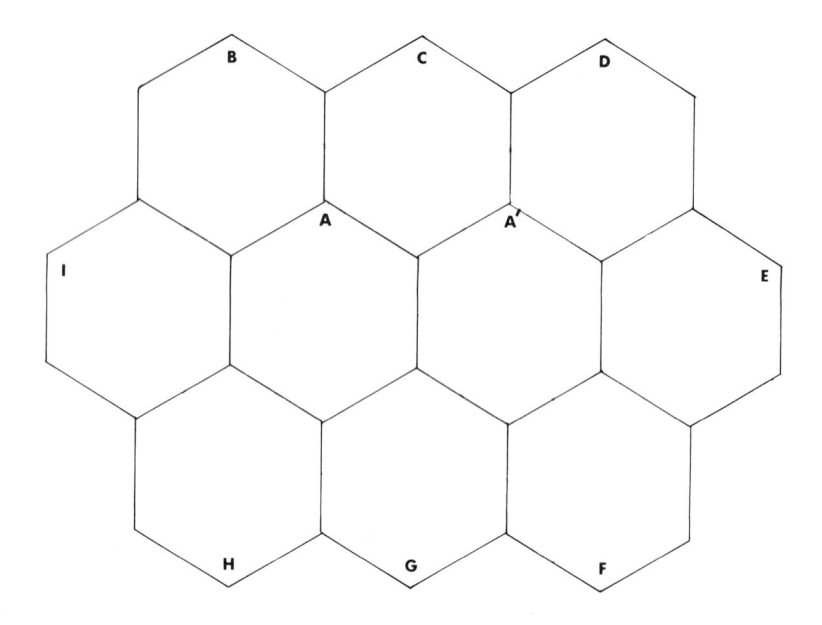

Exhibit 3. Outlines of bases of pyramids to show relatively independent relationship of pyramid A to surrounding pyramids. Spokes and vertexes of pyramids, as well as superstructure and curvature, visible in Exhibit 1, have been eliminated.

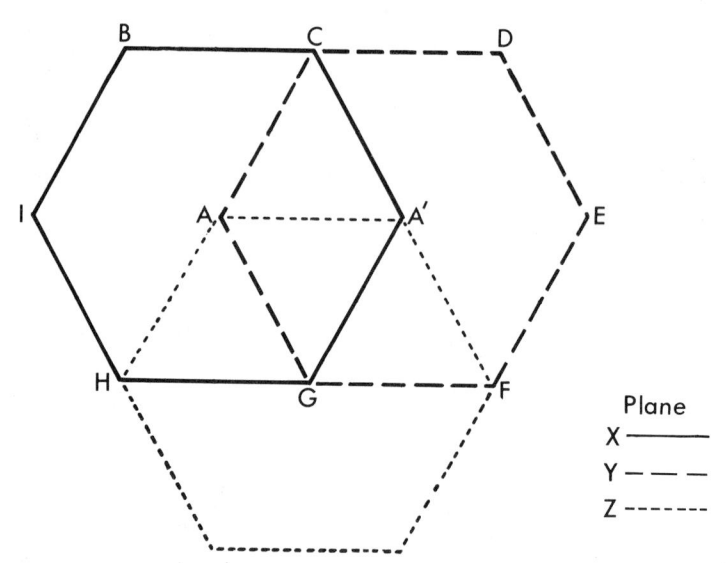

Plane
X ———
Y — — —
Z - - - - -

Exhibit 4. Planes X, Y, and Z. Outlines to show interdependence of three hexagonal planes of the superstructure. Underlying pyramids are not portrayed, but they correspond to those in Exhibit 3 and are identified by labels at the points of their vertexes.

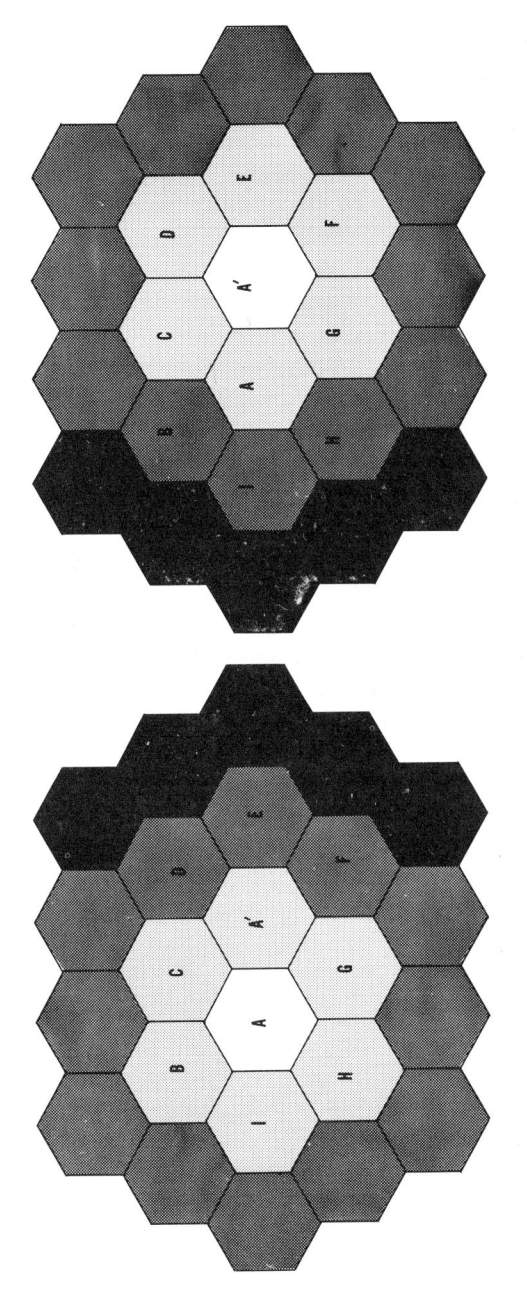

Exhibit 5. Focus pyramids A and A'. Shading in outlines of bases of pyramids to show effect of changing light (focus of attention) from pyramid A to pyramid A'. Amount of light in pyramids C and G remains the same; while that in other adjoining pyramids decreases or increases, depending on whether focal pyramid is A or A'.

outline the sides and bases of the triangles that make up the hexagonal planes, but the "faces" they outline are empty space. It is these features of the six faces of the pyramid, with the superimposed spokes of the superstructure (the plane) that, when viewed from certain angles, give the impression that the pyramids have 12 faces and that the faces of one pyramid are different sizes and shapes from those of other pyramids, and from one another. The 12 various shaped faces only *seem* to exist; they are not concrete constructions; and they are different in size, shape, and proportion only as they are viewed from different angles or perspective.

The Lighted Pyramid

An aid in visualizing the seeming 12-sided structure of the pyramids would be to think of a single light placed inside an otherwise unlighted dome and just within the base area of the focal pyramid. This device would, of course, serve also to maintain identity of the unit selected as the focal pyramid. When viewed from the outside, the lighted pyramid will stand out boldly, and the adjacent six pyramids will be highlighted (Exhibits 1 and 5). More distant pyramids will be faintly identifiable, with fewer and fewer features being identifiable as the pyramids become increasingly remote from the light. So, too, for the visibility of the hexagonal planes of the superstructure. The center of the plane described by the spokes radiating from the vertex of the lighted pyramid will be readily identifiable as it extends from the vertex of one adjacent pyramid to the vertex of another adjacent pyramid. Just as features of pyramids more distant from the lighted pyramid will be less distinct, so the features and identities of any one hexagonal plane will be less visible as they became distant from the lighted pyramid. It is easy to visualize the effect of moving around to view the structures from different angles. This is true, especially of the effect on sizes and shapes of the pyramid faces, and also of the effect on the shadings of the varicolored glass of the faces.

The Dome Examined From a Distance

One way to approach examining the structure of the geodesic dome is to think of standing at a distance and beginning the examination by focusing on a single pyramid (see Exhibit 5). The examiner would then allow his eye to move out radially from the focal pyramid, to examine adjacent structures and to trace interrelationships and connections among them. The focal pyramid might be designated as pyramid A, and the six adjoining ones, pyramids, B, C, A', G, H, and I. Whether examination is made in daylight or by the device of the light in the base of the focal pyramid, the same features may be noted, although they are perhaps more easily envisioned when the focal pyramid is lighted.

Effects of Varying Focal Pyramids

With the light within the base area of pyramid A, the surrounding pyramids—B, C, A', G, H, and I—will be highlighted. Of particular interest is the effect created by changing the light, and thereby the focal point, to the base area of pyramid A'. This, of course, highlights the six adjoining pyramids: A, B, C, D, E, and F. In other words, regardless of whether A or A' is the focal pyramid, pyramids C and G will receive the same amount of light, albeit from different angles. Other pyramids adjoining either A or A' will receive differing amounts of lights, and it will come from different angles.

With either pyramid A or pyramid A' selected as the focal pyramid, they will share the base boundary of one of their triangular sides and the two triangular faces that are common to the hexagonal plane X and Y of the superstructure which is formed by the spokes radiating from their vertexes (see Exhibits 5 and 4). In addition, pyramid A will be related to the four other triangular faces of plane X, which are not shared with pyramid A'. While, in turn, pyramid A' will be related to the four triangular faces of plane Y that are different from any related to pyramid A. With either chosen, they will retain some commonalities, but the other closely related facets will be different, depending upon which pyramid serves as the focal point.

If the examiner views the dome from a distance and attempts to allow his eye to move outward to examine structures in concentric circles about the focal pyramid, he will soon be aware of three phenomena:

Three Optical Phenomena

1. He finds that he is unable to pursue his examination in a completely equal radial pattern. Instead, he moves tangentially outward in the direction of one particular radius.

2. He finds it difficult to keep in touch with his original focal pyramid and to identify relationships of it to other units as he examines them. He becomes involved in describing relationships among various other tangential structures, rather than relationships of the structures tangential to the focal pyramid.

3. He finds himself moving to other units to be examined, leaving incomplete the examination, and even the identification, of some facets of the tangential pyramids and their superimposed hexagonal planes. As he proceeds to examine a larger and larger area of the total structure, the relationships to the focal pyramid become more difficult to identify. It requires more and more detail to trace the increasingly complex relationships; lines become blurred and then faint, until they disappear over the curvature of the dome.

Two features of the geodesic dome make it an apt analogue to the problem-defined:

Two Types of Units— No Starting Place

1. The dome is made of two types of identically sized and shaped composite units.

2. There is no identifiable starting or culminating place for constructing the dome.

One type of unit is readily distinguishable from the other, and each, throughout the entire structure, always bears the same relationship to the other type of unit. Another aspect of the first feature is that all units of either type are of equal importance to the total structure: no one unit is more important than any other unit of its type, and neither type of unit is more important than the other. In relation to the "no starting place" feature, the dome does not have a keystone, as does an arch, nor a vertex, as does a pyramid. At first, this may seem to contradict the analogy to the problem-defined since, to develop the problem-defined, the advice has been to work from a focal point, the crux of the problem. But, as the definition of problem develops, as the many closely related irritations are identified and their relations to the focal irritation elaborated, it becomes clear that the crux, rather than being identified by some particular inherent feature, is identified by an arbitrary decision of the investigator. The process is analogous to the standing-at-a-distance examination of the dome and selection of one pyramid as the focal one from which examination will be begun and to which surrounding structures and units will be related. Or the process and effect may be thought of as the arbitrary selection of the pyramid within whose base the light will be placed.

Abstract Super-structure Supports Concrete Structural Units

Other structural features of the dome also pose apt parallels in terms of elaborating the many facets of the problem-defined. They are the structures of the pyramids, with their solid faces, and the overlying structure of the hexagonal planes, with their support far-reaching and with each extending to many individual units of the underlying structure. The observable elements of the problem (the irritations and the persons, places, and processes) can be viewed as parallels to the pyramids. The speculations and discussions of the theories serving to explain the existence of the irritations and supporting suggestions for actions may be viewed as the units and framework of the superstructure.

The concrete observable elements of the problem-defined are particularly analogous to the pyramids constructed of solid materials. The abstract speculative elements of the problem are analogous to the airspace units of the planes. The theories and speculations are thoughts, not observable elements, just as the "faces" of the hexagonal planes of the superstructure are not observable; yet both provide indispensable support to the concrete units of their respective total structures.

The analogy of the problem-defined to the geodesic dome does not provide for absolute parallels in all aspects. Yet there seem to be enough parallels to use the dome as a model for envisioning, figuratively, the elements of the problem-defined and their interrelationships, and for developing concrete structures (constructs) to serve as bases for mental visualization of various relationships among many of the elements of the problem-defined.

One man's model, however, often becomes another man's Procrustean bed. The student should not allow the concept of the problem-defined suggested as analogous to a geodesic dome to become for him a Procrustean bed. Rather, he should take from the analogy the parallels that are meaningful to him and not try to make all suggested parallels fit into his thinking or his thinking fit all suggested parallels. For some students, the general analogy and most of the specific parallels will help in providing concrete visualization of various elements of the problem-defined and the various means for handling them. For others, the concepts will only add to the burden of attempting to fit all the pieces together in the process of defining the problem. As a basis for deciding whether the model of the geodesic dome is a help or a puzzlement, the student should consider the following suggestions:

One Man's Model, Another Man's Procrustean Bed

1. If he finds it difficult to fit the conceptualizations acquired in the study of the seven components of a problem-defined into the framework of the geodesic dome;

2. If, when he completed the study of the seven components, he felt that he was ready to attempt to define his problem;

3. If he now finds himself confused and uncertain about what he had formerly thought he understood;

4. If he does not readily envision the suggested parallels between elements of the problem-defined and the units of the geodesic dome;

5. If he once felt sufficiently confident of his understanding to start writing the definition of his problem, and now begins to lose that confidence as he tries to envision the suggested parallels;

6. IF THE STUDENT EXPERIENCES ANY OF THESE THINGS—

   a. He should omit study of the sections below where the analogies are delineated;

   b. He should not try to conceptualize the analogy of the geodesic dome, with the many suggested parallels of elements in the problem to units of the dome;

   c. He should move to developing his definition of problem on the basis of his understandings and conceptualizations gleaned from the study of the seven components.

The purpose of the following section, then, is to reidentify various concepts introduced in the delineation of the seven components of the problem-defined, and to discuss them in other detail. Through tracing parallels to the geodesic dome, some of the concepts introduced in the discussion of the seven components will be clarified. In addition, further information and thinking will be introduced to help the student understand the many concepts appertaining to the definition of problem.

Drawing the Parallels

Next to the general analogy between the problem-defined and the geodesic dome, perhaps the most meaningful specific analogy is one that relates to the crux of the problem. The crux of the problem, it will be remembered, is the focal point around which the definition of problem will be developed. It is the specific irritation the investigator would like to do something about. The many considerations relating to the crux of the problem may become graphically clear to the student as he notes the parallels to the specific pyramid chosen to serve as the focal point from which to examine the dome. He will recall the intricacies of the structural materials and the structured units, with their many attachments, and the relationships of particular units to adjacent and to remote units. All aspects of these intricacies and the structures composing them may have parallels in elements in the definition of problem. Perhaps the most significant is the influence of the specific pyramid selected as the focal point for the examination, and what happens when the point of focus is moved to another pyramid, even an immediately adjoining one.

The influence of the selected pyramid on the units that will be highlighted in the examination and on the direction the examination will take has its parallel in the influence of the particular irritation selected as the crux of the problem-defined. The influence of the "crux" irritation will be to highlight closely related irritations and the facts and theories introduced to explain the existence of the problem and to provide suggestions for its possible alleviation.

A Natural Crux

From the discussion of Component 1, in which a real, live story exemplifies the irritation about which the investigator wishes to do something, the student may have the impression that there is a natural crux for the problem as it will be defined. He may think, too, that the crux will naturally be the basic problem or the irritation about which he feels most keenly, or that, from the real, live episode, there will evolve an obvious crux for the problem. Yet some of the discussion of 1A's definition of problem suggested that the crux of the problem may have been arbitrarily selected. There were the discussions of differences that might have occurred had 1A focused on behaviors of personnel rather than of patients. Many aspects of these differences can be made more explicit through the analogy between selecting a particular pyramid to serve as a focal point for examination and selecting the irritation that will serve as the crux of the problem-defined.

Selected Crux

Two approaches for examining a geodesic dome are parallels to two approaches to defining a problem. This visualization will enable the student to begin consideration of many concepts about selecting the crux of the problem-defined. The selected crux is the specific irritation—the precise phenomenon—about which the investigator elects to contribute knowledge through his contemplated research. The planning of a research design cannot progress beyond the first component in the first step until the precise irritation that will be the central, focal concern of the investigator has been explicitly identified. The need for an explicit crux is illustrated in descriptions of irritating elements in 1A's problem and the proposals relating to how different irritations might have differing influences on direction and plan for the study. To return to the analogy, the focal pyramid is arbitrarily selected as a point from which to examine the intricacies of the geodesic dome. The selected crux is arbitrarily chosen as the irritation from which all elements of the problem-defined will derive and to which all will be related, however distantly. The discussions for clarifications will proceed along the lines of two approaches.

In one approach, the individual examining the geodesic dome from a distance parallels the individual attempting to define a global problem. In the second approach, the individual intrigued by the intricacies of the unit structures of the dome is the parallel of the person who views his problem in relation to one specific irritation.

Two Approaches

The individual with the global problem is impressed with the many pieces of the structure but, since his attention is on the total structure, he is unable to maintain focus on, or to describe precisely, the composition and structure of a single unit. As a result, he is unable to describe lucidly its relationship to other units of the structure, adjoining or distant. This individual, when faced with another type of architectural structure—one composed of many different materials structured into many sized and shaped forms and with many different types of connections—might readily identify a starting place and be able to describe the structure. But, when faced with the geodesic dome, with essentially only two types of materials, three shapes and four sizes of forms, and only two types of connections, he is unable to a focus on a single unit so as to fully describe it and its relationships to all other units that compose the whole.

Global Problem

On the other hand, the person with the specific irritation approaches his examination of the dome by seeking out the smallest structural piece and exploring until he has identified explicitly the smallest structural unit. From this point, he goes on to identify its relationship to adjoining units of equal composition and structure. Then he identifies all ways in which the units are related to each other, and ways in which adjoining units provide relationships for the focal unit with units more distant from it. In examining a single unit and its attachments and relationships to other units, the examiner becomes aware of structures and relationships held in common by two or more units; this, in turn, helps him to envision the support derived from certain structures by two or more interrelated units. He becomes aware that, if he were to examine in detail the structures and relationships of a unit adjoining the one he began to examine, he would be examining some of the same units as well as some units and relation-

Specific Irritation

ships not shared by the two. As soon as he realizes that adjoining units can share some common relationships and yet have some individual ones, he can move rapidly toward viewing the total structure of the dome, with understanding of all that composes it and of the relationships and effects of all structural units and connections among them.

The detailed visualization of the two approaches serves two purposes: (1) It provides a concrete portrayal of the value of beginning the definition of problem with a real, live episode. It is hoped that it will serve the student with the global problem to understand the possibility of such an approach. (2) It illustrates the distinction in the process of developing the *components* of the definition of problem and developing each *step* of the design for the investigation. Although there will be modest revisions in supposedly completed steps as later steps of the design are planned, delineation of each step is essentially completed before the next step is begun. In contrast, there will be movement among various components as the definition of problem is developed. The analogies of the elements of the problem-defined to the units of the geodesic dome may be described in further specificity. To the degree that specificity of parallels serves, and with cognizance that rigid parallels would be illogical, Component 1 may be thought of as parallel to one face of a pyramid. Component 2 serves as parallel to a single pyramid; in this component, the selected crux of the problem will be specified. Component 3 would be parallel to a group of pyramids, each sharing a base-bar with six adjacent pyramids and related to other pyramids by connections established by the superstructure of the hexagonal planes.

Movement Back and Forth Between Components

Content of Components 2 and 3 will stem from Component 1. The real, live story will provide identification of several closely related irritations. From among these the investigator will identify his primary concern, the crux around which he will explore the elements composing his total problem. In Components 2 and 3, he will identify related irritations and other elements pertaining to them. As he proceeds, he will find himself describing elements that lead him away from matters closely related to his central irritation and elaborating one of the closely related irritations. In analogy, he will move from describing all faces of one pyramid to describing those of an adjoining pyramid. (1A may readily have moved from concerns about relationships of fear and knowledge as reflected in patient behaviors, to concerns about reasons that staff were not assisting patients to ambulate.) When the investigator finds he is moving away from his selected crux, he should move back to think again about the irritation as he identified it in Component 1 and to determine whether, now that he has examined some closely related irritations, he wishes to explore them further or, alternatively, to focus on the originally selected crux. Whichever decision he makes, many of the elements that he described in his tangential explorations will be pertinent and appropriate portions of his problem-defined.

It is not really possible to identify the crux until the first three components have been explored to some degree. To identify one irritation as the crux without exploring other potentially crucial irritations is to rush toward solution from an incomplete base. Further, the need to move back and forth among the various components, in order to develop adequate bases for the problem-defined and for the design for the investigation, strengthens the admonition that the narrative of the problem-defined should not be presented in distinct sections labeled with the titles of the seven components. The components have been identified to help the student to think through and identify, in an orderly fashion, all elements pertinent to his problem. But the components are not meant to be—they cannot be—perceived each as a distinct whole or entity.

The real, live story will make it possible to identify several closely interrelated irritations. From the parallel of identifying the focal pyramid to selecting the desired crux, it is clear that several of the irritations must be subjected to some preliminary explorations before it is possible to determine the one that will be used as the crux of the problem-defined. And, whichever of the closely related irritations is selected, the others will be supporters of it; it, in turn, would support any of the other irritations, had one of them been chosen as crux. Furthermore, the selected crux will have many elements in common with other irritations, and elements identified in early explorations of various potential cruxes will be pertinent to the problem-defined around the selected crux. The parallel of examination of the entire dome to elaboration of the total problem-defined makes it obvious that the selected crux will determine the direction and content of the total problem-defined. In fact, it will influence the entire investigation, as the student will eventually discover.

Commonalities Shared by Interrelated Irritations

It is, therefore, pertinent to consider in some detail several of the factors that influence the selection of the specific irritation—the crux—from among the many interrelated ones that compose the problem. A very primary factor will be the real, live episode that gave rise to the awareness of an irritation. As mentioned earlier, it would seem that there should be a "natural" crux of a problem; that, once the irritation is identified, so is the crux of the problem. But there are situations in which the very basic problem is something about which nothing can be done, or about which the investigator cannot hope, or does not wish, to do anything directly. Further, there may be the situation of the global problem where the investigator has difficulty in identifying a single irritation from among the many inherent ones. In these or other instances, rather than there being a

Factors Influencing Selection of Crux

Example 1B and Crux of Expediency

single and obvious crux, the investigator must choose the particular aspect of the problem on which he will concentrate.

The following is an example of a situation where the selection of a crux other than the basic (first delineated or first felt) irritation was dictated by circumstances. In a psychiatric nursing study, the primary concern was that patients were not entering into socializing activities. Among the closely related, concomitant irritations was the fact that nursing personnel were not assisting the patients to socialize. The investigator's primary irritation derived from concern for the patients' behaviors; it was patients' conditions he would have liked to do something about. But such changes may evolve slowly and require long periods of consistent care, and he would not have been able to wait for the changes to become observable in the time available to him to execute his study. Therefore, with theories of the interrelationships of particular elements composing his problem serving as his base, and knowing that information about one irritation could provide information about closely related ones, he identified certain behaviors of nursing personnel as the crux for his problem. He endeavored to learn something about their behavior that would serve as a basis for producing change in this behavior, which in turn could be expected to effect change for the patients. The justification for pursuing such a line of investigation stemmed from theories and knowledge learned by others about effects of various actions of persons who associate with withdrawn patients, and on awareness that knowledge that contributes to one aspect of a problem may well apply to intimately related aspects. In this situation, the investigator could not search for direct information about the irritation with which he was most concerned. He therefore decided to settle for seeking related information, confident that this, too, would make a contribution to the broad problem of his concern.

Regardless of which of the two irritations—failure of patients to socialize or the failure of personnel to assist patients to socialize—was chosen as the crux, investigation of either one could have been expected to lead to information about the other. One irritation is intimately related to the other and, as the problem is defined around one crux, the second irritation falls into an immediate tangential area, like the pyramid adjacent to the focal one. In this example, as in 1A's study, findings from a study focused on behaviors of nurses would be expected to effect changes not only in nurses' behaviors but also in the patients' situation. Many of the suggestions that would compose Components 5 and 6 will involve interactions between elements of the selected crux of the problem and those of the closely related irritation. Indeed, a study related to patients—what happens to them, and their responses to care or neglect—may very well include nurse behaviors as part of the study. They certainly will enter into several components of the definition of problem.

But, in this example, it is also clear that the identities of the two potential cruxes would lead to quite different elements in the compositions of all components except the first one in the problem-defined. In Component 2, had the crux been the patients' failure to socialize, the identities of members of various disciplines and the patients' families, with their observed interactions with the patients, would have been introduced. The physical setting of the patients' daily hospital environment, with the apparent influence on patient behaviors of various elements within the setting, would also have been included, as well as descriptions of various institutional policies related to patient activities and routines. On the other hand, had the crux been personnel failures to assist patients to socialize, concern would focus mostly on nursing personnel: the categories of personnel, with qualifications and responsibilities for patient care assigned to them. There would be descriptions of personnel policies, supervision, work setting, and other elements related to motivation and promotion of work.

In Component 3, if the crux were patients' behavior, experiences of others and theories that might explain the behavior would focus on non-socializing behaviors of patients, with many concepts deriving from the literature of abnormal psychology and mental illness. If the crux were the failures of nursing personnel to assist patients to socialize, "experiences of others" would be those focused on nursing personnel in patient care settings similar to those in which mentally ill patients receive hospital treatment. Similarly, the theoretical material would relate to why personnel fail to interact with patients in a manner calculated to assist them to socialize; the theories would derive from the literature of sociology, cultural anthropology, and normal psychology.

The comparisons could be continued for each component in the definition of problem, but this brief and oversimplified presentation of differences in component elaboration promoted by differences in crux should illustrate the large influence of the specificity of the crux. Whatever the particular irritation selected as the crux, there will be many commonalities among the interrelated irritations. Focus on one individual irritation, however, will dictate the need to highlight factors that might have been of secondary importance had a related irritation been selected as the crux of the problem.

Essentially, the original observation that gave rise to an irritation (a problem prompting study) may provide for identification of several irritations, while the particular irritation selected as the focal point for scientific inquiry is determined by arbitrary selection by the investigator. The selection of the crux of the problem is influenced by many things, and the particular irritation selected markedly influences all subsequent elements in the investigation.

The cue to the crux of the problem is the thing that the investigator

Extensive Influence of Crux

Knowledge About Specific, Applicable to General

Step 1: Definition of Problem

wishes to "do something about." The crux selected for study, for various reasons, may be a closely related irritation, rather than the matter of most direct and immediate concern. Pertinent circumstances may be inherent in the problem itself, as in the example of the nonsocializing patients. Or the influencing circumstances may involve such factors as ability or interest of the investigator, or even such prosaic ones as time or money. These examples indicate that the selection of a crux, when it is other than the basic irritation, is usually influenced by several interrelated factors, rather than by a single factor. There is a useful test for identifying the crux of the problem: The crux is the specific irritation the investigator identifies as the one he will try to "do something about" through research to reveal new knowledge about it.

Distractions

Besides the legitimate reasons for selecting as the crux an irritation other than the one of greatest concern to the investigator or the one about which he was first aware, there are reasons that may be classed as distractions from the basic interest. In almost all instances, the distractions derive from the human foible of wanting a quick answer, a prompt solution to a problem. This often happens when the problem involves human behavior in circumstances where some individuals would be readily identified as victims in the situation.

Placing Blame

A natural reaction to an irritation is to endeavor to relieve the irritation; where humans appear to be being victimized, a seemingly natural reaction is to place blame. Observations lead to identification of an irritation but, before the total nature of the irritation has been fully recognized, thoughts move to placing blame as a ready means for relief. In 1A's study, for instance, the natural reaction was to propose that no one was helping the patients to understand about early ambulation, followed by suggestions as to what should be done to help patients. This type of thinking takes precedence over immediate concern for the patients' problems and pursues the line of what should be done and who should be doing it. A concomitant of this thinking is the inadvertent perception that the irritation, the "something about which something must be done," is what personnel are failing to do. In actuality, what any one group of personnel is failing to do is only one element in the situation. For 1A's problem, failure of nurses to instruct patients was one single irritation in the complex of the problem of patients' being fearful and not performing early ambulation activities.

Placing blame may not only lead the investigator away from his primary concern but, as will be illustrated in 1C's work (pages 54 through 60) placing blame may even blind the investigator to the primary concern. In behaviorial science problems, however, there are many irritations that do not involve individuals as victims or give rise to blame-placing: where the irritation of the investigator is curiosity or "wanting to know," as in studies of why persons behave as they do or how children learn; or where the investigator wants to find a better way, such as in studies to test various teaching methods or new highway patterns. Yet, even in these instances, there frequently will be distractions from the crucial irritation.

In all instances, the distraction derives from the urge for the quick or "obvious" answer. And the effects are the same. They cause the investigator to veer unwittingly from his primary concern and lead to confusion in defining the problem and in planning later steps in the research. Or they lead the investigator to omit development of Components 2 and 3. He will fail to identify and explore a variety of interrelated irritations, and he will move on to hasty, incomplete, and inaccurate development of Components 5 and 6. A problem so defined will cause persistent uneasiness and fail to provide needed ideas and information throughout the entire investigation.

Urge For the Quick Answer

If the investigator, when thinking of Components 5 and 6, finds that he can propose only one or two suggestions for actions that might contribute to creating some aspect of or an approach to the ideal of Component 4, he should look to his Components 2 and 3 to determine whether he has identified and discussed a number of irritations closely related to his selected crux. And if he finds himself at a loss when he comes to Steps 4 and 5, Defining the Terms and Identifying Data, he might well return to his definition of problem. He should consider, in particular, elaborations of closely interrelated irritations, to determine whether he succumbed to distractions from his central concern. Again, parallels could be drawn between elements in the process of examining the geodesic dome by extending outward from a focal pyramid, and elements in the process of defining the problem by moving outward from the focus of a specific irritation.

Effect of Distractions

The fact that the dome rather than the geodesic sphere was chosen as the point of parallel, it will be remembered, was because a sphere is a complete and closed entity, whereas a dome, like a problem, is never a "naturally" complete geodesic structure. The omission of identification and elaboration about many elements composing the problem-defined may be thought of as another parallel. On examination of the dome, it is assumed that the units on the side away from the lighted pyramid are there, but they need not be examined, identified, nor described to provide the examiner with an understanding of the essential structure of the dome. So it is with the problem-defined: as elements become more distant from the focal irritation, they need not be included in the elaborations.

Far Side of the Dome

Parallels to these ideas about structures on the other side of the dome may be seen in the recommendation to omit personal speculations from Component 3 and to delineate them in Components 5 and 6. The parallels apply, also, to Component 7.

Units of the Far Side in Various Components

In Components 5 and 6, the investigator limits proposals to those of his own or his discipline's concern and interest. Essentially, as he recognizes that potentially related facts and theories become only distantly supportive of his suggestions and concerns, he discusses them in less detail. These elements in the problem-defined may be thought of as the structures and units more distant from the lighted pyramid. Elements potentially related, but not mentioned at all, are analogous to units on the other side of the dome. In Component 7, as an analogy to the superstructure, the investigator, in effect, makes specific the perspective from which he is viewing the structure. He identifies the particular spokes (theories and facts) composing the hexagonal planes and their relationships to the various pyramids he will examine. He describes the various apparent influences of the spokes on the sizes and shapes of the faces of the pyramid to which they are attached. The components and structural configuration of the hexagonal planes, of course, are parallels to the facts and theories that the investigator perceives as explaining the irritations. Just as elements from other components remain implied (parallels to structures on the far side of the dome), so many of the facts and theories of Component 7 are left without full elaboration or are left implicit (as parallels to superstructure units on the far side of the dome).

Parallels to Optical Phenomena

These considerations of the observable phenomena that are part of actually looking at a geodesic dome, along with the examination of individual structured units and relationships among them, form a very apt parallel to the development of the problem-defined. As figurative parallels, for instance, to the three phenomena that occur as a dome is given detailed scrutiny, such as the inability to move outward in concentric circles of equal radii, and others (page 31), the student, as he elaborates elements of his problem, will move to more distant tangents for some elements than for others. He will not describe, nor even mention, all potentially related elements; some elements will be elaborated in detail; others, seemingly, will be left hanging. Some elements will be only tenuously linked to the crux of the problem, and many remotely related elements will be left implied—they are on the other side of the dome.

Which Facet to Which Plane

The analogy of the problem-defined to the geodesic dome also makes clear that it is very difficult to identify a single, specific hexagonal plane of the dome. The immediately adjoining units seem to run into and become part of it, or its parts seem to become portions of adjoining planes, as indeed they are. Similarly, one theory may explain several observed elements in the problem, and several theories may be pertinent to explaining a single observed phenomenon. Just as the triangular components, which support several related structural units and which serve as unit-components of two or more planes, are not duplicated in the structure of the dome, so theories that pertain to several observed phenomena need not be delineated repeatedly in the definition of problem.

A Geodesic Dome

One hexagonal plane supports several pyramids, and several planes may be identified as providing support for a single pyramid. So it is when developing the elements of Components 5 and 6. One suggestion and its elaborations lead to identification of one closely related to it, and to another and another. No single facet of a plane is ever the property of one plane alone: it is a unit of other planes that may encompass it. Further, no single triangular facet can be completely independent; it serves to compose a larger unit, which, in turn, is a unit of a still larger unit. (Big fleas have little fleas/ Upon their backs to bite 'em;/ Little fleas have lesser fleas/ And so *ad infinitum*. Paraphrase from Jonathan Swift.)

The inevitable evolvement of the complex of interrelationships among the elements of the problem-defined makes it imperative that the investigator complete elaborations of all proposals and concepts relating to a single element before moving to describe a closely related element. If he does not complete delineation of all facets of a single proposal of Component 5, this should be by choice, based on awareness that he is moving to another element and has a reason for doing so. Among his reasons for doing so may be that theories supporting the one proposal provide support for the newly introduced element, or that theories to provide the rationale for the element have been delineated earlier and their pertinence for the element under consideration may be left implicit.

For a dome, it takes careful scrutiny to determine to which composite unit a single facet of a plane will be ascribed. For a problem-defined, it may be equally difficult to distinguish the precise element that is being elaborated when particular rationale and supporting theories are being described. Frequently, it is unnecessary to make these relationships explicit. Nonetheless, awareness of possible vagueness about implied relationships can serve the investigator as a guide to possible sources of difficulties in clearly conceptualizing various facets of his problem or of describing them so that others may envision them as he does.

To put it another way, because of the blurring of boundaries between facets of one plane or between facets of adjoining planes, it is not necessary to be rigid about identification of boundaries or of precise elements to which any one concept or suggestion is related. Few will pertain to only one element or to a single definable unit of the problem.

Which Theory to Which Suggestion

But the student should be aware of the potential for blurring so that he can understand what has happened when he suddenly finds that he is far off on a tangent and getting farther from his selected crux with each new idea. He can correct this by tracing back to identify where he stopped elaborating about one suggestion and anticipated results, and started focusing on another suggestion. He can then complete the discussion of the initial suggestion or, deciding that it has been sufficiently elaborated, make clearly explicit the new suggestion and complete the discussion of it. He will, of course, decide to which of the closely related suggestions the seeming digression is most pertinent.

Seeming Changes in Size, Shape, Shading

The seeming existence of 12 facets in a pyramid and their seeming changes in size, shape, and shading provide another parallel to the blurring of boundaries between components, to relating theories to one element and soon finding them relating to another, and to sudden awareness of having moved from discussion of one element to discussion of another. The 12 facets only seem to exist; they are not concrete constructions, and they change in size, shape, and proportion only as they are viewed from different angles. So with many proposals of relationships of theories to suggestions for actions and anticipated results: they may yield varied constructs, depending on the perspective from which they are viewed. There are many illustrations of these concepts throughout the planning of research. One lies in the proposal that the definition of problem may be limited by interest, concern, and capability of the investigator. His interest and concern will influence the number and character of suggestions that will be proposed, the number and character of anticipated results, and the number and character of various theories elaborated to support the proposals. The angle from which the investigator views the elements of the problem will influence the composite units identified, along with the size and shape of the facets and the shadings of each facet.

Ideas in Clusters— Example 1A

Descriptions of elements, particularly those in Components 5 and 6, tend to evolve in clusters. One idea suggests another and another. Each will be explored and described in full, or at least in some detail. Finally, all seemingly closely related ideas will be exhausted, and the investigator will turn to another tack. This is similar to his having examined all pertinent faces and shadings of faces of one pyramid and now moving on to consideration of another pyramid—either one adjoining the focal pyramid or one attached by a spoke (theory or fact) of the superstructure. For example, 1A may have discussed elements related to ways to make early ambulation easier and less painful for the patient. She will have discussed elements related to effects of ambulation and failure to ambulate, including pathophysiological considerations of greatest import for patients with abdominal and thoracic surgery. She will have considered elements in the physician's responsibilities for patients' actions. She will have presented ideas about family members assisting patients to ambulate. She will have posed various suggestions about nurses teaching patients. Each major area of consideration will have been explored through discussing a cluster of closely related and pertinent suggestions and anticipated results.

As the researcher goes on with the planning and writing of the definition of problem, he will frequently pause to consider whether one detail or another *needs* to be included. After a few episodes of indecision, followed by (1) deciding that the detail is not needed, (2) writing other ideas, and then (3) finding that, in order to make a later idea clear or to show its relationship to the whole, he needs what he earlier had decided not to include—after a few experiences, he will learn that it takes less time to write a particular detail at the time it first seems pertinent than it takes to make the decision about whether or not to write it. Once written, he has it and is not repeatedly plagued with needing it and not having it. A good rule is: if a detail seems pertinent, write it! It may well be needed later and, if it is not, it can be readily deleted. Following this rule will save time and frustration in the long run—and defining a problem is a long run!

When in Doubt— Write It!

The potential overlapping of pertinent materials among various components, especially among 3, 5, and 6, can serve to remind the researcher that, although distinct components of the problem-defined may be identified, the narration of the definition of problem should not portray the seven components as independent sections. They are not independent, either in format or in the flow of the narrative of the many elements and their interrelationships.

Components Not Independent Units

Here again is an analogy to identities and interrelationships among individual structural units of the geodesic dome. The reason for identifying the seven components is to remind the student of major categories of elements that appropriately are components of the problem-defined and need to be developed in an orderly fashion. The planner should avoid *listing* various items as a part of the definition of problem. Elements in the setting, questions to which answers will be sought, or theories potentially pertinent to the problem are all appropriate components of a problem-defined, but they should not be in list form, save in the outline developed to guide the writing of the definition. A listing, in other words, should be viewed as the assembling of supplies at the work area. These supplies do not become a part of the problem-defined until they have been attached into their place in the structure. This calls for a precise identification of the other structural components to which they will be attached and a description of the nature of the attachment. The latter will elaborate the purpose served by the particular structural material as it relates to the adjoining structural materials and to the total structure.

Listings, No! Full Development of Ideas, Yes!

In the definition of problem, each idea should be woven into a narrative, through elaboration of the idea and its relationship to other ideas and to the whole. An idea should not be dismissed with mere identification. This is particularly applicable to questions suggested as guides to identifying information that might be sought through investigation. Before these questions can serve as guides to potentially pertinent information, it will be necessary to think through the kind of information that might provide answers to the questions and the potential sources for that information. The questions can serve to stimulate and organize thinking, but the thinking should be part of the narrated definition of problem, not something that may be left until later in the design planning, with the vague hope that it will not be so painful then. The thinking-through process will be equally painful whenever it is undertaken, but when done as part of defining the problem, its results can serve to make later planning easier and, incidentally, less diffuse.

Example 1A

For example, 1A may have identified the questions:

1. Why must patients perform early ambulation activities?
2. Why are patients afraid to move following surgery?
3. What early ambulation activities should be taught:
   To patients with abdominal surgery?
   To patients with thoracic surgery?
4. What information do patients need to know?
5. Who is responsible for teaching patients?
6. How can patients best be taught?

These questions and many more were pertinent to the irritation as 1A first recognized it. For the person knowledgeable in the area, the questions suggest information related to the problem. They do not, however, make information explicit nor do they indicate relationships among various elements of the problem and information about it. Furthermore, they do not identify precisely the information the researcher has in mind—all of which will be needed for development of later steps in the design and execution of the study.

Ideas, Questions, Suggestions, Answers— Elaborate

Questions do, of course, have a place in the development of the definition of problem. They can serve a very useful purpose in promoting thinking about the definition of the problem, but they are useful only if types of information needed for answers are logically thought through and delineated. The few questions noted above indicate the detail of the definition of problem. To be fully useful, delineation of potential answers must be a part of the research plan. The delineation will be no more difficult to do and will serve best when it is part of the definition of problem. After describing in Components 5 and 6, a number of suggestions pertinent to several major areas, the investigator will recognize that he is finding commonalities among many anticipated results. This is particularly so in relation to ideas supporting and appertaining to rationale for suggested actions. There, he will be describing ties and relationships between proximal and distant composite units of the dome. At this point of frequent commonalities, he may propose the suggestion that he believes is the action most likely to make the greatest contribution to alleviation of the problem. That is, he will introduce the action that he may expect to effect during his investigation, with the objective of revealing knowledge as a contribution to alleviation of the problem.

A Geodesic Dome

The final portion of the definition of problem should indicate the direction the investigation will take. To do this, the planner elaborates in greater detail about the particular suggestion he sees as most likely to make a major contribution to alleviation of the problem. The detail will include discussion of the elements composing the suggestion and their relationship to those elements identified as composing the selected irritation. In this section it would be appropriate not only to draw from observable elements in Component 3, but also to reiterate some of the theories from various sciences. The investigator will delineate how these theories provide ideas leading to the suggestion and serve as rationale for executing the proposed suggestion. He should also explain how they provide support for the anticipated results. This portion of the problem-defined will include the elements of Component 7.

Movement to Closure

For example, 1A may have suggested any number of actions to be performed by members of various disciplines that might serve to provide information to patients, with anticipated alleviation of the problem of nonambulation. She may have proposed use of many teaching techniques and media, and she could well have justified each suggestion with established theories and experiences of others as support for her proposals. She may also have proposed various outcomes for suggestions to alleviate the problem, such as that patients would have fewer postoperative respiratory and circulatory complications and less incisional pain, that hospital stay would be shortened, that patients' coughs would be more effective, and others. Indeed, her definition of problem does delineate facts and related theories about all of these suggestions. But her study had to be limited to what could be accomplished within the scope of a masters thesis and to her own competence in executing the investigation. Therefore, the culmination of her definition of problem was directed toward the suggestion that nurses might provide instructions for patients. She described the content of the instructions, the techniques and timing of the teaching: a simple instruction sheet with stick-figure drawings that she proposed would enhance the patients' understanding. Similarly, she limited elaboration of possible outcomes to those that could be reasonably expected to stem from teaching done by the nurse. She proposed that patients who were taught preoperatively and had reinforcements of the instructions early postoperatively could be expected to ambulate earlier and more frequently and to cough more effectively than patients not so taught. She supported this proposal with many learning theories and theories from physiology and psychology. The theories that excessive stress interferes with learning and that fear immobilizes were the primary bases for her suggestion. To indicate the significance of her study, she described the anatomical relationships and physiological processes affected by the surgery and the physiologic effects of early ambulation in preventing complications. The detailed construction

Example 1A

of this particular facet of the larger problem culminated in the development of the hypothesis that generalized and identified the facet of the problem to be studied, pointing the direction and serving as the focal point of the information-seeking investigation.

The concept of the culmination of the problem-defined being the development of the hypothesis which, in turn, is the focal point of the investigation, should not be confused with concepts about the crucial irritation as the focal point for the definition of problem. Distinctions in relation to these two focuses will be made clear in the discussion of Step 2.

Recapitulation

Essentially, then, the early delineation of the definition of the problem will identify many elements closely related to the original irritation. Preliminary explorations to determine what is known about each of the elements will yield suggestions about the ways in which the various elements are interrelated and their roles in the problem's existence. At this point, the planner will recognize elements within the setting of the problem, several of which may be considered irritations in themselves. Each of these will be evaluated against the planner's original concern and in relation to his particular interest and ability to execute a scientific inquiry, with the objective of selecting the specific irritation to be pursued. Once the crux of the problem has been identified and selected, all exploration and description of related ideas and knowledge will be directed to describing the problem in its setting and its effects, to explaining the phenomena of the problem, and to suggesting actions that might be taken to alleviate it. Accompanying the suggestions will be facts and theories that provide a rationale for the validity of the suggestions.

REVIEW OF LITERATURE

The facts and theories that validate the merit of the suggestions are derived from thinking through the application of what others have learned and thought about the problem. In essence, they are the section of the research usually referred to as the "review of literature." The format used to present this review may be arbitrarily chosen by the individual investigator. It would, however, seem easier to visualize the intimate relationship of these materials to the problem to be studied, if materials from the literature are used throughout much of the definition of problem, rather than being reserved for a different, or possibly separate, section. A fine example of a review of the literature being interwoven throughout the section devoted to definition of the problem may be found in the report of a study by Godfrey, where she titled the particular section: "The Problem in Its Context." [4]

Review of Literature

The researcher reviews the literature for many purposes and during various steps in his investigation. When a problem has been recognized, it is reasonable to search the literature to determine whether others have faced the problem and what they may have learned, thought, and done about it. Indeed, before the student turns to his teacher, he should first attempt to learn something about his problem for himself. His most direct and fruitful source is the literature. Just as search of the literature has a role in Step 1, so it will be used for particular purposes in other steps of the research process. Rather than a detailed delineation of the use of the literature here, description of this task will be limited to identifying the major purposes of a review of the literature and to making some recommendations that may save the beginning researcher a few time-consuming, trial-and-error experiences.

Adjunct to Several Steps

Essentially, the literature is reviewed for three major purposes:

Reasons For Review of Literature

1. To learn what others have learned, thought, done, and reported about the problem
2. To learn more about particular elements in the problem
3. To learn about techniques and tools which may serve requirements of the investigation.

The first purpose has been alluded to in the discussion of the various components of Step 1. This should be the only purpose in the early search of the literature. Expending time on the other two purposes before the problem has been defined in detail may well be time wasted—at least, as far as advancing the goal of the investigation is concerned. Particular elements with which the researcher will be concerned cannot be identified until the problem has been defined in detail. Identification of appropriate tools and techniques is dependent on those particular elements.

These facts will become clear in the discussions of later steps; they are mentioned here only to caution the student not to rush on to the solution before defining the problem. The procedure for reviewing the literature is similar, regardless of the purpose to be served, and it is one that all college students learn, long before they start using the writings of others to assist them in executing research: know your library, use the card catalogue, use indexes and library guides, and seek assistance from the librarian and others. Among some "simple" practices commonly overlooked by beginning researchers are the following:

Hints

1. Use bibliographies accompanying the reports of research of others studying the same or a related problem. Make an early judgment of the value of the bibliography submitted by a writer (quantity does not always indicate judicious selection). Check all entries related to the problem at hand.

STEP 1: DEFINITION OF PROBLEM

2. Be lavish in the use of bibliography cards. Shed traditional nurse frugality in use of supplies and dare to leave a major portion of a card unused. Limit notes to a single entry on a card. The complete bibliographic information for any one reference need appear on only one card: for succeeding ones, use author and journal abbreviations or develop a personal code.
3. Learn early the format for bibliographical entries used in the manual of style for theses and dissertations accepted by the faculty of your college; then enter all bibliographic notations on your cards in the approved manner. This will assure ready relocation of the reference and will save many hours of later checking.
4. Skim a reference to determine its revelance for your immediate concern and to judge the type of relevance. A part of this judgment should be a decision about the type of notations you will take from the reference: a brief evaluative note, a summarizing paragraph, a sketchy outline, or detailed notes, including direct quotations. Double-check all quotations for accuracy to obviate the frustrating need for later rechecking.

Annotated Bibliography

Allusions to and direct quotations from various references will appear throughout the research design and in the final report. Ideas gleaned from the literature will be incorporated in the definition of the problem, including the delineation of the theoretical framework. Many research reports present a separate section in which ideas and findings of others as they relate to the problem at hand are discussed. An excellent example of this may be found in An Investigation of the Relation Between Nursing Activity and Patient Welfare.[5]

A subtle, most interesting, and remarkably effective way to present the findings from related literature is to use judiciously selected direct quotations in an annotated bibliography. This requires careful study of the references to determine the words of the writer that best express his ideas pertinent to the investigator's concern. Scholarly judgment is necessary to select quotations with direct implications for the problem at hand. But the striking aspect of this presentation is the intriguing aptness of many of the quotations in their relevance to, elaboration of, and support for the points being made by the investigator. Presumably, some of the interest in this type of presentation is due to the elimination of stilting and repetitious "He-said-thats" found in many reviews of the literature. The direct-quotations annotated bibliography, on the other hand, presents some of the authors' best expressed ideas, couched in their own phrases, and enhanced by the intriguing subtlety with which they relate to the problem under examination.

Review of Literature

The beginning writer of research reports often asks: "What should go in footnotes?" Footnotes may be used to serve three major ends:

1. Acknowledge the source of the idea
2. Cite authority for ideas or information
3. Report information or explanations which will be of interest to the reader, but would interrupt the flow of the ideas if placed in the text.

Footnotes

Lest the student, overly conscious that "there is nothing new under the sun," hesitate to claim any ideas as his own, here is one guide: new ideas that have not yet become general knowledge should be credited to the originator, but ideas that have reached textbooks have become part of the public domain and perhaps have been widely enough disseminated as to not require acknowledgment of source. There may be exceptions to this rule-of-thumb, but if the student finds the same idea expressed in two textbooks by different authors, without one crediting the other, he may feel safe in omitting an accrediting footnote.

When to Give Credit

This does not mean that textbooks will never be cited in footnotes; they will frequently be used by the student who wishes to strengthen his presentation by citing authorities whose opinions he esteems and believes will be esteemed by his readers. Here, again, the student must assert confidence in his own abilities and not succumb to the timid, unscholarly practice of excessive citing of authority. He should avoid two obvious excesses: footnotes citing authority for every idea expressed, and footnotes citing numerous authorities for any one idea. There can be no absolute guides for appropriate use of footnotes to cite authorities, but it may help if the student tries to put himself in the place of his expected readers. He should try to anticipate the questions they may ask, the information they may want, or the information which he believes will be helpful to them.

Anticipate Reader's Interest

This latter consideration is perhaps the most important. Writing is done for others; writers wish to impart information to others; writers should have ideas about what it is they most wish to tell to others. Needless to say, if the writer is a student, the report a course assignment, and the anticipated reader the teacher who will ascribe a "grade," the footnotes citing authorities may be different from those presented by a researcher reporting to peers.

As in the other two purposes for using footnotes, some intuition is required in making judgments about the content of footnotes used to present information that would interrupt the flow of the narrative if included in the text. Related to this is the question of materials to be placed in an appendix. Some subscribe to the concept that materials "too lengthy" should be placed in an appendix, but this seems of little help. In both in-

Limit Explaining Footnotes

stances, the need for intuitive judgment is paramount. Perhaps the best guide in relation to explanatory footnotes is: *use as few as possible.*

1. Consider first the possibility of expressing the idea so that it relates closely enough to the text to be entered as a part of it.
2. If the above is not appropriate, consider the use of a parenthetical statement.
3. If neither of the first two will do, yet it will help the reader to have the information at this point, then resort to the explanatory footnote.

Examples of these three alternatives often occur in discussions of tables or charts:

1. "In Table N, the findings are . . ."
2. "The tabulated data (Table N) reveal . . ."
3. "The tabulated data reveal . . ." (with the information about the table placed in a footnote).

Each of these methods is correct, yet the first seems to be the least interruptive of the flow of the narrative.

With each succeeding step in the process of scientific inquiry, the student must make the decision about when he has done sufficient planning to justify his moving to next steps. This same philosophy applies to the review of the literature. The student must decide when he has sufficiently explored the literature for information about various elements in his study to justify incorporating what he has found into his plan and moving to the next steps.

THEORETICAL FRAMEWORK

The development of a theoretical framework is frequently considered as a distinct entity within the research design. But rather than thinking of this as something separate and entire in itself, it should be recognized that, as Components 3, 5, and 6 are being developed, the varied units that will be used in construction of the theoretical framework are being identified. In Component 6, particularly, selected units are being built into the structure of the problem-defined. This is not to say that the theoretical framework will not be recognizable as an identifiable element. Rather, since the theoretical framework is an integral part of the problem-defined, it should be recognized as an element (or network of elements) in the problem-defined, instead of as an individual step in the total research process. One reason for this proposal is that although the theoretical framework could be pulled out to stand alone, the problem-defined cannot stand without the theoretical framework. And, although the theoretical framework could stand alone, it would have little meaning without the specifics of persons, places, and processes of the problem.

The theoretical framework provides one of the most direct parallels to components and structured units of the geodesic dome. What others have learned, thought, and done about the problem (the facts and theories gleaned from the literature) are the elements in the problem-defined that parallel the spokes and hexagonal planes (the supporting superstructure) of the geodesic dome. The structural materials themselves, the structured units into which they are built, and their relationships to each other and to the units they support—all have their parallels in Components 3, 5, and 6. In addition, some are highlighted in Component 7.

Theoretical Framework: Superstructure of the Dome

Indeed, it is helpful if the planner very explicitly identifies the theoretical framework of the problem; nurses in particular need to consider this seriously. So far, nursing research efforts have resulted in, at best, tenuously related bits and pieces. Not until nurse researchers devote extensive time and effort to developing the theoretical framework structures of each problem investigated will new information revealed through research develop into a unified body of nursing knowledge.

Develop Integrated Body of Knowledge

The concept of *a unified body* of nursing knowledge, however, is a myth. There will never be a complete, unchanging, finally established body of knowledge to serve nurses. Nonetheless, nurses should strive to identify knowledge that is meaningful to nursing and to develop integrated patterns of the bits and pieces so identified. To the extent that each nurse researcher assumes responsibility for exploring widely and thinking deeply about all elements and their interrelationships encompassed in the problem under study, and then takes time to make them explicit early in the process of her study—to this extent will nurses develop unified, integrated, usable bodies of knowledge. It will be through the explicitly described relationships to nursing concerns that the bodies of knowledge will be available for all to use in their nursing practice.

The primary reason for the beginning researcher to develop the detailed definition of problem is to assure herself that she understands the many elements composing the definition of her problem and the potential meanings and interrelationships of each. In thus serving her own needs, she serves a second aim: the presentation of information and suggestions for applications in nursing situations. The accomplished nurse researcher might well consider this second purpose as her primary aim, viewing her elaborate definition of problem, which encompasses varied and extensive pieces of information and detailed explanation of potential meanings for nursing, as her primary concern. She might well address her report to the nurse practitioner. If she were to do this, to think that she is directly serving nurse practitioners who will read and use the information and reasoning she presents, she will achieve two major contributions to nursing

Problem-Defined to Serve Nurse Practitioner

in a single undertaking. She will have developed a usable definition of the problem she plans to investigate and, equally important, she will have made an early contribution to knowledge readily available to practicing nurses. And, by directing her discussion to nurse practitioners, she will have eliminated a goodly amount of research jargon from her writing and thereby helped clarify much of her own thinking.

In their first research efforts, nurses looked to behavioral scientists for assistance. They might now very well again seek this sort of help in developing their theoretical framework. The social scientists are in the forefront of researchers who are disciplining themselves to the patient, time-consuming effort of making explicit theoretical frameworks, of schematically portraying the numerous elements and their multiple interrelationships encompassed in the problem-defined. Nurses seeking the assistance of social scientists in this respect, however, must remember that the early assistance offered by social scientists led nurses to explore the concerns of the social scientists, not of nurses. Nurses now are sufficiently sophisticated researchers to take what is meaningful to them for studies of problems of intimate concern to nurses and to avoid problems more suitably and competently studied by members of other disciplines.

The development of a theoretical framework as a part of the definition of problem poses another problem that will confront the researcher throughout the entire investigation and one that confronts all researchers at all points in all research they will ever do. It is to decide when one step is sufficiently complete to warrant moving to the next one. When have all possible elements been considered? To sufficient depth? With adequate theorizing about interrelationships? The answer is, of course, "Never." At some point, however, the investigator must decide to move forward with his inquiry.

RECAPITULATION THROUGH EXAMPLE 1C

Example 1C elaborates one student's experience with the development of her definition of problem and also illustrates several critical aspects in the process of defining the problem.[6] Various aspects are elaborated, while explicit elaboration of others would be superfluous. The beginning researcher will empathize with many of 1C's feelings and much of her thinking; she may also learn a great deal from the single experience of one beginning researcher like herself.

Example 1C illustrates particularly well the variety of considerations and thinking that may be involved in selecting the crux of the problem. The first occasion on which 1C thought through her problem in a somewhat systematic fashion was when she was asked in class to identify a

Recapitulation Through Example 1C

problem (irritation) of concern to her. She began by stating: "My irritation is that school physicians are not doing their jobs." When asked to elaborate, she commented that children were neglected and school principals should make physicians do their work. When challenged to explain why she was concerned that school physicians were not doing their jobs, she protested that children had health care needs that were allowed to persist, with nothing done about them, for four and five years. If school physicians were doing their jobs, she contended, they would see to it that the children received care. This identification of a problem contains several elements pertinent to developing a definition of problem. The slightly more complete story will serve as a basis for their identification and discussion.

With only a few more probing questions, 1C told the following story of experiences, observations, and thinking that resulted in her first-expressed irritation. In response to the question, "What was the first thing you observed that made you start thinking 'something ought to be done'?" she referred to children doing poorly in school whose health records had identified them as having poor vision, limited hearing, infected tonsils, and other subacute disease conditions. The conditions had been identified by teachers and the nurse, and the diagnoses had been confirmed by the school physician three or more years earlier. The conditions had been reported to the parents, too. In many instances, the school nurse had visited the home to discuss an individual child's needs and to encourage the parents to seek medical attention for the child. But nothing had been done: the children had not been taken to a physician; the needs persisted; the children continued to do poorly in school.

The nurse had discussed the needs of particular children with their teachers, who deplored the children's conditions; they reported that they too had communicated with the parents and the school physician about them. The physician said he could do no more than identify the needs and inform the parents of the children's need for care. The parents offered the same excuses to the teachers as they did to the nurse. 1C proposed: "If the physician 'wanted to,' he could do something. He could *make* parents have the child cared for or he could *insist* on school and community programs that would provide for such children."

Obviously, there are several interrelated irritations in this story. Quite obviously, also, 1C identified several areas of blame: the school principal, the parents, and, most especially, the school physician. Part of her rationale for the latter was that the generally accepted authority status of the physician enabled him to do something; therefore, he *should* do something. Indeed, 1C had developed quite a mind-set on this idea, and it took considerable probing to help her move to a position about which she, as a nurse, could expect to do something. The probing included several shock

Blame

questions and admonishments, such as: "Why do you care how the physician does his job?" "What concern is it of yours, what the physician does?" "Remember, you are attempting to identify a problem about which you might expect to make some improvement, through study and revealing new knowledge. Do you expect to observe what the physician does with his time and then tell him how to do his job?" After she had expended some of her pent-up emotions on consideration of these and other questions, attempt was made to have her focus on what it was that irritated her: the very first stimulus to irritation. She was asked to describe the basis of her concern and the observations that had led her to think something should be done. What was it that she wanted to have changed? She persisted in identifying the behavior of the school physician as the irritation and the thing she wanted to see changed.

The Real, Live Story— Finally!

When pressed to describe one real, live episode that had started her thinking, she described visits made to the school healthroom by three children from one family. The children were aged 9, 10, and 11; each was a year or more behind in school progress; the health record of each revealed reports of poor vision for three or more years; none of the children had had medical attention for the condition. The nurse had discussed the situation with the teachers and had made a home visit. Nothing was done to help the children. She ended the story with a comment about the school physician neglecting his responsibility. She was reminded that, with her report of direct observation and experience, she had identified, as her basic irritation, concern for the children.

What the Investigator Can Help and Not Help

Because of her persistence in placing blame and proposing that the needed change was the physician's behavior, her story identified another factor in deciding about the crux of the problem to be defined: that is, the matter of elements in the situation about which the investigator may expect to be able to do something. 1C was challenged to describe elements of a study in which she might hope to influence the physician's behavior. Her response led to identifying a study whose primary purpose would be to gain knowledge relating to the nurse telling the physician how to do his job. Obviously, the possibility of acquiring the needed information was not very good; and, even if it were acquired, the nurse could hardly expect the new knowledge to be utilized by physicians.

At this point, 1C was ready to attempt to focus on the basic irritation —concern for the health of the children—and to identify many elements in the situation that would be the content of Component 2 of her problem-defined. This meant describing the physician's role in perspective and viewing it on a par with the many other elements contributing to, supporting, and impinging on the basic irritation. There was detail of effects of neglected health needs on the child's progress in school, his development in the family, his relationships with children in his home neighborhood, his future as an adult. These latter considerations, of course, are among the elements of Component 3: the problem in its largest universe, including theoretical considerations pertinent to the problem.

Further itemization of elements considered portrays the blurring of boundaries between Components 2 and 3. There was description of the school's program for meeting health needs of children, and of roles of the teachers, the nurse, the physician, the administrator, and the board members. Family provision for the child, including the many factors that influence the care provided, was described. Community provision for health care of medically indigent families was identified. Obviously, behavioral change on the part of any one group of persons involved in the original irritation could not be expected to do much toward alleviation of the problem.

Blurring of Boundaries

This does not mean that the original irritation did not provide a focal point from which to consider the problem, nor that it was a problem which a nurse could not investigate as a means for "doing something about it." Elaboration of Component 2 made it quite obvious that the selected crux of the problem could be the neglect of particular health needs of particular school children. 1C, as she had repeatedly observed and thought about episodes illustrative of this irritation, had concluded that the primary irritation was failure of school physicians to do their jobs. This was followed closely by the irritation expressed as the failure of the principal to make the physician do his job. Nonetheless, the real, live story made it obvious that the original source of concern was the neglect of the children.

Natural Crux and Concrete Observations

Among lessons to be learned from this is the fact that the original irritation provided a "natural" crux for a problem worthy of inquiry. Further, the "natural" crux stemmed from the true concern of the investigator, which, in turn, derived from concrete observations. The irritations first *expressed* by 1C were not derived from direct observations of facts; rather, they were interpretations of facts. It is true that the selected crux, the irritation around which the problem definition will evolve, may derive from interpretations of facts. But the researcher should clearly understand the relationship between the irritation prompted by interpretation of facts and the actually observed facts that gave rise to the thinking "something ought to be done."

Selected Crux and Interpretations of Observations

The most direct route to alleviating a problem will stem from defining the problem around the observed facts that gave rise to the first irritation. When an irritation arising from interpretations of facts is selected as a crux, it must be because various circumstances preclude direct investigation of facts surrounding the originally observed facts and the irritation they engendered. No such extenuating circumstances, however, dictated the need for 1C to pursue other than her original observations and irritation. Indeed, in her case, circumstances dictated against her pursuing the tangential irritations that had derived from interpretations of facts.

For 1C, identifying any of the closely related irritations as the selected crux of the problem would have led away from the original irritation and would have resulted in search for knowledge rather distantly related to the original concern. Among the ideas considered during the development of Component 2, and the search for the identity of the crux of the problem, would be: (1) The children had unmet health needs. (2) Many factors and persons were involved. (3) Extensive and varied information could reasonably be sought in attempts to alleviate the problem. (4) It would be possible to identify facets of the problem that could be investigated by one or more members of any one of the disciplines involved. (5) It would be possible to identify several facets of the problem-defined around the natural crux of the original irritation that could be investigated by a nurse. The most expeditious approach to alleviating a problem is to seek knowledge directly related to the basic irritation. A nurse, therefore, could pursue any one of several lines of investigation stemming from the original and basic concern—the neglect of health needs of school children. Under these circumstances, the only rational selection as the crux for the problem to be defined would be the original irritation; none of the closely related ones could be justified.

With this point reached, it was possible for 1C to move on to develop details of Component 3, wherein the experiences, thinking, and actions of others would be elaborated. Details of this Component and of Component 4 need not be outlined here. It may be seen, however, that the problem-defined around the natural and, in this instance, the selected crux could be voluminous. But if elaborations in Components 5 and 6 (suggested actions and anticipated results) were limited to suggestions for actions that the nurse might effect independently or might largely control, there would be some reasonable boundaries and an eventual stopping place for the definition of problem.

Attributes of Selected Crux

Defining the problem around the irritation occasioned by unmet health needs of school children illustrates several considerations pertinent to selection of the crux of the problem. Where there are many closely related and intimately interwoven irritations, and where the urgency of the problem leads the concerned individual to propose prompt solution, there may be resort to placing blame. Whether blame has played a part in identifying the irritation may be determined by questioning the source of the irritation and the process of its identification. Where the irritation has been identified through thinking about a situation, rather than through direct observation and experience of a situation, and where it has stemmed from a search for a cause for the observed irritation, it is possible that the identified irritation is tangential to the basic irritation.

Some attributes of an appropriate selected crux can serve as leads to selecting such a crux. The many closely related irritations should be examined to determine which possesses the following attributes: (1) The irritation stems from concrete observations that prompted thinking "something ought to be done." (2) The irritation is the one most urgently needing something done about it. (3) The irritation is one about which the investigator can reasonably expect to be able to do something.

An adaptation of the experience of 1C illustrates, in very limited detail, what might be encompassed in the exploration of a global problem. It is the failure to identify the crux of the problem that leads to the wandering, unfocused thinking of the student who has begun his approach to defining a problem by examining a global problem, or a problem with which he has had no personal experience. For example, 1C may have decided to explore the problem of "the unmet health needs of school children." Among the many areas she would then have had to consider would have been:

Derivation of Crux and the Global Problem

1. Health needs related to nutrition, hearing, vision, rest, exercise, immunizations, teeth, and others: lead to considerations in terms of (a) ages of children—preschoolers, early elementary, and adolescents; (b) care provided by parents and by community health programs; (c) the role of the teacher; and (d) the school's responsibility.
2. Psychological and social health-related needs, again in relation to ages of children and sources of responsibility.
3. Health care needs related to acute, subacute, and chronic illnesses.
4. Health care needs related to prevention of illnesses.

The above concerns are but a few of those that would have required consideration in attempting definition of the global problem of unmet health needs of school children. The items listed suggest considerations that stem, essentially, from observable irritations. Should the planner introduce potentially related theories, the volume and the scope of the definition of the problem would be staggering. It is also impossible to imagine selecting any one facet of the problem that might be pursued in order to reveal new knowledge that might help alleviate the problem.

It would be superfluous to elaborate further on this illustration of the potential effects of the lack of a specific crux around which to develop the definition of the problem. A hundred or more cruxes stemming from the global problem could be identified. Any problem-defined deriving from a definitive crux, identified in a real, live story, is too large to be solved through a single investigation—and any problem-defined deriving from a global problem fails to provide even a starting place.

The development of the definition of 1C's problem illustrates one further point that must be faced by the beginning researcher; this is that science is based on facts and that the scientist must be objective and must

Step 1: Definition of Problem

Researcher's Choices: Objectivity and Bias

utilize all the facts in the situation. He must not let personal bias enter into or influence his work. As has been proposed in relation to several areas and made explicit in the discussion of the "selection" rather than the "discovery" of the crux, the researcher *must* make choices. Is this necessity of choosing incompatible with the need for objectivity and utilization of all the facts? Several aspects of the problem of unmet health needs of school children make it quite clear that choice by the investigator is the only route to further action. If the problem-defined were fully elaborated around the crux of the irritation identified in 1C's original observation of three children in one family having unattended vision difficulties for three years, it would be obvious that dealing with all the facts is impossible in a single investigation. Furthermore, persistence by 1C in focusing only on the school physician or principal would have resulted in her being unable to secure needed data. The researcher *must* make choices, and his choices *should* be influenced by his own biases.

For the investigator to make choices as he defines his problem does not preclude objectivity in pursuit of his investigation. Objectivity is too often confused with honesty, and a negative connotation of bias is confused with interest or concern. The scientist must proceed in relation to his personal interest and that of his own discipline. He must be honest about the facts he uses, and he must be honest in including or accounting for all facts pertinent to his stated purpose. These admonitions are not synonymous with using "all" facts and denial of personal bias.

SUMMARY

The proposal that the problem-defined is composed of seven identifiable components, the detailed description of the many elements to be included in each component, and the interplay among the various elements in the various components leads students to shudder at the complexity and magnitude of the task of defining the problem. It is indeed a complex and large undertaking, and the analogy with a geodesic dome does not make it seem any less so. It is hoped, nonetheless, that the proposals that there are identifiable components and that various elements may be viewed as units, although dependent and/or markedly intertwined units, may enable the student to proceed with some degree of order, and may also help him to recognize and think about a beginning, a sequence, and an appropriate closing section for his definition of problem.

PURPOSES SERVED BY DETAILED DEFINITION OF PROBLEM

Perhaps the best way to conclude the description of the process of defining the problem is to suggest some of the purposes to be served by the detailed elaboration of the many facets of the problem.

1. It serves to ascertain and make explicit the crux of the problem to be defined and investigated.
2. It identifies and makes explicit factors that may—theoretically or in actuality—enhance, support, or maintain the problem.
3. It puts the crux of the problem into perspective with its related structure—with the total problem-defined.
4. It relates the problem to the larger, typical setting in which it occurs and to other problems in that setting.
5. It suggests varied avenues toward pursuit of potentially pertinent new knowledge.
6. It requires and stimulates speculative thinking about interrelationships of elements in the situation and of science theories that may serve to explain them.
7. It includes information for identification of relevant criterion measures and data to be used to accomplish the stated purpose of the study.
8. It provides a framework within which to hang findings from the investigation.
9. It provides bases for conclusions and recommendations to be derived from the findings.
10. It portrays the potential relationship of the "bit of knowledge" anticipated as an outcome of the investigation to other knowledge in the area of interest. It provides for contribution to the "body of knowledge" rather than adding one more bit to the many unrelated bits and pieces of knowledge.

REFERENCES

1. Couture, N. A. Planned Pre-operative Teaching of Early Ambulation for Patients Having Major Adominal Surgery. Unpublished masters thesis, Detroit, College of Nursing, Wayne State University, 1961.

2. Erickson, R. S. Informational Needs of Major Pulmonary Surgery Patients. Unpublished masters thesis, Detroit, Wayne State University, 1969.
3. Hanigan, D. Planned Pre-operative Teaching of Coughing, Deep-breathing, and Ambulating for Patients Having Thoracic and Upper Abdominal Surgery. Unpublished term paper, Detroit, Wayne State University, 1966.
4. Godfrey, A. E. A study of nursing care designed to assist hospitalized children and their parents in their separation. Nurs. Res., 4:52, 1955.
5. The Nurse Utilization Project Staff. An Investigation of the Relation Between Nursing Activity and Patient Welfare. Iowa City, State University of Iowa, 1960.
6. Grobe, S. Subacute Illness: Unmet Health Needs of Elementary School Children. Unpublished term paper, Detroit, Wayne State University, 1965.

STEP 2

STATEMENT OF PURPOSE
Determine the Focus for Study

TERMS DEFINED

Fact: A fact is an observable phenomenon.

Hypothesis: A hypothesis is the delineation of a relationship believed to exist between two phenomena; when substantiated by research, the statement moves to the realm of theory or principle.

Theory, Principle, Law: A theory, principle, or law is the delineation of a relationship between two facts that may be used to explain phenomena, guide actions, and predict results of actions.

Concept: A concept is a complex of ideas so united as to portray a large general idea. A concept may be essentially ideational, as the concept of liberty, or it may encompass concrete elements, as the concept of table; both of which involve a complex of ideas in contrast to a single idea (if such a thing as a single idea is possible).

Conception: A conception is the complex of ideas that portray a general idea for an individual. One person's conception of liberty may differ in some ways from that of another person, yet each would be examples of the concept of liberty.

Population: Population is the general group or category of entities under study; individual entities in the population may be animate or inanimate: animal, vegetable, or mineral. The population is represented in the study by selected subjects from whom the facts needed as data derive.

Seeming Repetition and Faulty Sequence

A great many concepts are pertinent to the meanings of the terms "hypothesis," "theory," "principle," and "law." The concepts relate to the use of these terms both in the research process and in the daily lives of people. As discussed within this chapter, these concepts will be considered in relation to their utilization by nurses as they plan and provide nursing care for patients, as well as there being elaboration of some particular conceptions of the meanings of these concepts for research. Because the many concepts and the extensive interrelatedness of them, there will be, unfortunately, a large amount of seeming repetition and many instances of return to a topic previously discussed. Efforts to eliminate this repetition have failed—probably because, as one concept is presented, other concepts must be introduced to help to explain it. In turn, one concept used to help explain another must be more fully elaborated in still other contexts. So, no matter what the sequential arrangement of the concepts, one not fully elaborated must be introduced to explain another and then must be reintroduced and more completely elaborated later in the sequence. Another explanation for the repetition lies in conceptions elaborated by various thinkers. Some will corroborate each other, while others will express differing conceptions. Essentially, most of the conceptions to be described will be those that have helped the writer to understand the concepts and to weave them into a pattern consistent with the meaning and use of the terms in science and related fields.

Four Major Subdivisions

The center and marginal headings should help to identify the aspect of the concept inherent in any one of the terms that is being discussed in any one subdivision of the section. There are four major subdivisions:

1. Discussion of more or less general concepts pertinent to the terms.

2. Elaboration of the meanings of the many conceptions as they are illustrated in one tested hypothesis.

3. Discussion of the attention that must be given to the many concepts as a hypothesis is posited.

4. Considerations of the development of statements of purpose that are not hypotheses but, rather, statements that identify the focuses for investigations in which no hypotheses will be tested.

CONCEPTS PERTINENT TO DEFINED TERMS

Fact

For the purpose of orientation to the research process, the definition of a fact that limits its meaning to the concrete, to the observable, will be used. The phenomenon may be grossly, directly observable; it may require instruments to facilitate observation, such as observation of a blood pressure; or it may be only potentially observable, such as an electron. Were the researcher exploring certain philosophical problems, he undoubtedly would extend his definition of fact to include nonobservable, revealed phenomena, the "eternal verities." These elements will not be included in the concept of a "fact" as it will be used in this text.

To enhance understanding and to serve as an anchor for the many and varied aspects of the concepts denoted by the terms—hypothesis, theory, principle, and law—excerpts from two widely published definitions of the terms are reproduced here, as highlights of attributes of the concepts. Although one set refers to the concept of hypothesis and the other to principle, the attributes listed for either are, essentially, applicable to both.

Attributes of Hypothesis Theory Principle Law

All hypotheses are hunches; not all hunches are hypotheses. A good hypothesis:

a. offers a possible explanation
b. adequately explains the observed facts
c. offers the simplest explanation possible under the circumstances
d. offers an explanation that is as complex as necessary under the circumstances
e. can be brought into agreement or disagreement with observations
f. is strong enough to compel inquiry
g. extends inquiry.[1]

A scientific principle must:

a. be a statement of a fundamental process, or a constant mode of behavior
b. be true without known exceptions within the limitations stated in it
c. be capable of demonstration or illustration
d. not be part of a larger principle
e. not be a definition
f. not deal with specific substances or varieties or with limited groups of substances or varieties.[2]

The term "hypothesis" is used to refer to various conceptions, even in reference to the process of research. The primary concept, of course, is the one referring to the delineation of a relationship between phenomena that is to be tested through scientific investigation. When used to refer to other concepts, the word takes on the meaning of what might better be termed "hypothesizing" or "hypothetical thinking." Those who use the term for such meaning explain that the thinking involved in developing all elements of a research design and its report utilizes a continuous sequence of hypotheses, which usually are unexpressed or implicit. Indeed, such is true of all thinking that involves development of ideas. This is what is

Hypotheses To Be Tested, Hypotheses and the Process of Thinking

referred to in the discussion of the definition of problem as theorizing: the thinking through of a great many possible interrelationships among phenomena and ideas, in attempts to understand and describe them and to develop patterns that will promote understanding.

By definition, such thoughts might be called "hypotheses," but the use of the word in this way seems to make for unnecessary confusion. Since the reference is actually to the process of thinking, and the terms "hypothesizing" or "theorizing" denote process, they are preferable. This would leave the terms "hypothesis" and "theory" to refer to precise statements delineating relationships that are to be or have been tested through research. Such limitation of the use of these terms, however, does not mean that for each hypothesis there would have to be an investigation. Rather, there would always be more than one hypothesis associated with any one scientific investigation: the main hypothesis to be tested, possibly several subhypotheses to be tested, and some proposed but not tested. In addition, there would be the hypotheses suggested by the findings of the study that would be recommended for future studies. Where the investigation is exploratory, there may be implicit hypotheses that guide some of the planning for the investigation, as well as those developed on the basis of the findings. Essentially, the justification for exploratory investigations is the development of hypotheses.

(These ideas about the use of the term are presented to help the student understand writings where the term is used to refer to the various conceptions, and to propose reservation of the term for "hypotheses" delineated with the specific intent that they be put to the test.)

Theory, Principle, Law— One Concept or Three

At the beginning of this chapter, theory, principle, and law were ascribed a common definition, yet many writers have postulated and "explained" differences between the meanings of the three terms. Because the student will be confronted with the supposed differences, in discussions about the terms and in their usage, many of these conceptions will be discussed, to help the student understand the concept denoted by each term and its meaning for research and for use of the findings of research.

Principle— Distinction From Theory

A principle may be distinguished from a theory in two ways: (1) by its linguistic origins in the Latin, Middle English, and Old French, with the Latin *principalis*, "a principle," deriving from the Latin *princips*, "first, chief, prince," which in turn was derived from the Latin *primus*, "first," and *capere*, "to take"; (2) by the concept inherent in several attributes ascribed to a scientific principle (see page 65), particularly those in "a," "d," and "f": a principle is prime, fundamental; it is not a part of a larger principle; it does not deal with specific substances or with limited groups of substances or varieties. The relationship delineated in a principle applies to all subjects of the substance identified in the delineation.

A principle, then, may be viewed as an encompassing generalization with extensive application.

Although a theory delineates the same relationship between two specific phenomena as does a principle, the former term is more limited in its application since it identifies specific subjects or categories of subjects involved in the relationship. A principle may give rise to innumerable theories or, conversely, many interrelated theories may lead to identification of a principle—that is, a generalization that applies to all instances described in the more limited and specific theories. *Difference in Scope*

For instance: "Cells deprived of nourishment and means of waste disposal will die." This generalization is prime, fundamental; a principle; it applies to all cells and to every possible means of deprivation; it applies to the cells in a blade of grass as well as the dermal cells in the skin. A theory deduced from this principle might be: "When blood supply is cut off, tissues will die." Here specific cells and particular means of nourishment and waste disposal are identified. This statement is not prime: it does not apply to all cells; it would not explain the death of a girdled tree, of an amoeba, or of a fish cast up on dry land. But the principle—cells deprived of nourishment and means of waste disposal will die—does explain all of these deaths. *Scope of Application*

Furthermore, this principle can serve to guide actions: should the wish be for a dead fish, it may be cast on dry land (the action); should the wish be for the fish to live, it should be allowed to remain in water (the action). The principle allows prediction of the outcome of the action: thus, it can be predicted that the fish cast on dry land will die (the outcome); the one left in its usual habitat will live (the outcome).

Structurally, a hypothesis, a theory, a principle, and a law are not different, one from the other; each delineates a relationship between two facts. Among those who perceive each term as expressing a unique concept, however, perhaps the most popular distinction is in terms of the weight of supporting data. (1) The delineation of the relationship in a *hypothesis* is based on few casual observations; indeed, it is a relationship only believed to exist. (2) The relationship delineated in a *theory* is based on an accumulation of planned and organized observations; the hypothesis has been tested, and organized observations have served to demonstrate that the relationship believed to exist does indeed exist. (3) A *principle* is supported not only by observations in a controlled experimental situation, but also from observations made when the principle is put to use in real-life settings; it is also supported by the fact that no exceptions to the stated relationship have been observed. (4) A *law* implies an exact formulation of the principle operating in a sequence of events in nature observed to occur with unvarying uniformity under the same conditions. Essentially, *Weight of Data* a law is a principle, is a theory, is a hypothesis, but each is distinct from the others on the basis of varying quantities of supporting data, with the quantity of supporting data increasing as we progress from the hypothesis to the theory, to the principle, to the law. In other words, the law enjoys a place of great confidence due to the duration and weight of evidence to support it. Principles are but slightly less respected. Theories are used as guides to actions, predictors of outcomes of actions, and explainers of phenomena, but they are continually being examined to determine the extent of their application and possible exceptions to them. All begin as hypotheses and move successively through theory and principle to become law, as evidence for their validity accumulates.

The foregoing outlines the commonly proposed distinctions, which seem to me to be artificial and not particularly useful, since there are exceptions to most of the defining statements. Archimedes' "law" of specific gravity, purportedly, was delineated on the basis of a single observation, while Newton's "law" of gravity has been supplanted by the "law" of quantum mechanics, and Einstein's identification of relationships between mass and energy and time continues to be referred to as the "theory" of relativity. The student should also remember that moving through the suggested stages from hypothesis to law does not change the relationship, structurally or functionally. The delineated relationship between the facts remains the same and serves the same purposes, whether viewed as theory, principle, or law.

Laws of Nature Not Created By Man

The relationships described in hypotheses, theories, principles, and laws are not created by man, but exist in nature. Man's role in their "development" is merely the recognition and precise description of the relationships. To describe the evolution of a theory is really to describe the sequence of thought processes as man has recognized relationships between various phenomena, with recognition of one leading to recognition of others. When Sir Isaac Newton was asked how he had "discovered" the law of gravitation, he replied, "By thinking about it all the time." The relationships between the various phenomena did not change as the recognition changed; the only change was in progressive recognition of various relationships.

The development of theories, principles, and laws does not follow a neat pattern of growth from the "infant" hypothesis, to the "child" theory, to the "adult" principle, and to the "sage" law. Rather, the movement may well be from hypothesis to law, with many principles and theories being deduced from the law. Therefore, if distinctions must be made between the concepts denoted by each term, they might best be made in relation to scope of application or scope of specifics encompassed by them, as in the example of the encompassing principle of the death of cells. Innumerable theories can be delineated from this principle, each

Concepts Pertinent to Defined Terms

identifying specific situations that support the principle, each making the principle explicit in a specific situation. This is what nurses do when they utilize this "principle" to plan care to prevent decubiti. Conversely, it would be possible to list many theories, each a generalization about the deprivation of nourishment to some organism or part of it, and to induce from these theories the principle delineating the relationship between nourishment and survival of living cells.

Two additional elements within the entire concept of relationships existing between phenomena in nature (call them theories, principles, or laws) should be considered. The first is consideration of the nature of the delineation of the relationship. The proposal that "a scientific principle must be a statement of a fundamental process, or a constant mode of behavior," seems to imply a cause-effect relationship. Indeed, as man uses principles to guide his actions, predict their outcomes, and explain his observations, he uses them as though they did delineate a cause-effect relationship. Because some long-standing theories have eventually been "disproved," and because some scientists apparently cannot tolerate being found in error, it has been proposed that there is no such thing as a cause-effect relationship between phenomena in nature but, rather, only co-relational relationships.

Cause-Effect Relationship

This is safe: we know that there are many relationships among phenomena that are co-relational and are not cause-effect. We know, also, that where a cause-effect relationship exists, there will also be a co-relational relationship. This is tantamount to insisting on swinging the pendulum full way. Certainly, proposing that there are only co-relational relationships is safe, and proposing cause-effect in many relationships is risking possible error. But to insist on complete immunity from possible error by contending that there are no cause-effect relationships in nature, and then to use any number of theories to explain observations, guide actions, to predict the outcomes—all with cause-effect connotations—it seems to be aspiring to the assurance of purity and faultlessness through proclamation, while at the same time risking possibility of error through actions because of expediency.

The knowledge of co-relational relationships, where these have been identified, can serve the same purpose as the knowledge of cause-effect relationships: to explain phenomena, guide actions, and predict outcomes. In the first instance, the relationship is that, where one phenomenon exists, the second also exists; in the second, it is that, as one phenomenon changes, the related one will change in a known manner. For example, it is known that when the temperatures of substances in contact with water change, the temperature of the water will change, and that as the temperatures of adjacent substances rise, so will the temperature of the water. This relationship may be stated in co-relational terms, but most persons

Co-relational Relationships

using the principle are more likely to see it as a cause-effect relationship.

On the other hand, many identified co-relationships will probably not be used very often. For example, a positive correlation has been established between the phenomenon of amount of complaint of pain and the degree of pain reported, and the number of siblings of the individual suffering the pain. It is unlikely, however, that knowledge of the relationship between these two phenomena will ever be greatly used to guide actions or to predict outcomes, or even to explain observations. It illustrates, however, the existence of a relationship to which cause-effect would hardly be ascribed. It may serve, too, to illustrate that where cause-effect cannot logically be ascribed, where observations provide no more than evidence of co-relationship, the theory should not be used to explain observations in cause-effect terms, or to justify actions that imply a cause-effect relationship. This does not mean that co-relational relationships are not useful and that understanding then should not be pursued with the same diligence as cause-effect relationships. Rather, the discussion is offered to help the student understand the difference between them.

Relationships Delineated Operationally

Another type of theory, distinguishable by the nature of its delineation, is one that delineates relationships operationally. Here, one of the phenomena in the relationship is not observable and probably never will be. Yet the relationship so delineated does serve to explain phenomena, to guide actions, and to predict outcomes. Theories that delineate relationships operationally can usually be identified by the fact that most of them are not expressed in single declarative statements, but rather in elaborations of the several concepts composing them: for example, Freud's theory of the ego, the id, and the superego. These phenomena have not been observed, and it is not expected that they ever will be. Yet theories about their relationships to other phenomena have been delineated and the theories serve to explain observations, guide actions, and predict outcomes.

Another example is the theory of the filtrable virus. Long before the development of the electron microscope enabled man to observe the organism, the existence of the virus was posited and its relationship to diseases delineated. Of course, this theory had precedence in the germ theory of disease posited by many and fully delineated by Koch. Still another familiar theory of this nature is the one delineating the relationship between genes and hereditary characteristics. It may be noted that most theories that explain observations operationally seem to lean toward the concept of cause-effect, rather than co-relational, relationships between phenomena. For further discussion of the concept of operational delineation see Step 3, pages 102 and 113–115.

The Term: Delineation

It will have been noted that, in the definition and in the many references to the concept of theory, the term "delineation" is used. This term is intended to serve as a reminder that, for a statement describing

Concepts Pertinent to Defined Terms 71

the relationship between two phenomena to be classed as a theory, principle, or law, it must do more than merely declare that the two phenomena are related; it must delineate the character and circumstance of the relationship. Three of the attributes ascribed by Feibleman (page 65) to a hypothesis apply equally to the substantiated hypothesis when it has moved to the realm of theory, principle, or law: (b) adequately explains observed facts; (c) offers the simplest explanation possible under the circumstances; and (d) offers an explanation that is as complex as necessary under the circumstances. These and other attributes of a good hypothesis certainly imply more than a mere declaration of the existence of a relationship between phenomena.

The attribute, "A good hypothesis is strong enough to compel inquiry," seems to be self-evident, in that the hypothesis serves as the focus for the inquiry in which it is involved. Nonetheless, in consideration of the extensive work involved in research, the student should be aware of this attribute. The purpose of research is to test hypotheses, and only as a hypothesis is "strong enough to compel inquiry" will the researcher be stimulated to pursue the many details required by the task of the testing. Statements that might be posed as hypotheses and yet could hardly be expected to compel inquiry illustrate two weaknesses: *Good Hypothesis Compels Inquiry*

> Nurses living on the east side of town change jobs less frequently than do nurses living on the west side of town. *Example 2A*

> When the basic courses in associate degree and practical nursing are combined, duplication in teaching will be avoided and the liberated instructor will have more time for individualized student instruction. *Example 2B*

To the first, one might comment: "So?" One might propose that "if" there were no scarcity of nurses, an employer might want to know this so that he could hire nurses from the east side of town and thereby ensure a small turnover of staff. Perhaps; but still the proposition hardly seems of such compelling interest as to warrant a full-blown scientific inquiry.

In relation to the second example, the proposed outcomes to the suggested actions are so obvious that there could be little interest in pursuing a study of the proposed relationships. Obviously, if two courses are combined into one with two groups of students attending the classes of the single combined course, there will not be duplication of teaching and, obviously, an instructor who does not have to teach a class will have more time for other things. This example illustrates the need to identify the purpose of an investigation in terms of the exploration that can be expected to yield the most information related to the problem under study. It also illustrates the appropriateness of sometimes pursuing an exploratory, descriptive study rather than testing a hypothesis. The statement of purpose finally developed to provide focus for an investigation of one facet of the problem was:

Example 2C The purpose of this study is to explore the feasibility of combining basic nursing courses of an associate degree program and a practical nursing program in terms of outcomes for students and in terms of utilization of instructor time and particular competencies.

These examples suggest that interest and obviousness are two criteria that might serve to judge whether a hypothesis is strong enough to compel inquiry. The beginning researcher should be aware of these criteria: the two examples given were early attempts of beginning researchers to state hypotheses.

Not All Hunches Are Hypotheses Other attributes of a theory, especially the one that states that it "must be a statement of a fundamental process, or a constant mode of behavior," will help the student clarify his thinking in relation to various materials in the literature that can be very confusing. The crux of the confusion is identified in the proposal that "all hypotheses are hunches; not all hunches are hypotheses." The student's confusion will arise as he reads reports where the researcher has identified, as the hypotheses tested by the study, statements that do not encompass the attribute of process or mode of behavior, nor do they delineate a relationship between two phenomena. Indeed, these so-called hypotheses are frequently hunches about the existence of a single observable phenomenon: that is, they are statements identifying potential facts.

It is hard for the student to reconcile such statements with his understanding of two attributes of a hypothesis: (1) when it has been substantiated through research, it moves to the realm of theory; and (2) it can be used to explain phenomena, guide actions, and predict outcomes. The report may declare that the "hypothesis" was substantiated, that indeed the phenomenon does exist as the researcher had suspected. Further, the report may suggest actions to be taken in the light of the newfound knowledge. But the student is unable to understand how the confirmation of the existence of a fact can serve to suggest action, and there is nothing in the original statement to identify the fact that can serve as a base for predicting the outcomes of proposed actions.

Communication could be enhanced and confusion lessened if the term "hypothesis," when used to refer to the focus of a scientific inquiry, were limited to a statement that delineates the relationship between two phenomena; better yet, if the term "hypothesis" were limited to a concept that, if substantiated by the investigation, would enable the hypothesis to move to the realm of theory, principle, or law. A statement of a hunch about the existence of a single phenomenon or fact, even if substantiated by scientific inquiry, cannot move to the realm of theory, principle, or law; it, therefore, seems a misnomer to identify such a statement as a hypothesis.

Concepts Pertinent to Defined Terms 73

This is not to say that such statements cannot serve as focuses or guides for scientific investigations. There are innumerable situations in which it is entirely appropriate to investigate the possible existence of one or more individual phenomena and to enlarge knowledge about their nature before positing relationships of one (suspected) phenomenon to another. It is because such investigations are both appropriate and valuable that it is proposed that the statement of focus for a scientific inquiry might take one of three forms, as discussed a little later in this chapter.

Research to Reveal Facts

The student is once more reminded that the purpose of research is to reveal new knowledge. Some have proposed that the purpose of research is to reveal new knowledge "through testing hypotheses." The final phrase, "through testing hypotheses," seems too limiting to be descriptive of all research. Yet the idea does have merit in terms of research undertaken for practical purposes: that is, when the reason for undertaking a particular research project is to reveal new knowledge for the sake of improving a product or a practice. This is usually referred to as applied or practical research, and certainly the most direct approach is through testing hypotheses. Nonetheless, even with the ultimate aim being application of the information gleaned from the investigation, the immediate purpose of any investigation is gleaning the information. How the information is used is outside the scope or concern of the investigation. And incorporating the phrase, "through testing hypotheses," into the purpose of research overlooks the fact that many scientific investigations are carried out to reveal new knowledge about individual facts, without attempting to test their relationships to other facts—in other words, without testing hypotheses.

Applied or Practical Research

The proposal that research yields knowledge through testing hypotheses does, however, have considerable meaning for nurses who profess to base nursing actions on principles. Any distinction as to whether the nurse bases her actions on the limited and more definitive "theory" or on the fundamental "principle" is perhaps merely semantic quibbling. What is important is that the nurse knows how to use delineations of relationships known to exist between phenomena (as demonstrated through research) to provide a basis for her nursing care and to improve her practice.

Nurses Base Actions on Principles

The nurse may better understand the use of principles, if she thinks of the process of identifying the relationship that the principle delineates. Though not invariable, the process usually begins with observation of the interrelationship between two phenomena in a particular setting. There may be repeated observations of individual illustrations of the relationship. From these observations will be evolved the generalization about the relationship and the circumstances of its occurrence. The generalization (the hypothesis) is then tested against many observations of a similar nature in similar circumstances. (The testing must not be in the identical setting

Development and Use of Principles Follow the Same Process

or circumstances, else the reasoning of substantiation would be circular.) Once the generalization has been demonstrated as indeed describing an existing relationship, knowledge of the relationship can be used to guide actions in individual situations. The process is cyclical: from specific, individual instances; to a generalization about all like cases; to use or application in specific individual cases. The nurse, as she uses a principle to guide her actions, follows the same cycle, beginning with specific and moving to general and back to her specific. In other words, she begins by considering the outcome she wishes to achieve for her patient as a result of the care she will provide. Having identified the desired outcome for her specific patient in her particular setting, she searches her knowledge to identify the principle that encompasses a phenomenon related to her desired outcome. Then, her knowledge of the relationship of the desired outcome to the second phenomenon identified in the principle, and her knowledge of the nature of the relationship as delineated by the principle will serve as a base to guide her to a specific action, and she can predict the outcome to be expected from her action.

Use of Facts; Use of Principles

Understanding of the process of using principles as guides to actions helps to clarify a related concept pertinent for nurses caring for patients. Nurses find themselves troubled about the role of facts versus principles as they are used as bases for nursing actions. Some perceive principles, since they are observable phenomena, as facts. Indeed, if a fact is an observable phenomenon and the two interrelated phenomena in a principle can be observed, a principle may be considered a fact, and some have so defined it. But if no distinction is made between a fact as a single observable phenomenon and a fact as an observed relationship between two phenomena, then there seems little point in using the two terms "fact" and "principle." Actually, the rationale for referring to a principle as a fact seems to be that the relationship has been demonstrated to exist; therefore, it is a fact. The trouble here is a confusion or a difference in the meaning of the word "fact." What is meant is that the existence of the relationship has been demonstrated to be true: that is, fact is equated with truth and not with an observable phenomenon.

This is a matter that has long plagued nurses. They have purported to base actions on principles, but few are able to identify principles and fewer still are able to describe their use of principles as they plan and provide care for patients. Few can explain their rationale for selecting one principle over another as a guide to action in a particular situation. They have not been helped, moreover, by the many books whose titles indicate that their content is devoted to identification (listing) of "principles" basic to nursing care of patients. Many of these books do not even define the term "principle," and none that I have seen is consistent in the characteristics of statements presented as principles. Instead, there is a mingling of statements delineating relationships between phenomena and statements identifying single phenomena, with no indication that one statement is different in any way from another.

This elaboration of the nature of a principle and its distinction from a single fact is intended to help nurses identify the nature of the various elements of knowledge they possess and to know how each may be used in planning care of patients. Thus, the nurse should know that principles can serve her as guides to identifying appropriate actions and to predicting the outcomes of her actions. But she should know, too, the role played by independent facts. Only as she knows the many independent facts about her patient—facts known from her educational background and from her immediate observations of the patient—can she select the principle(s) on which she will base her action.

For example, the nurse may be caring for a patient who has had a gastrectomy and for whom intravenous fluids have been ordered. The nurse observes that the patient shows many signs of dehydration (each sign is a single observable phenomenon). She knows from his record that he had been hemorrhaging before coming to the hospital, that he had been dehydrated on admission, and that he had had IV fluids preoperatively to help treat the dehydration—all single observable phenomena: facts. On the basis of her knowledge of these facts, she would have thought about changes that she might be able to effect for the patient—about the outcomes of care she might provide for him. Thinking in terms of specific symptoms, and having chosen, first, to relieve the symptoms of dehydration, she would search her knowledge to find a principle that would identify a phenomenon related in a causal way to the phenomenon of adequate body hydration. She might think, for instance: "The most expeditious way to get fluids into the body manifesting symptoms of dehydration is by intravenous infusion." (The thought processes of the experienced nurse are so rapid that she is scarcely aware of them. But they are conspicuous in the inexperienced nurse, particularly when each successive element of thought is elicited by a question from the instructor.) Having determined the principle identifying the phenomenon related to the desired outcome, the nurse would then expect to run the intravenous fluids at the maximum rate of flow ordered by the physician.

Example: Nursing Care of Patient with Gastrectomy— Facts Principles

About six hours postoperatively the nurse observes, in addition to the symptoms of dehydration, that the patient's pulse and respiration rates have increased, his breathing has become somewhat labored, and there are sounds of moisture in the respiratory passages not relieved by deep-breathing and coughing. Consequently, she would now focus her attention on a need that she would recognize as having priority over the need for relief of dehydration. She would search for a principle that would explain the phenomena of the signs of pulmonary congestion, which would, in turn, lead her to action based on a principle other than the one that led to maximum flow of the intravenous fluids. Operating on the principle that rapid intake of fluid can result in failure of equal absorption by all tissues, with pulmonary tissues absorbing an excessive amount (leading to pulmonary edema), she would now run the intravenous fluids at the least rate of flow ordered and, in addition, would notify the physician of the patient's condition.

These examples illustrate the role played by single facts in the process of planning care for patients through identification of applicable principles. Without such knowledge of facts, appropriate principles could not be selected to serve as guides to action or predictors of outcomes.

Descriptive Proposition: "What" Happens; Explanatory Proposition: "Why" It Happens

Still another conception of components is essential for a statement to be classified as "hypothesis." The preceding illustrations and discussion have portrayed a statement that might be classed as a "descriptive proposition": a statement that describes *what* occurs in the relationship between two phenomena. There are those who contend that a statement, in order to be classified as a hypothesis, must link a descriptive proposition to a general proposition that will explain *why* what happens happens. It may be assumed that, where an investigator has fully defined his problem and proposed the many theories pertinent to it, he has provided the general proposition that would serve to explain why the relationship he proposes may be expected to exist. He will, in his definition of problem, have presented general propositions meant to serve as the rationale for his proposing the relationship. He may not have definitely included an explicit, applicable concept in the statement of his hypothesis.

For example, the hypothesis developed for 1A's study might be classed as a descriptive proposition:

Example 1A

Major abdominal and thoracic surgery patients who are given planned preoperative instructions about early ambulation and receive reinforcement of these instructions the day after surgery, in comparison with similar patients who are not given planned instructions, perform early postoperative ambulatory activities more frequently.

The statement is limited to describing *what* occurs in the relationship. The definition of problem, however, included an account of the influence of fear on learning and the knowledge that persons under stress conditions perform actions more readily if they are familiar, rather than unfamiliar, actions. From discussion in Example 1A, it would seem that the theory that fear can be dispelled by knowledge is the one that prompted the researcher to propose the hypothesis she did. She might have introduced the statement of her hypothesis with the proposition: "Because knowledge eliminates the unknown that can produce fear, it may be expected that. . . ." Such a statement would not only explain *what* might be expected to happen as a result of the teaching, but it explains *why* it might be expected to happen. When a hypothesis, so constructed, is substantiated and moves to the realm of theory, the explanatory clause may be dropped from the statement. Although the knowledge of why one may expect the outcome does contribute to understanding and may well modify the manner, scope, and content of the action, the descriptive proposition alone can, in general, serve as a guide to action and predictor of outcomes, as well as explaining observed phenomena. And indeed, the *what* portions of hypotheses, when substantiated through research, become the *why* portions of future propositions.

It is recommended that the beginning researcher focus on the descriptive proposition as a stated hypothesis for testing. The rationale for so doing is twofold: (1) the many steps of the research process can be learned in relation to the more simply tested descriptive proposition; (2) most relationships that nurses will delineate in a descriptive proposition will have their explanatory base in theories from sciences in which nurses have limited backgrounds; to demonstrate a relationship between the explanatory theory and the descriptive proposition would require the nurse to acquire the background of knowledge in the pertinent science. This second reason for limiting considerations in this book to hypotheses that are descriptive propositions may seem to limit, if not negate, the value of the entire presentation. Many propose that, if students are to be helped to understand the research process, they should be helped to understand all of its components. On the other hand, the majority of nurses who will learn "something" about the process of research seek this knowledge in order to understand and utilize materials produced through research conducted by others. Most will not pursue formal education beyond the masters degree and most will not become researchers.

Beginning Researcher and Testing Descriptive Propositions

It is to this majority, therefore, that this book is addressed, with the aim of helping them to understand the research process but not of providing them with background sufficient for them to become independent researchers. A student can acquire a feeling for the process of research and an understanding of the many steps in the process if he has the experience of executing the steps in the development of a plan for a study that would be within the scope of possible accomplishment during an undergraduate honors or a masters program of study. If he were asked to develop a design for a study that would require acquisition of a background in another science, or require even extensive consultation related to another science, the scope of the undertaking would be beyond the limitations just mentioned.

Research Within the Scope of the Curricular Program

To test a hypothesis that includes delineation of the explanatory general theory would require collecting observations of the explanatory phenomenon's occurrence in a contiguous relationship with the occurrence of the phenomena of the descriptive proposition. To illustrate: had 1A attempted to test the hypothesis suggested above, with the inclusion of the explanatory clause, "Because knowledge eliminates the unknown that can produce fear . . . ," she would have had to measure the amount of fear experienced by her subjects and determine whether, indeed, the patients who were taught experienced less fear than those who were not taught. She would also have had to determine whether there was a relationship between amount of fear and type and amount of ambulatory behavior.

Testing for Explanatory Phenomena

A study that attempted to reveal the theorized relationship of the relief of fear, as an explanation for the influence of the teaching, would also have required that the researcher acquire background knowledge in the area of the phenomenon of fear: its influence on behavior and on learning. In addition, she would have had to learn ways to measure fear in various settings and under various conditions. Such an undertaking would have been quite beyond what she could have undertaken as a part of her masters program; whereas, by doing the limited study, she not only provided support for the hypothesis delineating the *what* of the relationship, but she secured from the patients indications about which of the explanatory theories proposed in the definition of problem seemed most likely to offer explanation of *why*. Her findings can thus guide a future researcher to a more direct path for identifying the explanatory theory related to the relationship demonstrated by her study.

To carry the illustration from 1A's study another step, it is quite obviously desirable to attempt to identify a relationship with an explanatory phenomenon, since the effect of the teaching (better postoperative ambulatory behavior) may have been due to some "cause" other than relief of fear. Indeed, in her definition of problem, 1A suggested various reasons that the teaching might be expected to produce the posited effect. Among the reasons were the physical practice of the activities, the foreknowledge of what would be expected, the very personal attention received in the teaching, or understanding of the importance of the activities. The study revealed that the teaching *did* make a difference in the activities performed by the patients, but it did not provide definitive information about whether the difference was related to amount of fear or to some other element.

Actually, 1A did not ignore explanatory phenomena completely, but she did not commit herself to precise measurements of them. She interviewed patients after the four days of observation of activities, and some of the patients' comments suggested various reasons for the effects of the teaching. Among them were: "It helps to understand what you will be expected to do," "I was less afraid to move," "Knowing did not make it less painful, but it was easier to stand the pain because I knew I was helping myself." The definitive, precisely measured findings of the study *did* confirm a limited bit of knowledge: teaching patients results in better postoperative ambulatory behavior. The findings did not, however, identify a reason for the result. Actually measuring the amount of fear, however, would have made it possible to relate the findings from this study to broader propositions: (1) knowledge (of the unknown) reduces fear, and (2) fear immobilizes. Or, it might have been learned that there was no difference in the amount of fear experienced by the two groups, and some other reason would have had to be sought to explain "why" teaching resulted in better ambulatory activities.

The foregoing may very well remind the student of the truism that research raises more questions than it answers, and that one investigation can examine only a very limited facet of any one problem. It also demonstrates that it would never be possible in one study to illustrate the presence of all causal and all explanatory phenomena in a given situation. Admittedly, the more research that uses previously established theories to reveal relationships that explain *why* for the observations of *what* occurs in the relationship between two phenomena, the better organized and the more extensively useful will be man's knowledge. Nonetheless, studies that must be limited in scope are useful in providing information about the what, and each such study provides a base for more definitive speculation as to the potentially associated general theory that will explain the why. Essentially, the processes of the two types of investigations do not differ other than in their complexity. Where one or more explanatory phenomena are included, the process must include planning for and collecting observations of the occurrence of those phenomena. There are necessarily many more elements to be integrated into the plan and execution of such a study. Each added phenomenon makes it considerably more complex than an investigation where only the *what* relationship between two phenomena is observed.

Rationale for Limiting Scope of Proposition to Be Tested

From this stems the rationale for recommending that the student researcher with limited time for study undertake a study that attempts to investigate relationships among phenomena that identify only *what* happens in the relationship, and not a study that extends the investigation in an attempt to identify the *why* of what happens.

This does not mean that beginners should never undertake such extended investigations. Among the several conditions that might make it entirely reasonable for the beginner to engage in such a study are: (1) where the potential explanatory theory is of particular interest to the student, and he wishes to learn more about it, (2) where measurements needed to account for the explanatory phenomenon can be readily obtained—that is, a measurement device has been developed and is relatively easy to use, and (3) where the student may be sharing an investigation with others—either fellow students or instructors. The student should

When Student Tests for Explanatory Phenomenon

always be encouraged to pursue an investigation as sophisticated as possible within the realm defined by the factors of interest, time, capability, and others.

Attributes Illustrated in a Tested Hypothesis

A discussion of the tested hypothesis may clarify the meaning and rationale of the many attributes of a hypothesis and describe further the relationships between theory and practice. The hypothesis posed by 1A, which delineated her hunch about relationships among certain phenomena in the patient care situation and which served as the focus for her investigation, will serve our purposes here and later in the discussion of the accomplishment of Step 2. The hypothesis was substantiated, albeit in a study of very limited scope, and may now serve as a principle on which to base nursing practice. The delineation of the relationship between two phenomena (planned preoperative instructions and the patient's performance of postoperative ambulatory activities) explains observed variations in patients' performances of postoperative ambulatory activities. The nurse may therefore be guided in her actions by the statement: she should provide abdominal surgery patients under her care with planned instructions about ambulatory activities before the operation and reinforce the instructions on the day following the surgery. The theory allows her to anticipate (predict) the results of her actions. She may expect that patients so instructed will perform postoperative ambulatory activities more frequently than they would if not so instructed. The theory explains the nurse's observations about patients, it can serve to guide her actions, and it allows her to anticipate the outcomes of her actions.

Adequately Explains Versus Not Deal With Specifics

For still further clarification, let us consider, in turn, the several attributes of a theory as they are portrayed by 1A's theory. Some of this discussion could wax into a "Sic et non" (Yes and No) proposition, but acceptance of seemingly contradictory attributes as counterbalances eliminates a feeling of skepticism. For example, "a good [theory] adequately explains the observed facts" may be considered counterbalanced by "a scientific principle must not deal with specific substances or varieties or with limited groups of substances or varieties." If only the former were considered, it might have been desirable to have made explicit in the statement the specific ambulatory activities, such as coughing, deep-breathing, turning in bed, getting out of bed, and so forth. Or the exact instructions to be provided patients might have been made explicit. When the latter are brought into the picture, it becomes clear that these specifics are beyond the scope of the statement of a principle.

Simple as Possible— Complex as Necessary

The scope of details made explicit in the statement of a principle are dealt with in other notations of characteristics of a principle: "a good [theory] offers the simplest explanation possible under the circumstances" and "a good [theory] offers an explanation that is as complex as necessary under the circumstances." In compliance with the first, 1A identified the patients to whom the theory applies as "major abdominal and thoracic surgery patients" without identifying specific surgical procedures or elaborating patient characteristics. She identified "planned preoperative instructions about early ambulation" without giving detailed and specific instructions for patients anticipating particular operative procedures. She indicated that the activities would be performed "more frequently," without specifying particular frequencies on particular days for patients with particular surgical treatments. It is known that these various elements will vary with different patients and in relation to the types of surgical procedures sustained by them. As for any generalization, all episodes encompassed by it are, essentially, alike, yet no one is exactly like any other. A theory is a generalization that encompasses all episodes similar to those described in it.

Similarly, in relation to the second attribute, "an explanation as complex as necessary," 1A identified the population to whom her theory applies as "major abdominal and thoracic surgery patients." This identification, as part of the hypothesis that served as the focus for her investigation, served to limit the scope of her inquiry. As an element of the principle established by her study, it identified the particular patients for whom preoperative teaching might be expected to result in more frequent early ambulatory activities—major abdominal and thoracic surgery patients, not other surgery patients—and thus serves nurses who will base their practice on it. This is not to say that other patients would not experience similar results, but the theory, as stated and tested by 1A, does not encompass predictions about others.

Parallel of Attributes in Hypothesis and Principle

A second feature illustrating details required by the complexity of the situation is inclusion of details about the preoperative instructions: "planned" and "reinforcement of these instructions the day after surgery." 1A's casual observations apparently had led her to believe that "preoperative instructions" alone would not result in more frequent early ambulatory activities, but rather that these instructions must be planned and they must be reinforced on the day following surgery. Again, these details served to provide focus for the inquiry and, as elements of the principle evolved, they serve as guides to action by nurses who will base their nursing care on the principle.

The close identity of the hypothesis with the principle is emphasized again when the second and third attributes ascribed by Feibleman to a hypothesis ("adequately explains the observed facts" and "offers the simplest explanation possible under the circumstances") are compared with the second attribute ascribed to a principle ("must be true without exceptions within the limitations stated in it"). The details of 1A's hypothesis discussed above foresees the attribute of the principle concerning "the limitations stated in it."

Empirical Test

Furthermore, the fourth attribute of a hypothesis ("can be brought into agreement or disagreement with observations") is closely related to the second and third attributes ascribed to a principle ("must be true without known exceptions within the limitations stated in it" and "be capable of demonstration or illustration"). The requirement that a hypothesis be capable of being "brought into agreement or disagreement with observations" is, of course, validated by the investigation for which it serves as focus. The attributes that a principle "be true without known exceptions . . ." and "capable of demonstration or illustration" are validated as a principle is put to the empirical test; that is, the hypothesis is tested under controlled conditions wherein the proposed actions are executed or observed, and the suggested results are observed in a carefully planned, controlled situation. The observations will either agree or disagree with those delineated in the hypothesis being tested. If there is agreement, the hypothesis moves to the realm of a principle, where it will serve as a basis for practice. As practitioners utilize the principle as a basis for action, they will follow the suggestions delineated within it, but they will do so in a real-life situation, not in the controlled situation maintained for testing the hypothesis. Observations of results will be more casual than during the testing of the hypothesis, but they will be based on the expectations of results delineated in the principle. The principle will hold so long as practitioners observe no exceptions to the anticipated results of their actions and so long as they can perform activities based on the guidance of the principle—that is, demonstrate the principle with their actions and results of their actions. Although scientific inquiry may demonstrate that the relationship delineated in the hypothesis can be brought into agreement with observations and move the hypothesis to the realm of a principle, it must still stand the empirical test in real-life situations, and it will remain a principle only so long as it lives up to these two attributes.

The history of medicine is replete with "principles" whose status has fluctuated under the test of empiricism. For example, there are the fluctuations of the theory of the relationship of phlebotomy to the course of various diseases in man. This does not necessarily mean that the "principles" used to guide actions in medicine do not stand the empirical test, but rather that the empirical test may be the only test to which the hypothesized relationships are put. An example of this is the purported relationship between a baby's feeding schedule and his well-being. There have been eras of demand feeding and there have been eras of rigid scheduling—but, to my knowledge, there has been no era of scientific investigation of the relationship of type of feeding schedule to results for the infants being fed.

The foregoing may seem a rather lengthy "definition," but the discussion seems appropriate, since the many concepts pertaining to a hypothesis, its role in research, and its progeny explain the reason for doing research. Furthermore, the concepts provide direction for planning many of the steps in the design for a scientific inquiry. Although the focus has been on concepts pertinent to the hypothesis, some of the preceding discussion serves to explain the three forms that may be taken by the statement of the purpose or focus to guide an investigation.

STATEMENT OF PURPOSE

FOCUS FOR STUDY

The focus for study is identified in the single statement that makes explicit the purpose for which the study is to be conducted, the outcome to be sought. The statement of purpose may take one of three forms: (1) a hypothesis, (2) a question, or (3) a declarative sentence that begins, "The purpose of this investigation is to determine (identify, describe, evaluate, etc.). . . ." Actually, the latter phrase is implicit in the statement of purpose for any investigation, but it need not be made explicit when the statement takes either of the first two forms. Nonetheless, the student should be mindful that, by implication, his hypothesis reads: "The purpose of the investigation is to test the following hypothesis. . . ." Remembering that this is his purpose can help him to plan in a way that will lead to attainment of his purpose and prevent him from devoting time to matters concerned with the direct and prompt solution or alleviation of his specific problem in his particular setting.

The decision about which form to use for the statement of purpose is influenced by several important factors. Since substantiation of a hypothesis can be expected to provide the most readily usable information, the researcher should review his definition of problem to determine what hunches about relationships between phenomena are suggested to him. He may propose several hypotheses and then consider other factors before deciding on the hypothesis to be tested. There may be one or more phenomena whose existence he suspects, but about which he has sufficient doubt so that he does not wish to assume their existence and propose a hypothesis of a relationship with other phenomena. In such an instance, he may decide that the focus of his investigation should be determination of the existence or nonexistence of the suspected phenomenon or phenomena. He would then state the purpose in the form of a question, which would have the implied introduction: "The purpose of the investigation is to answer the following question(s) . . . ?"

The point may be illustrated by converting into questions the triple

Hypothesis

Question

focus delineated by Carter for her study.[3] She titled the statements, "hypotheses to be studied," but since each identified only a single observable phenomenon, they do not meet the criteria for hypotheses, as discussed on page 65. Posing a question as the focus for a study implies that there is sufficient information about the problem to permit formulation of a question, but not sufficient knowledge to propose hypotheses whose testing may be expected to yield meaningful information. The answer to the question would be expected to make a significant contribution to the knowledge needed as basis for positing hypotheses to be tested in subsequent studies. Implicit also in this decision is that information acquired as the answer to the question will permit the development of hypotheses to be tested.

Declarative Sentence

If knowledge is so limited that neither hypotheses nor questions can be proposed, then the purpose of the study must be identified as a search for definitive facts about some particular aspect of the problem. Here again, the facts sought would be expected to permit development of hypotheses for subsequent study.

Interest of Investigator

Since no single factor can determine the decision as to the form that the statement of purpose will take or the particular facet of the problem selected for study, it is impossible to ascribe a hierarchy of importance to the various factors that influence the decision. The particular interest of the investigator, however, will play a major part in the decision. This is especially true in relation to problems about nursing care of patients, since such problems will be composed of elements of concern to persons from varied disciplines. In the discussion of definition of problem, it was mentioned that the scope of the problem-defined could be narrowed by limiting elaborations to facets of particular interest to the investigator. So, too, the identification of the particular facet to be studied, and even the nature of the study to be undertaken, will be markedly influenced by the interest of the investigator: his particular social and scientific interest. For example, the problem of 1A's study could have led to an investigation by an educational psychologist of the influence of fear on performance or the degree to which fear is alleviated by information. Or it could have led a physiologist to study differences in peripheral circulation in relation to specific amounts of physical activity during pre- and postoperative periods. Each study would have been expected to reveal knowledge pertinent to the problem, yet each would have been very different from the study that 1A conducted. The interests of investigators can lead to quite different investigations, though the initial irritation is the same for all.

Potential Usefulness of Information

Another influential factor in the decision about the form of the statement of purpose is a judgment about the potential usefulness of information to be obtained from various lines of investigation. Indeed, this consideration may take precedence over the rule-of-thumb that the most pertinent purpose for doing research is to test hypotheses. For example,

Focus for Study

enough may be known about a particular facet of a problem to permit development of a hypothesis whose testing could yield meaningful information. But this potential information would be relatively unimportant when compared to information about the many elements in the problem about which very little is known. Under these circumstances an investigation expected to reveal many new facts in the situation might be indicated. New knowledge of inherent facts, in turn, would permit proposing hypotheses of greater potential meaning than a single one suggested on the basis of current knowledge. Discussion of Example 2N, page 96, elaborates this point.

In addition to the two rather scholarly factors—primacy of hypothesis testing and anticipated yield of information—other more prosaic but nevertheless real factors may influence the decision about the form the statement of purpose will take: for instance, the competence of the investigator, the time available for the study, the availability of consultant help, or the expense involved. One factor that seems to influence student researchers is a fear of hypothesis testing, as demonstrated by the fact that much research done by students takes the form of exploratory study. This attitude is unfortunate, since hypothesis testing is the most direct approach to knowledge that can guide actions and predict outcomes. Furthermore, exploratory studies are by far the more difficult to plan and execute. This will become progressively more clear as details are described for developing each successive step of research planning and execution. Suffice it to say here that no matter how formidable the planning needed to test a hypothesis may seem, it will still be easier than planning an encompassing exploratory search for facts pertinent to even a very limited facet of a problem. *Prosaic Factors*

Regardless of which of the three forms the statement of purpose takes, it must be specific about the identity of the facts to be observed, the setting in which the observations will be made, and the subjects to be studied. These requirements, along with the many attributes pertinent to a hypothesis, imply the need for great precision of statement. If one primary attribute in the process of scientific inquiry could be identified, that attribute must be precision: an important characteristic that differentiates research from problem solving. Precision is needed more in some steps of the research process than in others, but in none more than in Step 2: the statement of purpose. This can be illustrated by the sample hypotheses below, so stated that one seems to say the same thing as another. These hypotheses identify the marked difference that seemingly slight differences in statement can make to the anticipated study. *Precision of Statement*

The sample hypotheses used here were selected from some preliminary efforts of students. Lest the reader feel that such use represents criticism or disparagement of the students involved, let me say that these students, with few exceptions, went on to develop excellent designs. These examples *Stumbling First Steps*

Step 2: Statement of Purpose

were their first stumbling steps in putting something on paper, something concrete with which to work and learn. (Students are apt to think of research as a whole new field of exploration—and a strange one. They even express the feeling that they "will never be able to understand it." They should be reassured to hear that, in order to understand the first few steps, with the many new concepts that must be introduced, and to be comfortable about the language and concepts, they would have to know in the first five minutes of the course what they will learn in the first five weeks. Sometime during the first one third to one half of the course, students do find that *"Now it makes sense!"*)

Finally, should any of the students who composed these examples read them as they are presented here, it is highly unlikely that they would recognize them as their own. Each moved so far in her understanding, made such marked changes in her statement, and developed so many scholarly ideas about her entire undertaking that she would hardly recognize the long-since surpassed, stumbling first step.

Example 2D

The first example (2D) illustrates several considerations to be kept in mind by the investigator as he develops the statement of purpose. Among them is the fact that 2D's hypothesis, as stated, cannot be tested.

> If the professional nurse, in working with the patient who is to undergo his first surgical procedure which is elective, teaches, determining his level of understanding as she proceeds, what to expect pre- and post-operatively, then the patient will view that his anxiety has been decreased and he is more relaxed than if he had not received such instruction.

Unnecessarily Detailed

Quite obviously, 2D was greatly influenced by Feibleman's attributes of a good hypothesis. She "offers an explanation that is as complex as necessary under the circumstances." Indeed, the statement is unnecessarily detailed. Still, it can serve as a base for considering several things that must be kept in mind as the statement of purpose is composed. First, this statement might be cleared of at least one unnecessary clause by simply removing "determining his level of understanding as she proceeds." The clause identifies an entity of the teaching that may be left implicit or be accounted for in the plan for introducing the teaching in the experiment.

Impossible to Test

What is it about this statement that makes it impossible to test? The key to the impossibility of testing the hypothesis as stated is, of course, "his *first* surgical procedure." It would not be possible to determine twice how a patient would react to his *first* surgical procedure under the two circumstances described. In this step, as in all planning for research, the problem (the original irritation) should never be far from mind. It is not difficult to imagine 2D's original irritation: that patients are apprehensive about imminent surgery and about their conditions following surgery. The faulty construction of the proposed hypothesis does not mean that the real problem and the implied relationship of two phenomena cannot be studied. Unquestionably, it is possible to construct a hypothesis that can be tested and that will express the concept the student had in mind.

The original observations leading to concern about the problem can remind the investigator of the population that is to be subject to study. Rather than proposing the relationship between two phenomena in terms of *"the* patient," 2D's proposal could have been stated as pertaining to "patients who. . . ." This can lead to prompt identification of the population involved in observations leading to the concern about the problem. It also reminds the student researcher that the planned study will be concerned with patients (plural) and not alone with the patient (singular). A hypothesis is a generalization applicable to a category or class of subjects and not specific to a single individual subject.

Study Population

Now let us rephrase 2D's statement into a usable hypothesis for study:

Example 2Da

> Patients about to undergo their first surgical procedure, which is elective, who are taught by the nurse what to expect pre- and postoperatively, will be less anxious and more relaxed than patients who have not been taught.

Although many hypotheses to be tested by nurses will be of cause-effect relationships, a smoother sentence construction can be achieved by using either (1) "Subjects who" or (2) "When subjects" to introduce the statement, rather than "If subjects." The foregoing example, 2Da, is not a particularly good illustration, since the statement remains decidedly awkward. It is used, nevertheless, for two reasons. (1) The change from the original illustrates the value of the proposed introduction to the stated hypothesis. (2) It precludes the need to introduce still another hypothesis, whose sole purpose would be to illustrate the one point about the introductory part of the statement of a hypothesis.

If—Then When—Then

The 2Da hypothesis, in its final clause, illustrates another important point. Rather than delineating the relationship in a statement to the effect that teaching patients will result in "diminished" anxiety and "enhanced" relaxation, the statement is now in terms of comparing subjects who experience the teaching with subjects who have not experienced it; it compares differences in reactions to the surgical experience. The significance of the foregoing is that planning must be done in relation to two sets of subjects, so that comparisons can be made.

Final Clause— Commitment to Comparisons

Now let us analyze and evaluate, in terms of their pertinence as components of a hypothesis, the various elements in the 2Da hypothesis. "Patients about to undergo their first surgical procedure, which is elective, . . ." This identifies the particular population to be studied. The identification could not be "patients about to undergo their *first elective* surgery," because some may then have had prior experience with surgery, even though it was not elective (2D wanted patients with elective

Step 2: Statement of Purpose

surgery because, due to limited time and to the patient's physical condition or state of apprehension, it is not always possible to teach patients prior to emergency surgery.)

Evaluate Individual Elements of Statement

Patients are to be taught "by nurses." For the testing of the relationship between the two phenomena, this specification is not truly needed. Indeed, it could suggest that the study might, among other things, determine whether teaching by nurses would have results different from teaching by persons other than nurses. Examination of the entire statement, however, makes it obvious that the latter is not the purpose of the study. Rather, teaching "by nurses" is specified because of the particular interest of the investigator. "What to expect pre- and postoperatively" might have been left simply, "what to expect." But the addition of "pre- and postoperatively" makes more explicit the phenomenon, "teaching," including indication of the focus of the teaching. "Will be less anxious and more relaxed" identifies two related or resulting phenomena more specifically than if the phenomenon had been identified merely as "will feel better about the surgery." This sample hypothesis, then, illustrates points to be considered in delineating a hypothesis and the components necessary to ensure the attributes of a good hypothesis. It also includes the elements that are indicative of, and foretell certain facets of, the investigation that will be undertaken to test the hypothesis.

Detail in Hypothesis to Guide Study

The relationship between the phenomena in the above example might be stated in a somewhat less complex way and, should the hypothesis be substantiated, it undoubtedly would be thought of in a simpler construction: for instance, the statement might have been to the effect that "teaching patients what to expect pre- and postoperatively lessens their anxiety and promotes relaxation." It is strongly recommended that a hypothesis be stated in such a way that, substantiated, it need not undergo structural change as it moves to the realm of theory. Yet, in seeming contradiction, it is also recommended that the student researcher develop a hypothesis so precise and detailed that it will not only describe the relationship between the phenomena, but will also identify pertinent conditions about the two phenomena and about the populations to be studied. This suggestion is particularly applicable when the student is learning the research process through his first experience of developing a design for scientific inquiry, and when the study will be conducted within the scope of a senior paper or masters thesis.

For such a study, the population sample will be limited in number and necessarily in heterogeneity. For example, 2D limited her subjects to patients with intraperitoneal surgery. Her findings in relation to these patients might be generalized to all patients having major surgery, but only by analogy. Should the findings from her limited study indicate that her hypothesized relationships do indeed exist, further investigation with a

Focus for Study

larger sample of subjects would be warranted. A senior paper or masters study may be viewed as a pilot for a larger study. Essentially, then, it is not really a contradiction of the earlier guidelines—that the hypothesis should be so worded that, if substantiated, it can move to the realm of theory without structural change—to suggest that the student researcher so construct the statement of purpose for his study, even a hypothesis, with explicit details. The suggestion applies equally to all statements of purpose. Though some details may be dropped from the statement if the hypothesis becomes a theory, the concept of the proposed relationship between phenomena will not change.

> Private duty nurses who receive a planned orientation are better able to give nursing care which is satisfactory to patient, physician, and self than are private duty nurses who do not have an orientation.

Example 2E

Some of the points to be made with this example will be clearer if the initial irritation is first summarized. 2E was a private duty nurse, new to the city. She was concerned about various distressing experiences she had had, all of which seemed to stem from the fact that she had not been oriented to the hospital or patient care unit when she went to a hospital new to her. Her lack of knowledge of means for securing equipment, of policies, and of physical setting led to delays in patient care, ranging in seriousness from mere inconvenience to actual danger for the patients. The imaginative nurse can readily fill in many details of this problem.

A knowledge of the problem is, however, not needed to identify two major flaws in the precision of this statement of hypothesis. One has to do with the knotty problem of the identity of elements to be compared and exactly what is to be measured. The second flaw in this statement actually leads to the first and demonstrates failure to think through what actually is the phenomenon of concern. What is it that irritated the investigator? What, basically, would she like to see changed? The hypothesis as stated directs attention to comparison of two groups of private duty nurses and indicates that the phenomenon to be measured is the ability of the nurses to give satisfactory care. But, in actuality, 2E was not concerned about private duty nurses' *ability* to give nursing care, although her hypothesis stated ". . . are better able . . ." Furthermore, as a student researcher and as a nurse with limited background in psychology, she would hardly feel qualified to pursue a study requiring measurement of ability. In addition, since the purpose of research is to test hypotheses with the objective of providing theories that will guide actions and allow prediction of outcomes of actions, it would seem wasteful of time and energy to test a hypothesis positing a relationship between an orientation program and nurses' ability to give satisfactory care. Substantiation of such a hypothesis would provide only the prediction that nurses were *able* to give satisfactory care; it would not allow, except by inference, prediction

Elements Being Compared

that nurses *would* give satisfactory care. Sometimes a statement of such a relationship is all that current information will allow, but in this instance, a more precise statement of the hypothesis might be:

2Ea Private duty nurses who receive planned orientation give nursing care that is more satisfactory to patients, doctors, and themselves than care given by nurses who do not have an orientation.

Or another statement might be:

2Eb Care given by private duty nurses who have a planned orientation is more satisfactory to patients, doctors, and the nurses themselves than is care given by nurses who do not receive a planned orientation.

In each of these delineations, the mere construction of the sentence places the focus on comparing the nursing care given by two groups of nurses. Here, too, nurses are to be compared to nurses in terms of the care they give—and this is true. Yet examination of the original and revised statements makes it obvious that one directs attention toward something *within* the nurses, and the other toward something the nurses do extending to others outside themselves. The direction of attention can be very meaningful to the beginning researcher, who needs all the help he can get to identify exactly what he must do to accomplish his study. To test the first proposed hypothesis, 2E would have had to seek facts about the nurses themselves; for the latter two, she could consider facts about nursing care. (The import of this distinction will be elaborated, at least by implication, in Steps 3 and 5.) It will be noted, also, that these proposed statements end with the comparative clause that would be unnecessary to express the posited relationship, but that can be helpful to the beginning researcher as he plans later steps in his design.

Example 2F, 2Fa Students who have positive attitudes toward mental illness will enter into more therapeutic nurse-patient interactions, either by initiating them or by responding to patient initiations, than will students with negative attitudes.

Nurse-patient interactions involving students with positive attitudes toward mental illness are more therapeutic than are interactions involving students with negative attitudes.

These two statements, 2F and 2Fa, apparently positing the same relationship between phenomena, might lead to two quite different investigations. Again, it is a matter of precise statement as to what facts are to be compared. In 2F, there is no way of knowing whether the intent is (1) that nurse-patient interactions will be *more therapeutic*; (2) that, of the interactions that do occur, *more of them* will be therapeutic; or (3) that there will merely be a *greater number* of therapeutic interactions. In 2Fa, however, there is no question about what will be compared. These examples illustrate what might be called the "dangling comparative," and the difference made by the answer to the question: "More than what?" They illustrate, too, the difference in the measurements that will be required in the two investigations, a point to be elaborated in Step 5. "More frequent" therapeutic interactions could require only a two-point scale to judge whether an interaction was therapeutic or not; whereas "more therapeutic" would require a scale that would measure degrees of being therapeutic. This exemplifies how the researcher must think ahead in his planning and how the precise delineation of the hypothesis can markedly influence major elements of the investigation.

> When hospitalized children receive small items of food from home they will have better appetites than when they do not have this food.
>
> Hospitalized children who receive small items of food from home will eat more of the food of their regular meals than children who are denied these items of food from home (or: than children who do not receive food from home).

Example 2G— 2Ga

The chief point here is the direction that each statement would give to the ensuing study. 2G indicates that, in the experiment used to test the hypothesis, the children who will be the subjects studied will serve as their own controls. That is, measurements will be made of their appetites during a period when they are not allowed to receive food from home; they will then be allowed food from home, and second measurements will be made. 2Ga, on the other hand, divides the children into two "equal" groups, one of which will receive food from home, and the other of which will not. Measurements will be made of appetites of children in each group, and comparisons made. Essentially, the same relationship between the same two phenomena would be tested in each study, and findings from one would, in general, be applicable to the other. While there are some instances in which the selection of one or the other of such hypotheses may be made by arbitrary decision, this would not be true in this example, since several considerations favor the selection of 2Ga rather than 2G. It might be expected, for instance, that children who are hospitalized might be acutely ill on admission and therefore not have much appetite, and that they might improve in health in a few days' time and be ready to eat. Furthermore, during the first few days in the hospital, children might be upset because of separation from parents and because of the strange environment; after a few days they would make some adjustment to these things and would be expected to eat better. Therefore, it would seem unreasonable for children to serve as their own controls for testing the relationship hypothesized to exist between the two phenomena. The various reasons for deciding on one or the other of these hypotheses to test will be elaborated as part of Steps 5 and 9, where such planning is more appropriately done.

Subjects Studied Serve As Their Own Controls

Step 2: Statement of Purpose

Precise Identity of Phenomena

The two delineations, 2G and 2Ga, of the relationship between the same two phenomena illustrate a second condition in which the researcher must think ahead to concerns of a later step in the research process: the precise identity of one of the related phenomena. 2G identifies it as the child's "appetite," and 2Ga, as "eating more food." To measure the quantity of food eaten seems a fairly easy task, but measuring appetite is less simple. Considering that the hypothesis delineates the relationship between two facts, and that facts are observable phenomena, it becomes necessary to consider the observability of appetite. Appetite denotes a concept encompassing elements beyond the mere quantity of food eaten. This consideration will be more appropriately elaborated in Step 5. The point to be made here is the marked influence of the selection of words sometimes used interchangeably, and what is meant by precision of statement in a scientific investigation.

Example 2H

What kinds of emotional trauma in which types of preschool children result in what kinds of poor social adjustment or frank mental illness in adulthood?

This example, 2H, and 2I to follow are in the form of questions rather than hypotheses. They are used here, however, as illustrations of vagueness of statement and obvious impossibility of study built into a statement of purpose. Considerations of the question as one form for the statement of purpose are elaborated on pages 98 to 99.

Vague, Diffuse, Global

Obviously, 2H really had a problem! It would be somewhat difficult, however, to imagine the original irritation and some of its appertaining elements from this "statement of purpose," although this was possible in each of the previous examples. Indeed, this example reinforces the influence of a well-defined problem on the subsequent steps in a scientific study. 2H had proceeded to this step with only the briefest discussion of her problem; she had identified very few of the elements in it, and she had thought through none of the interrelationships of the various elements composing the problem. Though not all poorly defined problems will lead to so diffuse a statement as this, it would be most unlikely that such a statement would evolve from a well-defined problem. Obviously, before any attempt could be made to develop a usable statement of purpose, it would be necessary to improve the definition of problem. There is no way that this statement could be analyzed and amended to evolve an identification of a focus for a study. Nonetheless, the statement does illustrate two points to be considered as the researcher plans and makes decisions about the facet of the problem to be studied and the focus to be made specific in the precise, definitive statement of purpose.

The first point concerns the global nature of each concept identified in 2H: (1) what kinds of emotional trauma? (2) which types of preschool children? (3) what kinds of poor social adjustment? (4) frank mental illness? (5) adulthood? The student was actually proposing to ascertain *all* facts about *all* persons who would ever be emotional and social beings since, by implication, and in order to have useful information about what leads to mental illness, it would be necessary also to have information about what does not lead to it.

The second point is the impossibility of carrying out such an investigation, even if definitions could be developed to make the global concepts specific and concrete. An investigator could hardly expect to live so long: to observe emotional trauma in children and then to wait for them to become adults and manifest poor social adjustment. These points need not be labored; one more example will illustrate the latter point and remind the student of analyses he must make in evaluating his statement of purpose for preciseness of all concepts expressed.

Impossibility of Proposed Study

> Nondiabetic people have a conception of the kind of life a diabetic must lead; does this conception affect their willingness to accept teaching if they should become diabetic?

Example 2I

Although this example does not have the flaws of Example 2H, which evolved from incomplete definition of problem, it does have the rather obvious limitation of being impossible to study. It would be impractical to the point of absurdity to determine conceptions held by a sufficient number of persons before they were identified as diabetics. Again, it would be a matter of "living so long."

The Researcher Should Live So Long

Study populations are elusive: that is, subjects are lost over even brief periods of time. Investigators doing longitudinal studies who have begun with 5,000 subjects and have made elaborate provisions for retaining their subjects' interest in participation have ended up with fewer than 2,000 subjects at the end of a five-year period. Problems and precautions related to retention of study subjects are pertinent in planning Step 6 and are discussed in detail in most texts on "survey research."

The Elusive Subject

In summary, then, and in relationship to the development of a hypothesis as the statement of purpose for a study, some elements which the student must consider are: (1) his particular interest, (2) the value of testing hypotheses, (3) the currently available knowledge about the facet of the problem about which he plans to seek information, (4) his personal capabilities, time, money, and available assistance, and (5) preciseness of statement. These same elements, as well as the other guidelines discussed in relation to the delineation of a hypothesis, apply equally well to the other two forms in which a statement of purpose can be expressed: the declarative sentence, and the question. The foregoing detailed discussion was presented in terms of the hypothesis, however, because the student learning about research *must* learn about hypotheses and the role they play in scientific inquiry.

DECLARATIVE SENTENCE AS STATEMENT OF PURPOSE

Examples 2J and 2K, below, illustrate statements of purpose in the form of declarative sentences. Such statements reflect extensive study and thinking that produced detailed and well-integrated definitions of problems.

Example 2J   The purpose of this study is to examine factors related to fear and anxiety experienced by nurses who must provide care for tracheotomized patients, with the view toward identifying and describing the many and varied factors encompassed in the care, such as equipment, procedures, nurses' attitudes toward giving the care, number of patients requiring this care (frequency of opportunity for nurses to have experience in providing care), and results of care for the patients.

Example 2K   The purpose of the study is to explore the use of nursing care measures to promote comfort and prevent deformities of immobilized patients, with the view toward determining the types of measures used, the frequency of use, the relationship of type and frequency to patients' needs, and the types of personnel using various measures.

Nature of Information Made Specific   These two statements make quite specific the nature of the information to be sought. Along with the definitions of the problem, they provide the investigators with ready materials and guides for planning many of the later steps; they also serve as a useful base for developing the report of findings from the study. In addition, such statements of purpose indicate rather clearly the nature of the problem being investigated. They serve as ready references for determining the information to be sought and the degree to which the investigator achieved his purpose. The extent of the usability of these statements will be clear as planning for later steps in the research design are described.

Example 2L   The threefold purpose of the study is to identify health-related superstitions held by Negroes, which influence behavior in relation to health practices and to nursing care provided; to indicate those with particular meaning for the public health nurse; and to trace the sources of the latter superstitions.

Limits Built In   Example 2L identifies the particular facet of interest to the investigator, chosen from among the many facets in the problem of sociocultural barriers to communication and health teaching that are encountered by nurses who endeavor to help patients. In addition, 2L illustrates "built-in" limits of the study to be undertaken. The statement recognizes that the search for health-related superstitions with particular meaning for the public health nurse will involve identifying many health-related superstitions and that tracing all to their sources would be an extensive task. Therefore, it specifies that those of particular interest to the public health nurse are the only ones for which the search for sources will be made. This statement does not identify the nature of the problem as definitively as do Examples 2J and 2K; yet, there is a general indication of it, and this is perhaps all that should be attempted.

Actually, the identification of the broad problem of concern in the statement of focus is not the primary attribute to be sought for this element in the research design. The delineation of 2L does reveal certain tasks that will be a part of the investigation. Obviously, there will be the searching of the literature of the health sciences, of history, and of mythology, as well as interviews with patients and health personnel. In addition, the statement indicates that decisions will be made about each superstition in relation to its meaning for the public health nurse. Essentially, the statement indicates that the search for information will be a three-step process: (1) the identification of the superstitions, (2) the classification of the superstitions, and (3) the tracing of selected superstitions to their sources. It may be presumed that the investigator will extend her study to propose the potential use of the information for public health nurses, though this statement does not commit her to doing so. Some suggestions for potential use would, of course, have been described in the definition of problem. The omission of the proposal for potential use represents another limitation on the scope of the study. From brief consideration of the possible scope of study suggested by the statement and visualization of the problem from which the single facet for study was selected, it is easy to envision the continuing study that could engage a researcher in a lifetime of fruitful, exciting, and meaningful search.

> The purpose of the study is to determine whether identification foot or palm prints of newborn infants are valid and usable and the extent to which they actually are used and for what purposes.

Example 2M

Example 2M may at first seem to be the concern of the criminologist and not of the nurse. But since nurses are the ones who secure most infant identification prints, it seems entirely appropriate for a nurse to pursue the study suggested in this statement of purpose. This is particularly reasonable in light of the investigator's original plan, which had been to test a hypothesis about the relationship of a method for doing prints to the usability of the prints.

Example 2M is used here to illustrate the factor that influences the decision *not* to test a hypothesis but rather to do an exploratory study to secure information expected to make a greater immediate contribution to alleviation of the problem. The initial irritation was the observation that many infant identification prints done by nurses were mere smears of ink. As the definition of the problem developed, many elements composing the problem evolved, such as the skill of persons doing the prints, avail-

Exploration Preferred Over Hypothesis Testing

able equipment, variations in techniques, and a disturbing vagueness about reasons for doing the prints. Among the latter was: "Parents like to have them." Also revealed was the fact that more than half of the prints done were of such poor quality that they could not be used for identification purposes. Although the investigator was interested in testing techniques for doing prints and wished to determine whether palm prints could be made more usable than foot prints, she decided that determination of this information would be of little service if prints were not used for identification purposes. Therefore, rather than testing the hypothesis, she decided to pursue the exploratory study suggested in the statement of purpose, with the view to using the information obtained as a basis for deciding whether testing the hypothesis could be expected to yield information of value. In addition, the proposed study could be expected to yield not only information identified in the statement of purpose but also information that could make planning for testing hypotheses more definitive.

Example 2N

The purpose of this investigation is to determine ways to facilitate gastric tube insertion for patients in terms of emotional preparation and support, and in terms of actual techniques of insertion.[4]

Example 2P

The purpose of the study is to explore the rationale for the practice of giving daily cleansing baths to all hospital adult patients with the view to determining the relationship between the rationale for the bath and the individualization of patient care.

Statement As Brief As Possible

Examples 2N and 2P are statements of purpose that are about as brief as such statements can be and still identify the focus for a scientific inquiry. Yet each not only identifies rather clearly the information that will be sought, but also indicates relationships that will be sought among the findings. Each is so structured that the reader can readily surmise the nature of the original irritation and many of the elements in the problem. In Example 2N, the phrases, "facilitate gastric tube insertion for patients in terms of emotional preparation and support" and "in terms of actual techniques of insertion," suggest that the investigator was concerned about the emotional aspects of what is never a pleasant experience for patients, yet an experience that many perceive as a wholly physical one. This is an example of seeing more in a situation than many people see and recognizing that others must be helped to see the emotional as well as the physical aspects of the treatment.

Exploratory Findings and Selection of Hypotheses

Example 2N also illustrates, by implication, the value of pursuing an exploratory study prior to testing hypotheses. On the basis of her experience and that reported by others, 2N was able to propose several hypotheses with explanatory bases in physiological, anatomical, and psychological theories. Yet the testing of any one of the hypotheses would have required an extensive study and, with available knowledge, it was impossible to determine which of the possible hypotheses, if tested, might yield the most useful information. 2N therefore decided that the exploratory study would be the most direct route to identification of hypotheses that might lead to useful knowledge. The exploratory study, she reasoned, might very well identify a few hypotheses with considerable potential for useful information, from among the larger number whose potential could not be estimated with any degree of confidence without the new knowledge.

The generalizations made about Example 2N apply equally to Example 2P. Both portray a keen sense of concern for patient welfare, it should be pointed out: an empathy with patients and a desire to improve care of patients through providing knowledge on which to evaluate old routines and to plan for individualized care. Both statements are brief; any attempts to elaborate any point or points in these precise and definitively structured presentations could lead only to unwieldy sentences since, to preserve balance, elaboration of one point would require elaboration of several.

Revision, Completeness, Succinctness

Statements as succinct, yet as encompassing and useful as these, are not written on the first try, not even when the first try follows a thorough definition of the problem. Indeed, the final formulation of the statement of purpose may come only after planning has progressed through Step 8. This is not to say that the focus for study must wait for precise delineation until Step 8. Quite the contrary: it must be clearly conceived and stated before progress can be made in planning any of the succeeding steps, even Step 3, Definitions of Terms. The suggestion that final expression may come as late as Step 8, however, is to emphasize the fact that the sequence of the words, and the very precise words to be used, may not be identified until the investigator has become steeped in the extensive thinking involved in planning the entire investigation.

Analogy: How a Precious Stone Is Cut

An analogy might be the extensive consideration by the diamond cutter of all facets and potentialities of a large and valuable uncut stone. After preliminary examination, he formulates a gross plan and a vision of results. Then, through extensive and intensive study, he commits to memory every facet and angle, envisions every potentiality to result from the blow that will cut the stone. He becomes so familiar with the totality of the gem that he feels it a part of himself. When he has attained this awareness of the stone, he can then strike the single blow that will yield the exact gems he had envisioned. So the researcher, after the first writing of the definition of problem, formulates a relatively exact statement of purpose. After extensive and intensive study and thinking during the development of Components 3 through 7, he is thoroughly aware of all entities and their interrelationships in a study to be pursued. He is then able to delineate the precise statement that will identify the focus and content of that study.

Example 2Q

The purpose of this study is to determine what the physicians think individual cardiac patients should know in preparation for discharge from the hospital, what nurses think the patients should know, and what the patients actually know.

One Word Predicts the Total Plan

Example 2Q is like Examples 2N and 2P in its precision and succinctness of statement, but it is used here to illustrate an additional point: the marked influence of a single word. The word "individual" (1) predicts the sources of the various items of information to be sought, and (2) indicates that the information sought will be specific about particular patients and not vague and diffuse in relation to what physicians and nurses think "cardiac patients" in general should know. The focus of the study will be on what physicians and nurses say about individual patients, not what they might say about the vague, general, all cardiac patients. The implication is that information will be sought from Dr. X about Patient C; from Nurses RN, HN, and SN about Patient C; and from Patient C. We will not consider here the way these findings will be handled nor their implications, but it takes little imagination to envision some of the potentials. Not always can one word hold so much meaning, but here "the individual" really matters.

A QUESTION AS THE STATEMENT OF PURPOSE

The concept of a question as a statement of purpose seems contradictory from a grammatical standpoint, since a question differs from a statement in structure and intent. As a matter of fact, this contradiction applies in a research sense as well. Where a problem has been fully defined and it has been concluded that the largest contribution can be made through study to determine the existence of a specific fact, it is common for two or more related facts to be sought; these require delineation of two or more questions. Further, under the above circumstances, a single declarative statement could be constructed to describe the focus of the study. This situation is exemplified by Carter's so-called "hypotheses." (3) As indicated on page 84, each of her statements identified a single observable phenomenon, and might well have been couched as questions:

1. "[Do] patients on a psychiatric ward perceive patient-patient interaction as therapeutic"?
2. "[Can] the patients . . . communicate their perception of therapeutic patient-patient interaction"?
3. "[Have] the patients . . . entered into interpersonal relationships with each other"?

On the other hand, the statement of purpose to guide the study might have taken the following form (a declarative sentence):

> The purpose of the study is to determine whether patients in a psychiatric ward (1) enter into interpersonal relationships with each other, (2) perceive these interactions as therapeutic, and (3) are able to communicate these perceptions.

Such a statement would have identified the focus planned for the study. More detailed questions might have been delineated to identify or highlight the individual types of information sought.

The foregoing discussion leads to the recommendation that a question *not* be used as the statement of purpose. This is not because a question could not delineate the focus of a fact-finding study, but because a declarative statement can serve the purpose just as well. Further, using a question for this purpose might limit or make confusing the use of questions elsewhere in the study. Where a declarative statement is used, any number of questions can then be posed to identify and clarify particular information to be sought and to serve as guides to planning the observations and the organization, analyses, and report of the findings. But where a question or questions are used to identify the study's purpose, there is the need for repeated explanation as to which question is being discussed throughout the study report: one of the statement of focus questions? or a subquestion or one of secondary importance? So, there would seem to be little advantage to using a question for the statement of purpose of the study, and considerable advantage in not so using the question. But, regardless of the form used for the statement of purpose, the delineation must specifically identify the phenomena to be observed and the subjects to be studied, with careful attention to preciseness of terms used and concepts implied.

Reserve Questions For Detailed Planning and Organizing Findings

STATEMENT OF PURPOSE: NARROWS FOCUS FOR REVIEW OF LITERATURE

The statement of purpose is developed primarily to identify the scope and limitations of the study and to serve as the focus for the study. It also narrows the field of the literature to be explored. This latter and extremely useful purpose is the reason the investigator must resist developing the statement of purpose until the problem has been thoroughly defined and the literature explored broadly. Only after the investigator has learned what is known and thought about the many elements in his problem, and only after he has thought through the meaning and pertinence of the knowledge from the various fields for his problem should he consider

Resist Premature Development of Statement of Purpose

delineation of the statement of purpose. Not until then should he decide which particular facet of the problem he will study and delineate the precise direction and focus for his study.

Though the investigator must resist premature development of the statement of focus, there will nonetheless come a point at which he must decide that the broad exploration has extended far enough and the next step must be begun. At this point, he will have selected the facet of the problem to be studied and can limit his reading to literature directly related to that facet. After study in depth of materials pertinent to the facet to be studied, the statement of purpose will be delineated.

REFERENCES

1. Feibleman, J. K. The role of hypotheses in the scientific method. Perspect. Biol. Med., 2:339. Spring, 1959.
2. Henry, N. B., ed. Science education in American schools. *In* Forty-sixth Yearbook, National Society for the Study of Education, Part 1. Chicago, The University of Chicago Press, 1947, p. 31.
3. Carter, F. M. The critical incident technique in identification of the patients' perception of therapeutic patient-patient interaction on a psychiatric ward. Nurs. Res., 8:207.
4. Teranes, B. Patient Views on Nasogastric Tube Insertion. Unpublished masters thesis, Detroit, Wayne State University, 1967.

STEP 3
DEFINITION OF TERMS

TERMS DEFINED

Definition: A definition is an arbitrarily imposed description that allows common understanding.

Variable: A variable is a measurable or potentially measurable component of an object or event that may fluctuate in quantity or quality, or that may be different in quantity or quality from one individual object or event to another individual object or event of the same general class.

Independent variable: The independent variable is that phenomenon in the hypothesis that, in the experimental study to test the hypothesis, is manipulated by the investigator.

Dependent variable: The dependent variable is that phenomenon in the hypothesis that, in the experimental study to test the hypothesis, is not manipulated, but is accepted as it occurs.

Extraneous variables: Extraneous variables are all variables in a hypothesis-testing investigation that are not the independent variable, the dependent variable, or criterion measures of the dependent variable.

Criterion measure: A criterion measure is a quality, attribute, or characteristic of a variable that may be measured to provide scores by which subjects or things of the same class may be compared with respect to the variable. (The term is most frequently used in relation to a dependent variable, but the concept is equally applicable for any variable on which subjects are to be compared, described, or measured.)

Operational definition: An operational definition is a definition that uses observable processes, actions, or structural analogues (or explicit and detailed word descriptions of them) to describe concepts represented by the term being defined; an operational definition is an explicit description of a single entity or phenomenon considered to be a concrete referent of the term being defined, whether the referent be an object, a process, or an action; it specifically identifies a single entity or phenomenon to be measured to provide one component of a score of the variable or characteristic being measured and evaluated. Put more succinctly, an operational definition is a description or actual display of a process, action, or object suggested as an analogue or single representative example of what is meant by the term being defined.

CONCEPTS PERTINENT TO DEFINED TERMS

Definition of Terms For Use in Research

The concept that a definition is an arbitrarily imposed description that allows common understanding may helpfully be extended when the concern is definitions of terms to be used in research. The extension should add the concept that the definition is composed of three parts: (1) a dictionary or general definition, (2) a pertinent general definition, and (3) a for-instance definition.

These parts and the purposes they serve will be clarified later in this chapter, but two sets of concepts can be introduced here.

(1) The dictionary definition is a general definition: a generalization that fits all cases. (2) The pertinent general definition may be thought of as a *specific general* definition, a generalization that fits only specific cases. To avoid the antithesis of "specific general," this phase of the definition is termed the "pertinent general." It is still a generalization, but it narrows the definition to identify the particular interest of the investigator. (3) The for-instance phase of the definition identifies a single entity or phenomenon that is illustrative of the pertinent general is illustrative of the general (dictionary) definition. (A rose is illustrative of a flower is illustrative of an object of natural beauty.)

Illustration: Communicates

The three phases are illustrated in abbreviated fashion in the following example: The investigator plans to seek facts about nurses communicating. The term to be defined is "communicates."

1. Dictionary definition: to impart, pass along, transmit; to give, or give and receive, information, signals, or messages in any way. This definition could fit anyone and any means of communication: an automobile

salesman; a baseball catcher, coach, or umpire; a kindergarten instructor; an astronaut preparing for splashdown.

2. Pertinent general definition: A nurse talks and listens to patients, family members, and co-workers; gives instructions about treatments; writes nursing notes on patients' records; discusses patient's condition with physician. This identifies types of communications that are of interest to the investigator; it identifies the particular kinds of communications and the individuals involved.

3. For-instance definition: Nurse Y told Mr. Jones he was to go to X-ray; Nurse L answered visitor's questions about the patient's need for rest; Nurse J recorded in nurses notes, "Had a good night; no complaints." Here are examples of individual observable communicating actions or results of actions performed by nurses. They illustrate specific phenomena with which the investigator is concerned. As will be seen from later examples, the pertinent general and the for-instance phases of this definition would be markedly extended if communicating were the dependent variable of a hypothesis to be tested.

The second set of concepts needed by the student at this point consists of: (1) The dictionary definition will not necessarily include a complete citation from the dictionary, but only the portions pertinent to the investigator's immediate concern (see example of definition of nurse, pages 115 and 116). (2) Criterion measures and other variables to be observed or measured are identified in the pertinent general portion of the definition. (3) A single occurrence of a phenomenon to be observed will be identified in the for-instance portion of the definition. Either the pertinent general or for-instance portions may include multiple individual units of their particular class of units for the definition.

Here is another example illustrating the concepts of such a definition. The investigator is interested in determining relations between body temperature of patients and environmental temperatures. The term to be defined is "temperature." It may seem to a nurse that the meaning of temperature is sufficiently commonly understood as to hardly need defining. Yet, a set of temperatures reported in relation to a single patient at a single report period might be: room temperature, 78.4, 69.2; and patient's body temperature, 37.0, and 98.6. The differences in reported observations of the same two phenomena are due to the absence of the pertinent general and the for-instance phases of the definitions of the terms "environmental temperature" and "body temperature." There obviously was a "noncommon" understanding. For the environmental temperature, two individuals apparently ascribed different meanings to the pertinent general phase, while using the same for-instance phase. They both used a Fahrenheit thermometer, but they obviously measured different areas of environment. For

Illustration: Temperature

the body temperature, the two individuals used the same pertinent general meaning of the term, and each took an oral temperature. But they used different for-instances: one used a Fahrenheit thermometer and the other a centigrade thermometer. Another possible source of confusion lies in the fact that the nurse is aware of criterion measures of temperatures other than the thermometer. For example, there are measures, along with for-instances, such as the tactile sensation, "warm to the touch," or verbal reports, "It's hot in here" and "He is burning up." To preclude misunderstandings, the term should be so precisely described that any one knowledgeable person would make the same measurement of a single, representative occurrence of the phenomenon that any other knowledgeable person would. Temperature might be defined:

1. Dictionary: the degree of hotness or coldness of anything, usually measured on a thermometer. (This definition could apply to temperature of anything, any place, any time.)

2. Pertinent general: Body temperature—the degree of body temperature of study subjects, taken orally, observed and recorded by a nurse at six specified times of day. Environmental temperature—the degree of environmental temperature for study subjects, taken at a level 5 feet above the floor, within an 8-foot distance from the patient's head, observed and recorded by the nurse at the same times that the body temperatures are taken.

3. For-instances: A body temperature might be 97.2° Fahrenheit at 7:00 A.M., and the coincident environmental temperature might be 72.4° Fahrenheit.

It is entirely probable that the pertinent general phase for environmental temperature would be extended to delineate distances from sources of heat and draft. But the limited descriptions serve to illustrate the nature of the three parts of a definition of terms. The pertinent general identifies the particular attribute or quality of the phenomenon that is to be observed (measured). The for-instance phase identifies a single observation (measurement) and, in this instance, makes explicit the scale of measurement, the Fahrenheit scale. In some instances, the scale of measurement is left implicit. For example, in the limited definition of "communicates," above, the only scale of measurement that may be inferred is a frequency count. Identification of the investigator's interest in some particular qualities of communicating would lead to—indeed, necessitate—identification of other criterion measures and scales appropriate for classifying individual measurements. These concepts will be extensively elaborated in later discussion of this step and in Step 5.

It may have been noted that discussions of the first two steps of the research process did not include some rather common terms of research

Concepts Pertinent to Defined Terms

jargon. Actually, such terms as "variable," "data," and "control" were deliberately not used in the first two chapters. They were not essential to the discussion, and it seemed better to introduce them at the points where they become imperative for continuing discussion and where they are particularly pertinent. It may be argued that the concepts of independent variable, dependent variable, and data could hardly be more pertinent than to the discussion of the hypothesis. Yet the extensive discussion of the hypothesis does not really need these terms, whereas concepts about fact, theory, and principle *were* necessary for that discussion. It is now time, however, to introduce the words "variable" and "population," to define them, and to discuss the concepts of their meanings as they are used in the research process.

Omission of Jargon

The parallel listing below indicates the many terms that are used to refer to the independent and dependent variables:

Independent variable	*Dependent variable*
cause	effect
if	then
controlled	uncontrolled
antecedent	consequent
manipulated	accepted (come what may)
experimental	result
treatment	outcome
action	outcome

The list, although not exhaustive, includes the terms most commonly used and makes explicit the concepts of independent and dependent variable. It also suggests that in delineating a hypothesis it is logical to identify the independent variable first in the statement. This is not a necessary or unvarying pattern, but it adheres to the commonly held idea of action preceding outcome. It is logical, too, in relation to the experiment to test the hypothesis. In an experiment, the independent variable will be introduced first, followed by measurement of the dependent variable. On the other hand, when the hypothesis moves to the realm of theory and is used to guide actions, the process is reversed. That is, as a theory is applied, the desired outcome is determined first, followed by the identification of the action necessary to effect the outcome.

Essentially, there are three categories into which extraneous variables may be placed, controlled-for, accounted-for, and confounding, with only the first two of major concern for all studies. Those of greatest concern are the controlled-for variables: those variables that are apt to affect the dependent variable in a manner similar to the affect of the independent variable (illustrated in Example 3A, below). It should be noted that the designation is controlled-*for,* which should not be confused with controlled,

Extraneous Variables— Controlled-for or Confounding

one of the common terms used to refer to the independent variable. These extraneous variables will be controlled for, they will not be controlled or manipulated, per se. The reason for controlling for them is to eliminate the influence of potentially confounding variables.

Confounding variables, in turn, are extraneous variables that influence the dependent variable in the same way the independent variable influences it. Some classify confounding variables as those of prime concern, after the independent and dependent variables. But, if variables that are apt to confound the findings are controlled for, there will be no confounding variables, since their influence will have been precluded.

Studies of Humans: Are They Scientific?

Because there is little if any research wherein all potentially confounding variables can be known, let alone controlled for, the researcher must always be aware of the possibility of potentially confounding variables. This is especially true where research involves human beings. It has been asserted that, since it is obviously impossible to control for all variables "other than the one under investigation," no study of human beings can be classed as scientific. Many imply, or even state openly, that such studies should not be undertaken. Some persons feel so strongly about this that they refuse to accept the idea that the process and techniques of scientific inquiry are applicable in the study of human beings.

All would be better served if this semantic debate were abandoned, and the valuable time, effort, and intellectual energy were devoted to promotion of studies. Whether his studies be in the physical, biological, or behavorial sciences, let each investigator, following his own interest, pursue his own studies, using the processes of science to advance his work. Let all respect the work of others, and let them call it what they will—science, scientific inquiry, research, study—so long as they communicate a generally understood meaning. Let the purist concede that those who study problems involving human beings know that they cannot control for all variables. And let those who study problems involving human beings *be* aware that they cannot control for all variables. In all studies there will always be potentially confounding variables, but awareness of this can lead to planning to control for these variables. This, in turn, will either eliminate their influence or will permit accounting for the degree of their influence.

Extraneous Variables— Accounted-for

The second most important category of extraneous variables is the accounted-for variables, as distinguished from the controlled-for variables. They are those variables about which information is gathered during the study for the sake of gleaning additional information, even though it actually is not needed in relation to testing the hypothesis. Accounted-for variables differ from controlled-for variables in the amount of attention that must be given to each. Actually, accounted-for variables could be ignored, so far as testing the relationship between the two phenomena in the hypothesis is concerned. On the other hand, the controlled-for variables

Concepts Pertinent to Defined Terms

must be precisely identified, plans for controlling for them must be developed and executed and, in some instances, information about them must be gathered. Background information that is obtained on the subjects studied is frequently information about accounted-for variables. The purpose served by information about accounted-for variables is to enable more extensive analyses and interpretation of findings. Further comments about controlled-for and accounted-for variables and their relationship to the other elements in the investigation are best placed in the context of an example.

Example: Godfrey

The study done by Godfrey illustrates several points about extraneous variables. The hypothesis, as Godfrey delineated it, was: It is believed that separation at the end of the visiting period can be emotionally more comfortable for the child and his parents if the nurse is readily available to assist them during the visiting period and at the departure of the parent, and if she remains with the child 30 minutes after departure of the parent, provided she purposefully gears her nursing care toward assisting them in their separation.[1]

The subjects studied were "children on the pediatric ward who were between 2 and 6 years of age, who were oriented to the environment, whose parents were present during the visiting period, and who were at the second or later chronological day of hospitalization." "No attempt was made to match the groups according to age, sex, diagnosis, previous hospital experience, previous emotional adjustments, length of present hospital stay, or number of children in hospital room. It was hoped that the sampling of patients in both groups would be large enough to minimize these variables." "There were 23 cases in the control group and 27 in the experimental."[1]

These excerpts can serve as bases for discussing various points about extraneous variables. The independent variable can be identified as the "availability of the nurse during visiting and for 30 minutes following departure of the parent . . . with care geared to give comfort." The dependent variable is "emotional comfort for the child and parent." The report does not indicate whether Godfrey had considered "age, sex, diagnosis, previous hospital experience, . . ." and others as potentially confounding variables during the planning. It would appear that she may have. She did handle them as accounted-for variables, in that she recorded information about them. She also attempted to control for them to some extent, in that she used a modified random sampling method for assigning patients to each group, but the procedure proved inadequate for controlling for some potentially confounding variables.

Controlled-for Variables

The controlled-for variables in the Godfrey study can be identified as age, day of hospitalization, and number of patients in the room. Others might have been gravity of prognosis, in relation to the dependent variable for the parents; and previous hospital experience, for the older children. It does seem that the 2- or 3-year-old child may display greater emotional distress at the departure of the parent than the 5-year-old; that number of children in the room could influence the child's manifestations of distress, and that the parent's distress may be greater in the early days of hospitalization and where the child suffers from a possibly fatal illness. On the other hand, in the age group 2 to 6, it would not be expected that sex or weight of the child would influence his expression of emotional distress at the time of the parent's departure. Nor would either of these variables be likely to influence the feelings of the parents. There would therefore be no need to record information nor to attempt to control for the sex or weight variables.

Potential Accounted-for Variables

There are other variables that might have been of interest: for example, the number of days the nurse had provided care for the child and the number of times she had talked to the parent, the number of siblings and sibling position, the child's previous experience with separation from parents, and the preparation the parents had given the child for the hospitalization. The list could be extended, but one of Godfrey's objectives was to determine whether an instructor could carry out a scientific investigation while carrying a full-time teaching load. Each additional variable for which information is collected requires additional time-consuming work: defining the variable, observing and recording the information, and organizing, analyzing, and interpreting the findings. Godfrey failed to substantiate her hypothesis, and it may well be that failure to control for some of the variables was the reason. Details about her findings need not be reported here; suffice it to display selected findings on two variables:

TABLE 1. *Number of Children in Two Study Groups by Day-of-Hospitalization and by Age* [*][†]

VARIABLES		CONTROL	EXPERIMENTAL
Age:	2 yr	7	9
	3 yr	4	10
	4 yr	6	5
	5 yr	6	3
Hospital day:	2	7	7
	4	4	10
	8	6	3

[*] This table does not appear in the quoted report, but was constructed by the writer from the data in the report. The groups arranged for this table serve to illustrate points about accounted-for and controlled-for variables.
[†] Totals differ because only children in each specified group by hospital day are included.

Controlling for Variables

The differences in numbers of patients in the two groups show that the variables, age and day-of-hospitalization, were not equally distributed in the control and experimental groups. This point becomes meaningful when viewed in the light of Godfrey's report that, where one of these variables *was* equally distributed between the control and experimental groups, the hypothesized relationship of the type of care to the children's manifestations of distress was substantiated. Specifically, it was demonstrated that, among the 2-year-old children, who were almost equally distributed between the two groups (7 in the control group and 9 in the experimental) those who received the experimental care displayed less distress than did the children who did not receive the care. The same held true when the variable day-of-hospitalization was controlled for: children who received experimental care on day 2 (equal numbers of controls and experimentals) manifested less distress than children who did not receive the experimental care. From these and other examinations of the findings, it may be stated that these variables were confounding variables, and outcomes might have been different had they been controlled for.

CONTROLLING FOR VARIABLES

There are four ways of controlling for potentially confounding variables: defining terms, random sampling, matching, and analysis of covariance.

The first of these, defining terms, is used particularly in making specific the characteristics of the subjects to be studied and the setting or environment in which the study will be conducted. Godfrey controlled for age to the degree that her subjects were specified as children between the ages of two and six years. In other words, she "defined out" children less than two and more than six. Also by definition, she eliminated the first hospital day and children who were not oriented. 1A, in her study of early ambulation in surgical patients, controlled for complications that could interfere with early ambulation by defining them out. Controlling for a variable by definition is usually through elimination of the variable from the population studied, or by eliminating specific degrees of the variable, such as Godfrey's specified age limits.

#1 Defining Terms

Random sampling of the population and/or random distribution of subjects between the control and experimental groups controls for a variable through distributing it equally in the two groups. It is then assumed that any influence the particular variable might have on the dependent variable will be the same in each group. This means, then, that if the two groups differ in the measurements of the dependent variable, that dif-

#2 Random Sampling

ference cannot be due to the influence of the controlled-for variable; the latter, through random distribution, is equally distributed and would have equal effect in each group. Godfrey had hoped that her modified random assignment of patients to each group would yield an equal distribution of the variable, age, between the two groups. But it turned out that the distribution of this variable was different in the two groups. A more precise plan of randomization, including stratification or a sufficiently large sample, might have effected equal distribution. But truly random selection requires that a total sample be selected at one time and that the stratified randomization into the control and experimental groups be done before any data collection is begun. This was obviously not possible for Godfrey within some of the limitations of her study. Also, "a sufficiently large" sample can be exceedingly large. In Godfrey's work, it might well have had to be two or three times the size she had.

#3 Matching

Matching subjects in the two groups is another way to assure equal distribution of one or more variables in each of the two groups. Some statisticians reject this as a valid procedure for assuring equal distribution. Even with matching, they say, there will be differences, and it is impossible to match for more than a very limited number of variables. Others, however, consider matching on some variables the only reasonable way to proceed. Indeed, most researchers would agree that it would have been entirely reasonable and not too difficult for Godfrey to have matched patients on from two to four of the potentially confounding variables: for instance, on number of patients in the room and on day of hospitalization. Nor would it have been overly difficult to have matched for age and previous hospitalization. Granted, such matching would have taken considerable planning and would probably have prolonged the study by many weeks. The fact remains, nonetheless, that these particular variables could reasonably have been controlled for through matching.

#4 Analysis of Covariance

Analysis of covariance is a statistical procedure that can be used to account for the degree of influence of unequal distributions of potentially confounding variables. It is the availability of this measure that leads some statisticians to object to matching. As stated above, they contend that, even with matching, there will be differences and that since the analysis of covariance permits determination of the degree of influence of the differences, it serves little purpose to match. Even those who do advocate matching warn against over-reliance on this procedure and propose that, where feasible, analysis of covariance should also be used.

The student is referred to statistics texts for procedures and discussions relating to analysis of covariance and to other statistical concepts mentioned in this book. The researcher is also advised to consult a statistician early in the planning for his research. The first consultation might be before the completion of Step 5 and not later than the completion of planning for Step 9.

Summary on Variables

Essentially, then, there are three categories of extraneous variables, with the controlled-for variables being those of greatest concern to the researcher. These potentially confounding variables may be controlled for in four ways: by eliminating them or their influence on outcomes for the sample population, through assuring equal distribution in both control and experimental groups. Eliminating their influence may be done by "defining them out." Equal distribution of them in the two groups may be accomplished (1) through random sampling of population and random assignment to group, and (2) through matching. The degree of their influence in the groups may be determined through analysis of covariance.

Criterion Measures

The student is again reminded that research deals with facts. The researcher achieves his stated purpose through collecting facts, accumulating quantities of individual observations of phenomena, and through thinking synthetically and analytically about them. The researcher who is testing a hypothesis will accumulate facts about his dependent variable (outcome or effects). Most dependent variables are not themselves observable or measurable: for example, Godfrey's dependent variable, "emotionally comfortable," which is not observable, or 1A's "early ambulatory activities."

Some might maintain, of course, that these variables, especially "early ambulatory activities," *are* observable. But facts, if they are to be usable in scientific investigation, must be so precisely identified that any knowledgeable person would make the same measurement (observation) and report of any single representative phenomenon that any other knowledgeable person would make of the same phenomenon. These concepts will be elaborated in Step 5; they are introduced here only to explain the "nonobservability" and as a reminder of the need for precision in defining terms.

There is particular concern for defining the dependent variable, since criterion measures are identified in its definition. Both Godfrey and 1A had to define their dependent variables in terms that would identify the phenomena to be observed as examples of manifestations of the variable or some aspect of it. The examples of manifestations, of course, had to be attributes of the dependent variable relevant to the particular concern of the study and ones that would appropriately be selected as criterion measures. Each investigator ascribed a measurement for each phenomenon identified, with the view that the measurements would yield scores in the generalized concept of her dependent variable.

Criterion measures are identified in the pertinent general phase of the definition of terms, wherein the specific qualities, attributes, or characteristics of the dependent variable relevant to the interest of the investigator are identified. The nature of the measurements to be made are identified in the for-instance phase of the definition. This is where the specific nature of the rule, test, or scale as a whole, and of single units or items on the scale or test, will be identified, implicitly or explicitly.

Step 3: Definitions of Terms

For-Instances and Scale of Measurement

The for-instances will identify the nature of a single observation or measurement of any specific quality, attribute, or characteristic. The nature of the instrument of measurement (test, rule, or scale) will be specifically identified, or its identity may be inferred from the nature of the individual observations cited in the for-instances as representative of the measurements to be made. An example of identification of the instrument is the previous definition of the dependent variable, temperature (pages 103 through 104). There, the pertinent general identified precisely the attribute or quality of temperature to be observed. A for-instance was reported as 97.2° Fahrenheit, indicating a single measurement (observation of a single occurrence of the phenomenon), and identifying explicitly the Fahrenheit scale as the one to be used. In the example on "communicates," among criterion measures selected as pertinent to the interest of the investigator were: talking to patient, family members, and co-workers; giving instructions; writing reports. In the for-instances, individual observations (measurements) were identified in: (1) Told Mr. Jones to go to X-ray, and (2) Noted on Mrs. B's chart. . . . In this latter example, the nature of the measuring instrument is not made explicit, but it may be inferred that it will not be a scaling device. Rather, the "measurements" will be observations reported as descriptions of individual instances or occurrences of a characteristic of the variable. The score that any particular observation or "measurement" would yield may be inferred to be a frequency count of one. (These concepts will be further elaborated in Step 5.)

Where the dependent variable is a phenomenon of multifarious attributes, multiple criterion measures will be needed, and the pertinent general phase of the definition may be rather extensive. Among those particularly illustrative for nurses are such variables as infection, anxiety, and security. The latter is illustrated in the definition included in example 3B, pages 125 through 126.

Criterion Measures Variously Defined

The definition of criterion measure used here differs from that suggested by others who sometimes use it interchangeably with dependent variable. Some propose that *the* criterion measure is the dependent variable; others that the dependent variable is *the* criterion measure; some maintain both at the same time. Still others propose that a criterion measure is a score in the dependent variable. It seems illogical to equate a criterion measure directly with the dependent variable, since more than one criterion measure is usually identified for any one dependent variable. And, since few phenomena identified as dependent variables are directly observable (measurable), it seems equally illogical to define criterion measure as a score. Because of differences in perceptions of this concept so fundamental to the research process, the student is encouraged to examine the various discussions of the subject and to develop his own conceptualization of the various entities purported to describe and identify the nature of a criterion measure.

The conception of criterion measure presented here will become clearer with discussion of Step 5. Also in Step 5 (page 145), the criterion measures identified by Godfrey, along with the particular scores ascribed, are described. Another example of criterion measures is 1A's. She identified deep-breathing, coughing, turning, sitting out-of-bed, and walking as criterion measures of postoperative ambulatory activities. She used the frequency count, scoring one point for each time a patient was observed performing any one of the activities, as the measures (scores) of the phenomena.

An operational definition uses observable processes, actions, or structural analogues (or explicit and detailed word descriptions of them) to describe concepts represented by the term being defined. It is an explicit description of a single entity or phenomenon considered to be a concrete referent of the term being defined, whether the referent be an object, a process, or an action. And it specifically identifies a single entity or phenomenon to be measured to provide one component of a score of the variable or characteristic being measured and evaluated. The definition of operational definition may seem very involved, but once the elements composing it are clarified by explanation and illustration, it becomes evident that it is merely succinct and is really expressed in concrete terms. An operational definition is composed of two distinct elements: (1) a generalization in more or less abstract terms and (2) one or more for-instances in concrete terms, describing a process or behavior that can be observed. Essentially, an operational definition is similar to the proposed three-part definition to be used for defining terms, except that, where used in a general context and not specifically to define terms for scientific investigation, the pertinent general phase, which identifies a particular interest, would be replaced by a description of a general nature.

Operational Definition

For example, in the earlier definition of "communicates" the pertinent general would not identify the persons involved nor particular messages communicated. Rather, types of communication in general (writing, talking, gestures, signals), and types of messages (information, expressions of feelings or attitudes, commands) would be identified. An operational definition is generally used where a phenomenon is of such abstract and complex nature that detailed description, including analogues to it or actual, concrete, observable entities and phenomena are needed to identify it. This extensive description is needed if all persons hearing or reading the term are to attain a similar perception of the phenomenon.

Operational definition, however, can also serve a wider purpose. It is suggested here that researchers use the concept and process of operational definition to describe many terms that will be employed in particular connotations in their investigations. In so doing, they will identify not only concrete entities and observable phenomena in general, but will extend

Another Purpose

the definitions to identify pertinent general entities and phenomena. That is, they will identify elements of their particular interest and include for-instances of individual entities or phenomena that are examples of the phenomena of their specific concern.

Complete Opposites in Operational Definitions

There are two types of operational definitions that seem to be complete opposites: (1) the definition that uses concrete, observable phenomena to describe an abstract concept; and (2) the definition that uses ideational, nonobservable conceptualizations to identify observable phenomena. Both contribute considerably to understanding of the phenomena being defined and permit communication not otherwise possible. An example of the first type is shown in definitions of the word "gyroscope." About the only definition that could be expected to convey an understanding of the concept of the gyroscope would be an operational definition. A model of a gyroscope must be displayed and its functioning demonstrated in order to communicate a concept that would be commonly understood. Here the operational definition uses specific acts or processes to make an abstract concept understandable.

The second type of operational definition may be thought of as "something that works." When the definition is used in this context, its construction is essentially the reverse of the one just described. An example of the second type of operational definition is Freud's conceptualizations of ego, id, and superego. Here abstractions are used to explain observable processes and behaviors.

Interpretation, Misinterpretation, and Condemnation

It was in relation to a problem in electrodynamics involving the attempted definition of an atom that Percy W. Bridgman coined the term "operational definition." But scientists have attacked Bridgman's concept, maintaining that it is not workable. Actually, Bridgman proposed the term only to identify an idea he had hit on as he was preparing two advanced courses in electrodynamics. He discovered that he could visualize the concepts and present them to his students by describing the way electrons, protons, and other particles behaved in relation to one another and to the whole; that is, how elements of an atom worked (operated). This he referred to as explaining the nature of the atom operationally or by operational definition. That is all he meant. But the objectors protest that the definition of the nature of an atom cannot be so simple. It is not merely the acting and interacting of particles. The matters of time, space, velocity, contiguity, and many others must be taken into account. And they add that there is no way of identifying space between particles. The very act of attempting to measure the space causes the particles to move, and the space is never the same for any two instants in time. Therefore, the argument runs, the concept of an operational definition of an atom is an anomaly, and scientists should throw it out. Bridgman was willing to do so, since others had blown up the concept way beyond his limited intent.* Yet, the others did not throw it out. Instead, they have applied to it the term "operationalism"; they have modified it; and they continue to explain why and how it cannot work!

Such protests suggest that the terms "process definition" or "for-instance definition" be used to refer to a definition that makes a concept explicit through describing an example of how the referent works or performing an operation to demonstrate how the referent works, as in the instance of defining a gyroscope. On the other hand, despite the protests, it seems reasonable to retain the term "operational definition" and to use it as Bridgman envisioned its use. And that's what will be done in this text. The concept of operational definition, like that of criterion measure, will become clearer through the discussions of definition of terms and identification of data needed.

In summary, definitions of newly introduced terms, of whose concepts there must be common understanding in order to understand and use ideas appertaining to the process and rationale of defining terms for a study, have been elaborated.

DEFINING TERMS

The general concept of word definition calls for arbitrarily imposed descriptions that allow common understanding. Usually, to determine the definition of a *word*, one looks it up in a dictionary. In this book, though, the concern is with definitions of *terms*, but the concept of definition as an arbitrarily imposed description remains the same. There is a distinction, however, in the means for determining the description to be imposed. Although, even in defining terms, the researcher will do well to begin with the dictionary definition, he should then go on to impose and elaborate his own specific meaning for the term as it will be used in his study.

Word, Term

For instance, if a person were to look up the *word* "nurse" in the dictionary, he would find it to mean a great many things and to serve as a noun, adjective, and verb (active and passive). There are many contexts for each, ranging from suckling or feeding a child, to a worker ant, to conserving a highball. Yet this remains a commonly understood word.

*The Word: Nurse
The Term: Nurse*

---

* The student may be interested in reading one of the discussions about the concept: in particular, Bridgman's witty response to excited protestors who refused to understand or accept his simple concept: *The Validation of Scientific Theories*, Philipp G. Frank, ed. (New York, Science Library, Collier Books, 1961), pp. 45 to 83.

Regardless of the context in which it may be used, most readers would understand its meaning as intended and would not ask for further definition. On the other hand, for a particular study, an investigator might define the *term* "nurse" to mean: a man currently registered in any state in the United States to practice professional nursing and who has been registered for at least one year and not more than ten years, and who is working full-time as a registered nurse in an accredited general hospital. This arbitrary description markedly limits the meaning of the term "nurse" and eliminates most of the generally accepted descriptions of the meaning of the word. It makes specific the meaning it will have in the particular investigation.

"Right" to Define Terms— Better It Were a Privilege

The researcher has the right to ascribe any meaning he wishes to the terms he chooses to use. It might be better, however, if researchers viewed this as a privilege, rather than as a right. This would lead them to adhere more closely to generally understood meanings of the words and thus enhance their communications. Otherwise, they insist, in essence, that all readers adapt to *their* thinking and shift their own concepts each time they encounter particular terms in reading the research report. A fictitious example illustrates this point. For a study concerned with patients' failure to follow doctors' orders, the investigator defined the term "blind" to mean "any protest against following the physician's orders: whether overt, such as saying that he will not do his exercises, or covert, such as failing to have a prescription filled." Such a definition may reveal much about the investigator's feeling about patients who do not follow the doctor's orders. But it also requires a reader to adjust his thinking about the meaning of the word "blind" each time he encounters it in the research report. This fictitious example is not absurdly extreme; definitions of equal absurdity can be found in the literature. Fortunately, most investigators use their right with greater discretion. And, indeed, the right must be preserved.

To preclude esoteric definitions of terms, the investigator should start with the dictionary definition that most closely describes the meaning of the word as he will use it. He should then follow this with the specifics that will describe the meaning of the term as it will be used in the study.

Definitions of Terms From Definition of Problem

It is when he starts to plan Step 3, Definitions of Terms, that the student will first become aware of the usefulness of the work done in defining the problem (Step 1). If the problem has been thoroughly defined, then the meanings of most of the terms needing specific definition for the study will already have been described. For example, as 1A defined her problem, she described in detail the meaning of "early postoperative ambulation." She discussed the meaning of this treatment in relation to the anatomical structures and physiological processes involved, both in terms of the surgery and in terms of the ambulatory activities. When she came to defining the term, in Step 3, she had only to go to the dictionary to find the meaning of ambulation in its broadest, generally understood sense. She then turned to her definition of problem to identify the generally understood meaning of early postoperative ambulation. There she also found the for-instances to serve as the specifics for describing the meaning of the term precisely as it would be used in her study. The specifics would ensure that all who read the term in her report would know exactly what was meant.

Even though a thoroughly defined problem can provide immeasurable help, defining the terms can still be a time-consuming task. In research, the meaning of terms must stem from the problem of concern: they must be relevant. Nonetheless, the researcher can frequently save much time, and yet have a definition that will serve his purpose, by using a definition devised by others concerned with elements of the same problem or one similar to his. A fine example of the value of this procedure may be found in *Uninterrupted Patient Care and Nursing Requirements,* a study planned and conducted by a faculty group.[2] One term that had to be defined was "chronically ill." To define this would not be easy even for a single individual; for a group of nurses to agree on a definition of chronically ill would be virtually impossible. Fortunately for the progress of the study, the Commission on Chronic Illness had previously published: *Care of the Long-Term Patient, Volume II.*[3] This contained a definition that was the consensus of a group of people respected for their knowledge of the chronically ill. Although some of the faculty did not like parts of the definition, it was decided that no amount of trying would yield anything better—or, at least, anything more acceptable to every individual in the planning group. This is one purpose that can be served by using definitions developed by others.

Terms Defined By Others

Definitions developed by others can be helpful, too, in definitions of abstract terms, of those with vague, diffuse meanings, and of those terms that are very commonly used but rarely defined succinctly and precisely: attitude, anxiety, confidence, nursing, for instance. For such terms the same three-part process of definition as described on page 102 should be followed: dictionary definition, pertinent general definition, and for-instance definition. After introducing the dictionary definition, the investigator should examine how he used the term in the problem-defined. This examination may well lead to definitions that have been developed by others. Several would probably have been gleaned during the review of the literature and used to elaborate the problem-defined. Although definitions need not be presented in full in the definition of problem, reference should be made to them, and the sources should be listed in the researcher's bibliography.

Not all definitions from others will serve without modification. The definition must be pertinent to specifics of the problem to be studied. For example, one nurse investigator may be concerned with a problem of nursing care of geriatric patients and another with a problem of nursing care of premature infants. Both might have drawn from Henderson's "Nature of Nursing," in describing the various elements of their problems and in developing their definitions of the term "nursing care."[4] Yet, for a complete definition, each will have to draw from additional sources for the specifics that will make the definition pertinent to and usable in her particular investigation. In short, there is value in using definitions developed by others, but such definitions must meet the test of pertinence to the problem being studied.

Influence on Step 13: Recommendations

One further illustration may be given of the importance of definitions of terms and the value of adhering closely to the commonly understood meaning of the word. There have been numerous and often extensive studies of nurses' attitudes. Many have been concerned with attitudes of nurses toward direct care of patients, and most of these have used nursing students as subjects of study. Some have limited their work to developing measurements of the attitudes; others have attempted to measure changes in attitude. Almost all have limited their concerns to a single facet of the dual-faceted concept of attitude. They have attempted to measure postures, but have not extended their studies to consider the influence of the posture on consequent action taken by the individual. Their discussions of the concept, attitude, usually indicate their awareness of its dual-faceted nature. Most include the concepts of the physical as well as the psychological posture and the relationship of either or both to a consequent action. But then, in an effort to limit the scope of their studies, these investigators choose to define attitude by describing only the posture aspect of the concept. Either they do not refer to the consequent action, or they make explicit that the consequent action has no part in their study. This marked narrowing of a generally understood and broad meaning of the term illustrates, of course, the delimiting function of defining terms; this was undoubtedly the aim of the researchers who have used the limited definition. But the limitation they wished to establish, for the scope of their studies, could have been accomplished through an explanatory, limit-setting statement. The limitation thus made explicit would not have resulted in the imposition of serious limitations on other aspects of the study. The limitation imposed by the explanatory statement suggested above would be less than the limitation implicit in not mentioning consequent action in the definition used.

Attitude is most frequently and commonly defined to mean the composite or total complex of [a nurse's] feelings, ideas, interest in, and concern about direct care of patients. But when limitations such as those described above are imposed on this generally understood meaning, the unfortunate result is often a restricted list of recommendations presented as outcomes of the studies. This list predominantly includes proposals for further applications of the tools developed for measuring the posture aspect of nurses' attitudes toward direct care of patients. Among these may be recommendations for further testing of the tools, for possible adaptations of the tools for use with other populations, and—occasionally—for development of another tool: one that might be used to measure nurses' overt behaviors as they give direct care to patients. The new tool would be used concomitantly with the attitude measure in an effort to determine relationships between the attitudes as measured and the behaviors as measured. Such a recommendation does suggest thinking beyond the immediate limited studies reported. But the potential for recommendations would have been much greater had vision not been curtailed by the limited definition of attitude. Recommendations could have been extended to proposed studies of the relationships of nursing care behaviors to attitudes; they would not have stopped with the recommendation that an instrument be devised to measure the behaviors. And, without the limitations, there could be proposals about outcomes—in terms of patient progress and/or of nursing care behaviors related to identified attitudes. Many of the studies have potential as bases for further and exciting research, but the possibilities have not been envisioned. This lack of imaginative proposal may well have been due, in large part, to the limits imposed by a too-limiting definition of a term.

Many of the attitude studies referred to above have been good and valuable ones in many respects; this makes the limitations discussed all the more lamentable. The student interested in attitudes should read several of these studies as his first step in exploring the literature in the area. Among other things, he will learn a great deal about how to develop a definition of the term "attitude," and he will also learn of the extensive task involved in developing an instrument for measuring attitudes.

TERMS THAT MUST BE DEFINED

There will probably be more "terms that must be defined" in the planning stages of the design than appear under the special heading in the eventual research report. This is because many of the terms that must be defined in order to proceed with later steps in planning the design can be included as part of the narrative in either a completed design or the report of the research. In Godfrey's report, for instance, the only terms included in the section, "Definition of Terms," are "a week" and "child situation." Yet other sections of the report make explicit the meanings of many additional terms.

To identify terms that must be defined, the student should look first

In Design, In Report

to his statement of purpose. This must delineate the phenomena about which information will be sought, the subjects to be studied, and, usually, the setting. The statement of purpose identifies these entities in general terms. The definition of terms, however, makes each one specific and pertinent to the particular investigation.

Dependent Variable

When the purpose of the investigation is to test a hypothesis, the first term to be considered is the dependent variable. Where the purpose is to explore and describe, the terms that identify the phenomena about which information will be sought should be defined first. In the real world of beginning researchers, though, this latter practice is seldom observed. These phenomena are usually expressed in the most abstract terms, so the student delays the "hard" (difficult, solid, concrete) thinking required to define them until the very last. Some delay it until Step 5, and some until Step 8, Tools, which is the very last point since no work can be done here until the dependent variable has been explicitly defined. Some students view the definition of the dependent variable as the identification of it—possibly because they feel they have accomplished a great deal when they have done even that. Which, indeed, is true. But mere identification of the variable is not sufficient. The description of its meaning has to be so elaborate and so clear that, should two persons knowledgeable in the field read the definition and then observe the occurrence of a phenomenon fitting the description, each would identify the phenomenon as illustrative of the dependent variable. This explicitness can be assured by following the suggestions for developing a three-part definition. (1) Delineate the dictionary definition that most closely describes the meaning intended and pertinent to the proposed investigation. (2) Review the definition of problem to identify the generally understood meaning of the term (pertinent general definition) as it is used in the context of the problem under study. (3) Excerpt for-instances from the definition of problem: that is, specific observed behaviors or objects that illustrate the meaning of the term as it will be used in the study.

Independent Variable

The second term, or category of terms, to be defined is the independent variable, using the same process of definition as described for the dependent variable. Here, the question may arise—perhaps more frequently than in relation to the definition of other terms—as to how much detail to include. Once the definition is begun and for-instances identified, there may be a tendency to describe the independent variable in detail and to include its introduction to the experimental group. This should not be done at Step 3, although the definition should be sufficiently detailed that all will understand its specific meaning, the concrete referent. An adequate definition may be accomplished with illustrative for-instances; it need not include all specifics inherent in the concept.

Terms That Must Be Defined

For example, 1A defined her independent variable, preoperative teaching, as "a brief, informative, and factual discussion to inform the patient about postoperative ambulatory behaviors that would be expected of him; the content includes (1) definitive information about activities, such as coughing deeply, turning in bed, and walking; (2) the value of, and reasons and methods for performing the various activities; (3) discussion of the potential of pain and that medications would be given for relief of pain; and (4) assisting to practice the activities as they would be doing them after their surgery." (An outline of the plan for doing the teaching was developed as part of Step 9.) The definition provided sufficient detail and specifics for anyone knowledgeable in the field to fully understand the meaning of the term "planned preoperative instructions about early ambulation." The definition was all that was needed in Step 3 to permit planning subsequent steps.

Example 1A

Actually, the student need not be concerned about the sequence of defining terms. He needs only to identify all the terms that must be defined and proceed in any sequence that occurs to him. The reason for suggesting that the dependent variable be defined first, then the independent variable, is that it may help the student to avoid avoiding the hard work. This is comparable to the advice that he resist quick answers and early closure in defining the problem. Students can expend quantities of time and energy defining innumerable terms of secondary importance, many of which do not really need to be defined. But time is spent; work is done; there are pages of print to show for it—yet the dependent variable has yet to be defined! At this point the student is likely to explain to his teacher that he has struck a snag and cannot seem to move on with his planning. A query about the definition of the dependent variable will elicit various stammering sounds. Nonetheless, even in this there is good: from this point there is a starting place. There is but one starting place, and there is but one direction to go: the definition of terms must be completed. The student can no longer avoid defining the dependent variable; the hard work that was avoided by engagement in only slightly less hard work must now be tackled. The student who disciplines himself to define the dependent variable first finds the other definitions easier to do. In addition, he does not need, in his effort to avoid the hard work, to spend time in lengthy definitions of terms not requiring such specific identification in the investigation, or for which very simple definitions will serve.

Avoid Avoiding the Hard Work

For the definition of the population, a good place to start is the real life population of the student's early observations. But the entire definition of problem should also be reviewed, since the extended description of the problem may identify implications for a much larger population than the one represented by the individuals in the early observations. Or a decision

Population

may have been made that the problem may be better studied in relation to subjects of another population. Indeed, the final firm definition of the population to be studied should wait until the conclusion of Step 6. When the data to be collected have been precisely identified, the population can be specifically defined in relation to the potential sources of the data.

Criterion Measures of the Dependent Variable

While the investigator is defining his dependent variable, he will be identifying some criterion measures. They will be expressed in the pertinent general phase of that definition. Sometimes, the for-instances are at a level of concreteness where further definition is unnecessary. If the for-instances are not expressed so as to describe clearly individual observable phenomena representative of specific criterion measures, then these terms will have to be defined. For example, 1A's definition of early ambulation was: "a program of exercises, such as coughing deeply, turning in bed, and walking, which is started within twenty-four hours after surgery." She then had to define each criterion separately. This will be made more explicit in Step 5.

Personnel

Frequently, the individuals who will introduce the independent variable and other personnel involved in the investigation must be defined. This means that the investigator must make decisions about what to include and to omit. Over and above the categories of terms already noted as needing definition, the investigator should define such terms as he deems necessary in order to communicate clearly with others about his study. Clarifications sought by others may help him in this task. The fact that others ask to have a term defined or explained should alert the investigator to the possible need to define the term as a part of his plan.

Discuss Plan Any Time and Every Time Anyone Can Be Cornered

Anyone planning a research design should talk about it to anyone who will talk to him and every time he will talk to him. Of course, he would stop short of the point at which persons start avoiding him or suggest that they will be happy to see him after he gets the thing out of his system! Seriously, planning research should not be a solo project; an investigator needs ideas and leads from others. The need for formal consultation from persons in other disciplines whose special knowledges are needed is generally recognized, but much can be accomplished in discussion with the nonexpert who is merely interested.

Variables in Exploratory Descriptive Study

Where the statement of purpose is not a hypothesis, the same pattern of definition of terms must be followed. The particular phenomena about which information is to be sought are usually identified, in the statement of purpose, in general terms: frequently in terms of a high level of abstraction. For these terms, the three-part definition is appropriate, beginning with the relevant dictionary definition. Pertinent qualities, attributes, or characteristics (criterion measures) of the phenomena will be identified in a pertinent general phase of the definition. The definition will be completed by excerpting for-instances from the definition of problem that will describe individual observable phenomena, processes or objects, that illustrate the exact meaning the investigator has in mind for each particular term. Examples 2F through 2L, in Step 2, are illustrations. Thus, Examples 2F and 2G included for-instances in the statement of purpose. In each case, the definitions of these terms that would include description of observable phenomena would be comparatively simple. The identification of the specific categories of observations had already been done in Step 2. Example 2I, as well as 2J and 2K, is one where the investigator couched the identity of the areas about which she would seek information in quite abstract terms. She wished to determine whether "foot or palm prints of newborn infants are valid and usable and the extent to which they are actually used and for what purposes." The last two areas are less abstract than the first two. The investigator had to make explicit her meanings of the terms, valid and usable, in relation to her particular problem.

The investigator planning a descriptive study must also define terms that identify the subjects to be studied and the setting of the study. Just as in a study to test hypotheses, it is frequently desirable to make explicit the personnel to be involved. As the use to which these definitions are put is described in the discussion of later steps of the research design, their value and the rationale for doing them will become clear.

Essentially, the three-part definition is applicable for defining terms that identify phenomena that may have quite different referents in different contexts. For example, observable attributes for nursing care, as described above, would be rather different in the context of care for geriatric patients and the care for premature infants, even though the underlying philosophy and the general concept of nursing care would be the same. The student, however, must not be carried away by the concept to the point of, for example, defining the term, preschool-aged child, by developing the three-part definition for each element of the term, including "pre," and then combining them into a final description of the term as he will use it. The definition of such a term can be rather directly lifted from the definition of the problem. It will express the intent of the investigator, with concrete attributes of particular age in months and years which the investigator intends to be the boundaries of preschool age. His definition may include other attributes to make it a comprehensive description of his subject, such as wellness or illness, sex, sibling sequence, and others.

Don't Gnaw a Clean Bone

The device of the three-part definition should be used wherever it will enhance thinking and clarify description of the terms. The previous discussion of definition of criterion measures should assist the student in making judgments about terms that need the detailed three-part definition. Where his concern is with a variable on which subjects are to be compared, and the variable possesses multifarious attributes to be observed and measured, the three-part definition will ensure a description that will promote common understanding. When the variable is a concrete phenomenon for which commonly understood measurements such as age and weight have been established, a less complex definition lifted from the definition of problem will serve. The three-part definition should not be used where it leads to oversimplification: to gnawing a clean bone.

Narrative of Steps Versus Narrative of Design and Report

Written materials developed in the process of accomplishing the definitions, as a separate step, will differ from the narrative of the research design and of the report of the study. This means that there are distinctions between the format used for writing the steps and the format used for the design. For example, the design begins with a brief introduction that describes the essence of the complete plan for the study. The writing of the steps begins with the real, live story that is illustrative of the nature of the problem of concern. In the design, some terms may be made explicit in the running narrative without being listed under the heading "definitions of terms." But in the written steps, all terms that must be defined to make explicit their pertinence to the study will appear in the section so marked. This does not mean, though, that after the steps have been written, the investigator must then start from scratch to write the narrative of the design. In writing the design, he will lift, without change, most of what has been written in the plans of the steps and he will place the various units of planning in proper sequence in the design. The rationale for the two writings lies in the fact that the various individual steps of a design are not completely separate, independent entities in the outcome sought through the planning. Yet they can be identified as separate entities to facilitate development during the early planning.

The Recipe, The Ingredients, The Mixing

An analogy might be the relationship of the ingredients of any recipe to the product sought in collecting and mixing the ingredients. In order to have an edible cake, the chef carefully identifies each ingredient and mixes it into the batter in a specified sequence. Essentially, planning and writing the steps is the identification and preparation of each ingredient in turn. The writing of the design is the mixing of the ingredients. The completed design is the cake, whose quality will reflect the care with which the ingredients were identified and the skill with which they were prepared and mixed.

Example: 3A Vague, Unusable Definition

Some examples of varying degrees of completeness and usefulness may help the student visualize concepts about the adequacy of definitions. For instance, "Anxiety refers to a series of acts or operations which are the manifest results of a series of conditions," is an unusable definition. Although anxiety is a frequently used word and means many things to many people, this definition would hardly provide people with a commonly understood meaning nor identify precisely the meaning the investigator has in mind for the term as it is to be used in his study. It does not identify or describe attributes or characteristics (criterion measures), nor does it describe an illustrative manifestation (a for-instance). Actually, this definition could serve as well to describe the meaning of joy.

EXAMPLE 3B

To illustrate a definition of the term designating a dependent variable that will serve as a firm base from which to develop later planning, Example 3B is quoted directly from a design developed by a masters student.[5]

Statement of Focus (Hypothesis)

Children who receive care from nurses who are assisted to know the development of a child's concepts of death and to understand the dying child's ways of communicating his sense of dying are supported to a greater degree than those who are cared for by nurses not so assisted.

Supported, according to Webster, is "having courage, feeling confident, receiving help when needed, experiencing comfort, strength, and approval, being provided for, and sustained." A child who is supported will feel loved and understood. He will have courage and confidence in facing new and trying situations. He will feel secure, safe, and protected, because he knows the nurses and his parents are concerned about his welfare. He knows he is "cared for." *Definition of Dependent Variable "Supported"*

When a child is supported he will feel free to express, either verbally or through play, his fears and concerns about both his hospital experience in general and particular painful situations. Also through reassurance from someone he trusts, he will be less fearful, less anxious, will rest more comfortably, and worry less frequently. Support will aid in dispelling his doubts and apprehensions because he knows he has someone he can trust to answer his questions truthfully and informatively.

A child who is supported can depend on someone to recognize his needs and meet these needs consistently. For example, he will know what to expect in relation to treatments and procedures because he will receive explanations in terms he can understand. He will not have to face the unknown entirely in the dark.

The supported child will not feel as lonely and isolated as one who is not supported because he can count on having "his nurse" with him when he needs her. Even if it entails just sitting beside him, holding him, telling him his favorite stories, or playing with him. He can expect this warm personal contact at times when he is especially in need of it. For example, after his parents leave, and before bedtime when fear of the darkness is most apt to occur. He knows his nurse will look in on him frequently to see if he needs anything, without his having to call her each time.

He senses the relationship between his parents and the nursing staff and knows they trust and respect each other. He will have a positive outlook toward his illness, and knows he will receive assistance in setting realistic goals for himself. He feels independent because he is encouraged to carry out certain aspects of his care and is praised when he is successful. Also, he knows his behavior will be accepted. For example, when he is irritable and demanding due to pain and discomfort, he can expect his nurse to understand. He will develop new interests which will help in averting feelings of hopelessness and preoccupation with his illness. For example, he will be included in social activities occurring on the ward when his condition permits. A child who turns to his religion for assistance in coping with his fears, knows his nurse will understand this and assist him, for example, in saying his night prayers with him.

Examples 3A and 3B illustrate two extremes of explicitness of descriptions of observable processes or objects that portray the meanings of terms as they are envisioned by the researchers in relation to their pertinence for the proposed investigations. The detail to which the investigator in Example 3B thought through her definition of a term and the value of the work will be illustrated further in the discussion of Step 5.

REFERENCES

1. Godfrey, A. E. A study of nursing care designed to assist hospitalized children and their parents in their separation. Nurs. Res., 4:52, 1955.
2. Wandelt, M. A. Uninterrupted Patient Care and Nursing Requirements. Detroit, College of Nursing, Wayne State University, 1963, p. 2.
3. Commission on Chronic Illness. Care of the Long-Term Patient. Cambridge, Mass., Harvard University Press, 1956, Vol. 2, p. 5.
4. Henderson, V. The nature of nursing, Amer. J. Nurs., 64:8, pp. 62-66.
5. Murphy, H. M. Greater support of the dying child. Unpublished research design, Detroit, College of Nursing, Wayne State University, 1967.

STEP 4
ASSUMPTIONS

TERM DEFINED

Assumption: An assumption is a statement describing a phenomenon or condition that is accepted as being true on the basis of logic and reason.

The reason for accepting the conditions as true on the basis of logic and reason is so that the investigator may get on with the study he wishes to do, without having to stop to demonstrate that the stated conditions are indeed as logic or reason would lead knowledgeable people to believe them to be.

STATING ASSUMPTIONS

Step 4, in contrast to other steps, has no one best place in the sequence of steps. The investigator may identify assumptions that must be made explicit as he plans the statement of purpose, or he may identify some as he works through Step 5; he may even delineate some assumptions as late as Step 13. Regardless of when the assumptions are stated, they will be part of the planning from the time that the statement of purpose is finally established. On the other hand, they may not be made explicit at any time during the planning.

Most Assumptions Left Implicit

If scientific inquiry has more of one single ingredient than of any others, that ingredient is assumptions. All planning, all doing, and all analyses of findings are carried forward on an undergirding of assumptions. Most assumptions are accepted as self-evident. If questioned at all, they will be recognized as inherent in the performance of the many tasks of the researcher, and they will be accepted without request that they be made explicit. Most assumptions are allowed to remain implicit; they are not even identified, let alone described precisely or provided with rationale for their acceptance.

Explicit Assumptions

Few assumptions must be made explicit in any study; for many studies, none is needed. In determining assumptions that must be made explicit, the student should be guided by the same rule-of-thumb proposed in relation to determining the terms that need to be defined: that is, he should be alert to questions posed by persons with whom he discusses his planning. He should take note when such questions as "What do you plan to do about . . . ?" "How will you account for . . . ?" "On what basis will you . . . ?" are asked. When the questions do not refer to specific observable phenomena that he has already described or plans to describe, the investigator should ask himself whether he needs to account for his planning on the basis of an assumption. Does he need to state that he will accept a particular condition as being true—not because it has been demonstrated to be true, but because it is logical that it be true? Following are examples of assumptions pertinent to particular studies.

Examples: Implicit

1. Students will be willing to write the process recordings.
2. The patients will have pain following surgery.

Little information about these studies is needed to indicate that these assumptions need not be made explicit. The first one might apply to Godfrey's study. She was an instructor in pediatric nursing when she conducted her study; she planned to and did have her students provide nursing care for the study subjects and write process recordings of the episodes. "Anybody knows" that students would be willing to do the process recordings if requested to do so by their instructor—or at least that they *would do so*. Godfrey did not need to make this assumption explicit in order to move forward with planning her study. In the second instance, the study involved a test of the effectiveness of certain nursing measures in relieving patients of pain following major amputations. Planning could move forward without having to state the assumption; all would accept on the basis of reason that the patients would have pain.

Example: Explicit

3. Seniors in nursing education programs are able to recognize manifestations in patient behavior that are indicative of anxiety.

This, in contrast, is an assumption that needed to be made explicit. The investigator wished to secure information about anxiety in patients.

Stating Assumptions

She planned to have nursing students record observations of patients, and she did not wish to take the time to have the students demonstrate that they could correctly interpret various behaviors of patients as being manifestations of anxiety. It will be noted that the assumption includes the specification, "senior" students. Had the statement indicated "students," it might not have been acceptable as a valid assumption, since reason would indicate that freshman students would probably not be capable of such interpretation. Hence, the need for the investigator to state the assumption and to do so precisely.

Validity

The assumption just discussed suggests some of the considerations involved in deciding whether to state the assumptions or to leave them implicit. Although most assumptions may be left implicit, there is some value in recording them. The mere process of writing them down stimulates thinking about them and it sometimes leads the investigator to recognize that one or more of the assumptions is of questionable validity. If the stating of the assumptions does not result in recognition of questionable validity *a priori*, it may serve to test process and planning of the investigation *a posteriori*. If the study fails to substantiate the hypothesis, the investigator should first look to his assumptions for an explanation. His question should be: Was failure to substantiate the hypothesis due to proceeding on the basis of invalid assumptions? The answer to the question will not always explain the failure to substantiate the hypothesis, but the question should always be asked.

Assumptions Not Accepted on Whim

The investigator himself has the final responsibility for deciding on the assumptions that he will accept as being true and on whose bases he will proceed with his study. He will do well, however, to seek advice from persons knowledgeable in the field concerning the potential validity of the assumptions he wishes to accept. The decision to accept an assumption should not be arbitrary, unfounded, nor weakly based in logic and reason.

Test Validity?

An occasional investigator will include among the aims of his study that of testing the validity of particular assumptions. Many assumptions have all of the characteristics and outward appearance of hypotheses to be tested; the only distinguishing factor is that the investigator stating them has declared them to be assumptions. By so designating them in his study, the investigator implies that he accepts the conditions described as true, so that he may proceed to test his hypothesis. It then seems illogical for him to state that one aim of the investigation is to validate the assumptions. This is not to say that the condition described in an assumption may never be tested through research; many are subjected to such study. But when one is, its delineation becomes the statement of purpose for a study; it no longer can be called an assumption; it no longer is being accepted as true on the basis of logic or reason.

Nor should these comments be construed to indicate that findings from a study do not sometimes serve to confirm validity of an assumption. On the contrary, in some studies the findings of greatest importance turn out to be those that support the validity of one or more assumptions basic to the study. But in these instances, such an outcome is a happy coincidence, rather than the outcome resulting from the pursuit of a specified aim of the study. The investigator is sensitive to the potential for this outcome whenever he states assumptions, and he examines his findings in search of it. But since specified aim implies directed focus for the total planning for the study, and assumption implies acceptance without search for evidence, validation of assumptions as an outcome would not be a specified aim. These considerations provide one more example of the need for precision in the use of all words as studies expected to qualify as scientific inquiry are planned, executed, and reported.

Assumptions That Allow Planning

Two kinds of assumptions are appropriate considerations in any scientific study, but these are not appropriately listed in the major subsection titled Assumptions. One such type of assumption includes those made to enable the investigator to move on with the *planning* of the study. The investigator will assume that a sample population will be available for study; he may assume that he will receive permission to conduct his study in a certain institution; he may assume that he will be able to enlist the assistance of personnel to staff his project. These and many other conditions he may assume to be true as he develops his plan. Although his planning will proceed for varying periods on the bases of the assumptions, he must pause at intermittent points to determine for certain that the conditions he has been assuming to be true indeed are true. He must secure evidence that the conditions are as he has been assuming them to be.

Assumptions That Provide Rationale For Doing the Study

Illustrative of the second kind of assumption not listed as such are those that serve as part of the rationale for undertaking the study. These, in contrast to those that allow planning, are usually made explicit since they explain the timeliness and significance of the study. They are statements identifying the anticipated usefulness of the knowledge to be gained through the research. An example of such an assumption is:

> For future nurses, basic professional nursing education at university level is preferable to basic nursing education in a diploma program with subsequent university preparation.

This statement is a value judgment and therefore lacks the attribute of demonstrability essential to a hypothesis. Nonetheless, it undoubtedly was based on several component assumptions that would be amenable to testing, such as: Basic nursing education in a university in contrast to diploma education (1) provides a sounder educational base; (2) is more economical of time and money, (3) provides for more and earlier years of prepared service in the profession. Each of these assumptions can serve as a rationale for the study, but none would be necessary as a basis for getting on with the study.

Two devices may help the student in determining which assumptions must be made explicit. The first is the simple one of using reminder words. It is suggested that the subsection titled Assumptions always be introduced with the clause: "Assumptions *basic to pursuit* of *this study* are: ." Or, for variety: "The following assumptions are *basic to pursuit* of *this investigation*." The italics would not be used in the report; they are used here to highlight the reminder words, which should alert the student to ask himself: Are the assumptions basic to my getting on with the study? Am I accepting the stated conditions because, in so doing, I can proceed with my study? Am I accepting them because, otherwise, I would have to interrupt progress on my planned investigation in order to determine the existence of these conditions?

Basic to Pursuit of Study

The second criterion on which to judge whether the assumption must be stated in the subsection Assumptions is whether it must stand as an assumption throughout the entire study and into the report and utilization of the study findings. Must the user of the findings accept, on the basis of logic or reason, the conditions as stated in the assumption? This criterion eliminates all assumptions that underlie many of the planning steps; for example, the assumption that a particular sample of a population will be available for study. The investigator will have ascertained that this is a valid assumption long before the research is completed. Although it may be stated in a very early draft of the plan for the study, even there it would not be under the heading Assumptions and it would not be a part of the report of the investigation. The potential user of the study findings would not be required to accept the assumed condition; it would have been demonstrated to be true. Essentially then, if a condition accepted at some point on the basis of logic or reason does not have to be accepted on that basis by the eventual user of the findings, the condition need not be declared as an assumption basic to proceeding with the study.

Must Stand Through Study, Report, and Use of Findings

SUMMARY

Assumptions are statements of conditions that are accepted as true on the basis of logic and reason for the purpose of getting on with the study. Every phase of scientific inquiry proceeds on the basis of many assumptions, but few of these need to be made explicit in the "Assumptions" subsection of the report. The major criterion for identifying an assumption as such is whether it must stand as an assumption throughout the investigation and into the period when findings from the study will be used. If the eventual user of the findings must accept the conditions on the basis of logic and reason, then the conditions must be stated as assumptions basic to pursuit of the study. The investigator, as an aid to identifying assumptions that need to be made explicit, should note questions asked by persons with whom he discusses his plan of study. If they ask him to describe the basis on which he will account for the effect of a particular condition, this may identify a condition that must be made explicit as an assumption for all with whom he expects to communicate about his research, and for the clarity of his own thinking.

STEP 5
KINDS OF DATA NEEDED

TERMS DEFINED

Datum: A datum is a fact: a single observable or potentially observable phenomenon.
Data: Data is the plural of datum.

CONCEPTS PERTINENT TO DEFINED TERMS

As with many words taken directly from the Latin, there is controversy about datum versus data. For every authority who proposes that "data" may take a singular verb, there is one who proposes that the original usage be retained: that datum be used with a singular verb and data with a plural one. The "data is" school of thought seems to be winning in actual usage, though it is a bit difficult to understand why this should be so in the research field, where precision in thinking and statement is paramount. It seems most illogical for researchers to state: "The age, education, and income data *is* displayed in the following three tables." They would be quick to protest were the statement: "The blue, green, and white chips *is* equally divided among the three contestants." Furthermore, the research data about which such statements are made are usually very obviously plural. At any

A Datum Is; Data Are

rate, *datum* will be used in this text to refer to a single fact and *data* to denote more than one fact, and accompanying verbs will be in accordance.

If precise thinking is needed in planning any step in research, it is most needed when planning for data to be gathered. Yet this is a step that, in most discussions of research, is handled most glibly. Some texts mention the step between discussions of defining terms and developing data collection tools, with no more than passing mention that the investigator must first decide on the data to be collected. The discussions speak of gathering data, but few of them make explicit that data are gathered one by one. So let me make it clear:

Gathering Data: One Datum At a Time

Gathering data is the making and recording of observations—one observation at a time! Each datum is the recording of one observation of one single fact or phenomenon. Individual data are gathered one at a time, and an accumulation of them composes the data. Just as apples are picked one at a time, so data are gathered, one datum at a time. And just as an individual apple can be selected from among other apples in the container into which all have been gathered, so an individual datum can be drawn from the "container" into which it and other similar data have been gathered. Either an apple or a datum may be selected from the accumulation, to be examined individually or to be moved to another container. If a particular apple or datum were tagged with some identifying device before being placed in the collecting container, either could be identified from among its peers and could be traced wherever it might be placed. It could be followed through any number of handlings, even to conversions to other shapes—including the apple into applesauce or the datum into a mean score. The datum is a single fact.

DETERMINING KINDS OF DATA NEEDED

Analogy: Raw Data and Building Materials

Raw data are to the findings of a study what the raw building materials (sand, stone, nails, lumber) are to the finished building. This analogy illustrates many points in research planning. It can extend the concept of the individuality, singleness, and identifiability of an individual datum. Each division of the building—the foundation, the frame, the interior and exterior walls, the roof—is analogous to a variable in a study. Each type of material is analogous to the criterion measures or relevant attributes of variables. The particular sizes, shapes, and general composition of each type of material needed for the building will identify a single unit analogous to specific observations of units or occurrences of a particular criterion measure—each a single fact, an observable phenomenon, a datum. The needed number of each will be selected from among all members representative of each variable before the building is constructed. So with the data for any study: data representing more than one variable will be needed, and only certain representatives of any one variable will be pertinent to the study.

This analogy also illustrates the need, in research, to visualize beforehand what the expected outcome will be. Some persons fail to understand this requirement of the research process and propose that if the researcher already knows what information he will find, why do the research? The absurdity of this point of view is evident: unless the researcher has some fairly definitive ideas about what he expects to find, he cannot know what to look for. The builder who knows the kind of building he plans to build knows the kind of materials he will need for its construction and, on the basis of this knowledge, can identify each type of material that he will select from the variety of each type available. He will also have a fairly good idea of the number of units of each item that will be needed. The researcher must decide the types of variables—independent, dependent, extraneous—appropriate to his concern. He must identify the particular types of representatives of each variable that will be needed (the criterion measures),* and he must estimate the number of each type of the representatives that will be needed.

Visualize Completed Work Before Collecting Materials

The analogy can be carried still further. The expert builder estimates the needs for a particular building fairly precisely. He does not gather unnecessary quantities of any one type of material, nor quantities of types of materials not needed in the construction. The researcher should plan similarly. He should gather the quantity of each type of datum that he estimates to be necessary for the stated purpose of his study, and he should not gather types of data not needed for his study. This point will be elaborated further in Step 9.

Precision of Estimates of Materials Needed: Types, Quantities

The term "data" was deliberately not introduced any earlier in this text, to permit thorough consideration of it once it was introduced. The objective was to help the student to develop a full understanding of the meaning of the term before he makes it a part of his vocabulary. The knowledgeable student will use the terms "datum" and "data" with precision, knowing exactly the observable phenomena to which he refers each time he uses them. He will not use the term "data" with the vagueness and imprecision that has become part of the vernacular. Data are facts, but they are not just any and all facts, without regard to context or to precision of identity and measurement. In general usage, "data" refers to facts

Use of the Term "Data"

---

* Throughout this discussion, when reference is made to criterion measures, the concepts are applicable to qualities, attributes, or characteristics of all variables for which observations and measurements of individually manifested phenomena will be sought and recorded. The concepts apply not only to dependent variables, but to descriptive, accounted-for variables in the hypothesis-testing study and to descriptive variables in exploratory studies.

composing information on which decisions are based. In a research context, "data" refers to facts that are observations systematically collected with the view to supporting generalizations about the statement of purpose of the investigation.

Statement of Purpose Prerequisite to Identification of Data

The building materials of research are facts. The facts of concern to the researcher are those designated as the data: the phenomena to be observed, noted, analyzed, and interpreted. From the time that the statement of purpose is delineated, throughout the planning of the design and writing of the report, everything the researcher does will be in relation to specific facts pertinent to the purpose of his study. The first recognizable concern for these facts occurs during the planning of Step 3, when terms are defined. Many of them will have been identified as germane to the study earlier—during the definition of the problem. There they were considered as they related to the entire problem and, at that point, no decisions were possible about their later use in the research. It is not until the particular focus of the problem has been determined that decisions can be made about the specific facts that will be needed for the study. The determination of specific facts to be sought will be initiated with the defining of terms. Here, too, the attributes of variables potentially relevant to the investigator's interest will be identified. In Step 5, the facts that actually will be sought will be selected from among the many identified in the definitions of terms.

IDENTIFICATION OF DATA NEEDED

Definitions of Terms and Identification of Data

In general, the data needed will have been identified in the definition of terms. These data are observations of phenomena representative of the various germane attributes of variables of concern. If terms have been defined operationally, with for-instances of specific observable phenomena, the various data needed will have been identified. If terms were defined in abstract terms, without descriptions of concrete observable phenomena, then these descriptions will have to be developed in Step 5. Here is an example where thoroughness in the execution of one step saves work in a later step. Conversely, failure to complete a task in one step means that it will have to be accomplished in a later step.

In relation to identifying the exact data that will be needed, the analogy of the building materials can serve again. The builder will order the exact type of sand required. He will use a term or terms to identify the sand, which will denote to the supplier the chemical composition and size of granules. He will order exact stones, by size, shape, and composition; the exact nails, by sizes, lengths, and head-types; the exact lumber, by type of wood, length, width, and thickness. The researcher must identify

Identification of Data Needed

the types of raw data he will need and plan for the exact dimensions of each type of datum he will need.

Two other analogies can help illustrate the processes for determining the exact identities of the various data needed. The first situation is one where two persons are asked, "What are you going to do?" One person is interested, at the moment, in himself; the second person is interested, at the moment, in research.

Analogy: Ground-Ham-on-Rye

SELF-INTEREST

What are you going to do?
GET SOME NOURISHMENT

What nourishment are you going to get?
FOOD

What kind of food?
SANDWICHES

What kind of sandwiches?
MEAT

What kind of meat?
HAM

What kind of ham?
GROUND SMOKED HAM

What will one sandwich look like?
GROUND HAM ON RYE WITH LETTUCE AND MAYONNAISE

RESEARCH-INTEREST

What are you going to do?
GATHER DATA

What data are you going to gather?
FACTS ABOUT BEHAVIORS OF POSTOPERATIVE PATIENTS

What kind of facts?
OBSERVATIONS OF EARLY AMBULATORY BEHAVIORS

What kind of early ambulation behaviors?
WALKING

What observations of walking?
POSTURE

What measurements of posture?
VERY BENT, SLIGHTLY BENT, AND ERECT

What will one datum look like?
SLIGHTLY BENT

This may seem a long way to lunch, but it illustrates the point. The researcher must so specifically identify his data that any person engaged to collect them will know specifically the observations he is to make, the interpretations he is permitted or expected to make, and precisely how each observation is to be recorded.

If more than one person were to "get some nourishment," it is entirely possible that the variety of nourishments would be equal to the number of persons getting the nourishments—particularly, if each was unaware of the nourishments being selected by any of the others. One might bring a malt, another roast beef, another pancakes, and another lemonade. But when the nourishment is identified as food, those securing it would then narrow their selection to solid or semi-solid food. When the food is further specified as sandwiches, those getting the nourishment would bring food that included bread of some sort and a filler, and the sandwich would be plain, toasted, open-faced, closed, or triple-decked. The identification of meat eliminates peanut-butter, banana, squid, and nasturtium leaves, but still permits a wide selection of fillers. The objective is for each person to return with essentially the same type of nourishment. Each sandwich should be so like the other that the individual requesting the nourishment will make no distinction among them as he selects one to eat. If he specifies ground ham on rye with lettuce and mayonnaise, the chances are good that all sandwiches will be very similar to what he had in mind. Of course, variations are still possible. Should the self-interested, hungry person not be able to abide toasted dark rye, he will have to be more explicit in his identification of the specific sandwich he wishes.

Commonalities of Representatives of a Criterion Measure

Essentially, the identification of the specific nourishment involves identifying all possible commonalities shared by two or more individual units. Nourishment alone denotes something consumed. Sandwich identifies several commonalities, such as bread and filler; meat introduces still another commonality; and so forth. It will be recalled that it is possible to identify laws of nature because many phenomena occurring in nature are similar to other phenomena. A law of nature is a generalization about a relationship existing between two classes of phenomena. The individual phenomenon in any of the classes is very similar to any other individual phenomenon in the same class, yet it is always just a bit different.

The data for a study are the recorded observations of many representatives of each of the various classes of phenomena that are of concern for the study. In order that all data gathered as representatives of a class may indeed be members of that class, the characteristics that make it a member and without which it would be excluded from the particular class of phenomena must be described. The greater the number of characteristics, the fewer will be the representatives of the particular class of phenomena. For example, the characteristic, "dark rye," will exclude all sandwiches on light rye; "toasted" will exclude all sandwiches on untoasted bread; and "mayonnaise" could presumably exclude those with mustard or catsup. At least it would exclude those not possessing the characteristic, "mayonnaise"—and soon the individual making the request may go hungry!

The reader will recognize that the type of datum used in the parallel listing was from 1A's study. The facts or observations of behaviors of postoperative patients could have been identified as sleeping, requesting medica-

Identification of Data Needed

tions for relief of pain, refusing to look at wound, worrying, eating, and many others. Behaviors of early ambulation could have meant turning in bed, with or without help; deep-breathing and coughing; sitting in a chair; or walking. Walking could have implied observations of the number of times the patients walked, the distance walked, the length of time spent walking, willingness of the patient to walk, or posture when walking. Posture could be described in the three ways used (1A used stick-figure drawings to illustrate the three postures). The types of posture might have been identified as poor, fairly good, and good, in which case each would have been described or illustrated by drawings. They might have been identified by a symbol: A, B, C, or 1, 2, 3, which again would have had to be defined (the posture so described that each person observing a particular posture would identify it with the same term or symbol). When an investigator states that the data needed are observations about nursing care, he is identifying the data on a "food" level, and he must get it to a ground-ham-on-rye level. This is the significant point and the important concept to be understood from the analogy.

Data Identified at Various Levels: Food, Sandwich, Ham-on-Rye

Nursing care is apt to be of concern to many nurse researchers, and frequently some of the data needed in a study will be observations about nursing care. But there are perhaps as many types and attributes of nursing care about which studies will be done as there are types of buildings to be constructed. The builder must decide whether his materials will include steel girders or wooden beams; slate, shingle, or asphalt roofing; cement, terrazza, tile, or parquet flooring; and so on. Selection will, of course, depend on the identity of the building to be built. So the nurse researcher must decide on the types of observations of nursing care that are germane to the purpose of her study. What specifically is the type of nursing care about which the nurse wishes to obtain facts? Since the purpose of her study derives from the definition of problem, it is to the latter that the researcher must turn to identify the types of data needed. In the definition of problem, the nurse researcher will have described nursing care as it is and as she thinks it should be. Now, from the definition of problem, she identifies the specific observations to be made and the descriptions of data to be gathered. Her concern may be in terms of the nursing care provided or of the outcomes of particular care provided, as was 1A's concern. Interests of three fictitious nurse researchers may be used for illustration. One is concerned with problems related to small children receiving corrective therapy for clubfoot. A second nurse's concern is adults with mid-thigh walking casts, and the concern of the third nurse is stroke patients with lower-limb weakness. All may identify walking as a phenomenon to be observed in their studies. Yet, the measurements, the specific observations to be made, would be different in each study and different from those selected by 1A.

Ham-on-Rye Level From Definition of Problem

Illustration: Relevant Attributes Identified in Problem-Defined

As each researcher defined her terms she would look to her definition of problem to identify the many attributes and the many representative examples of each attribute inherent in the variables of her concern. And, as she planned for specific data to be sought, she would again check her definition of problem to find bases for selecting those data most relevant to her interest. Each of the three investigators cited above was concerned with nursing care related to ambulation activities. Each may have decided that walking was the particular ambulatory activity she expected to be influenced by nursing care. For each, walking was the variable to be observed and measured. Yet, the attributes or characteristics (criterion measures) of walking and the descriptions of representative examples of walking (for-instances) would, in all probability, have been different in each investigation. For the patients in the walking cast, the characteristic of concern may have been a swinging of the leg with outward rotation of the hip. For the stroke patient, concern would have been about foot-drop or use of body swing. Each of these specific types of characteristics and examples of them would have been described in the definitions of problems. They would be in each investigator's descriptions of her irritation, the possible causes of supporting elements in the problem, what she considered the situation to be, and what results might be anticipated for the proposed corrective actions. This again illustrates the contribution of the thoroughly done step to the planning of later steps. The problem thoroughly defined contributes to definitions of terms, identification of criterion measures, and specific units of each measure.

Criterion Measures and General Classes of Phenomena

The above differences can also help the student to identify the specific elements in relation to general terms. Performance of ambulation activities is the general phenomenon that is the central concern of each of the fictitious investigators, just as building materials is the general category of items sought by the builder. These categories correspond to the dependent variable where a hypothesis is to be tested, and to a major category of facts where the study is descriptive-exploratory in nature. One of the types of the general phenomenon, early ambulatory activities, for 1A, was walking. One of the types of the general phenomenon, building materials, for the builder, was cement. These general phenomena or classes correspond to the criterion measures or relevant attributes of the variables of interest to the investigator or the builder. One dimension of walking was identified by 1A "posture, slightly bent." One unit of cement, or one dimension of the specific type of material, might be "stone, 1-4 cm." "Posture, slightly bent" and "stone, 1-4 cm" each correspond to a single datum. Posture and stone would have been identified in the pertinent general of the definition of terms, and slightly bent and 1-4 cm, in the for-instances.

But, in these examples, another level of category or class for identification of the explicit nature of the observations (data) to be sought is introduced. The definition of terms identifies three class or category levels of the data:

1. The term being defined, which names the variable about which information is to be sought.
2. The pertinent general, which enumerates attributes of the variable.
3. The for-instances, which suggest individual representative occurrences of the various attributes of the variable.

One and frequently two additional levels are indicated for precise identification of some data. These levels are suggested in the earlier proposal that there is sometimes a need to define the criterion measures that have been identified in the pertinent general phase of the definition of the dependent variable: that is, a three-part definition of the attributes enumerated as being relevant criterion measures. In the examples of the criterion measures, cement and walking, "stone" is a class or category level between cement and one of its individual representatives: "stone, 1-4 cm." Likewise, posture identifies a category level between walking and the individual representative, "posture, slightly bent." But the analysis must be carried one step further to provide yet another level needed for orderly planning of the individual units of data to be collected.

There is need to identify the scale of measurement that will be used. In the examples, the builder used a centimeter scale to identify the desired diameter of the stones. 1A used the nominative scale, with a range from very bent, through slightly bent, to upright. The level of specific measurement is sometimes not described in so many words. Rather it is identified by implication in the level of individual data. For example, without explicitly stating that he was talking about diameters, the builder implies this in the identification of the individual representative: "stone, 1-4 cm." Yet, 1-4 cm could refer just as well to circumference or to radius.

Scale of Measurement

Needless to say, the identities of these category levels, too, will have been at least introduced, if not described in detail, in the definition of problem. The student is reminded again that imagination and judgment are needed when planning and executing all aspects of a scientific investigation. Suggestions for detailed planning are presented to help where they are needed. Not all details of planning are needed in all studies; for some types of data, for instance, the details describing five category levels of data are not needed. Identifications of data for 3B's study (pages 147 to 149) illustrate the usefulness of making explicit four levels. They also demonstrate the lack of need for greater explicitness. The researcher should describe as many and as few category levels as he needs to understand clearly what he is doing and to make clear to others what he has done. These concepts of identification of category levels for description of data are illustrated in the following analogy.

Analogy: Improving an Apple Crop

Working through a second sequence of the identification of data illustrates various types of individual data that may be appropriate to the needs of a study. The focus of the fictitious study is a hypothesis, roughly stated as: Use of fertilizer XYZ will result in an improved crop of apples. The dependent variable is crop; this is what the researcher seeks to change. In order to determine the data needed (the observations to be made) about the crop, it is necessary to first define the term "crop." The definition, in turn, would derive from elements in the definition of problem, and ultimately, from the original irritation. What bothered the farmer? What about his apple crop did he think could be improved? What did he want changed? Changed to what? Answers to these questions could lead to identification of the particular attributes of the apples that should be measured. These, in turn, lead to types of observations (the specific classes representative of the criterion measures) that should be made; then, the specific measurements that might be made. Finally, individual representative observations would be identified. Without knowledge of the original irritation, a frequent first guess about the meaning of crop is related to amount or quantity of apples, followed by guesses about their size. Without knowing the original concern or any of the related elements that would be identified in the definition of problem, the ambitious researcher might decide to seek observations about many attributes of the crop of apples: their quantity, size, color, quality, etc. Yet the farmer's only concern, it might turn out, was the amount of juice in the apple. So it would be senseless to observe for all the other attributes when the only effect the farmer was interested in was the juice content of the apples.

Suppose, however, that the farmer believes that everything about his apples could be improved, and an ambitious salesman has convinced him that a single fertilizer, XYZ, will do the job. It may then be presumed that in the definition of the problem, the various attributes of the apples and of the total crop will be described as they now exist, and the particular elements of the fertilizer enumerated. The potential effect of each element will be described, and these descriptions will serve as bases of for-instances in the definition of the term "crop," identification of the criterion measures, and the specific classes or types of facts to be collected. Among them will be the following, listed under category level headings:

I VARIABLE: Crop (specifically, crop of apples)

II CRITERION MEASURE	III SPECIFIC CATEGORY	IV SPECIFIC MEASUREMENT SCALE	V APPEARANCE OF ONE DATUM
1. Quantity of apples	a. volume	a. 1. bushels 2. pecks 3. carloads	a. 1. 5.6 per tree 2. 22.4 per tree 3. 1.6 per 100 trees

II CRITERION MEASURE	III SPECIFIC CATEGORY	IV SPECIFIC MEASUREMENT SCALE	V APPEARANCE OF ONE DATUM
	b. weight	b. 1. pounds 2. tons	b. 1. 358.4 per tree 2. 17.9 per 100 trees
	c. number	c. frequency count	c. 1,075.0 per tree
2. Size of apples	a. diameter: 1. stem to blossom 2. largest between stem and blossom	a. centimeters	a. 1. 9.8 2. 12.1
	b. diameter 1 and 2 as above	b. inches	b. 1. 3.5 2. 5.0
	c. circumference 1 and 2 as in 2.a., above	c. centimeters	c. 1. 75.2 2. 117.2
	d. circumference 1 and 2 as in 2.a., above	d. inches	d. 1. 12.0 2. 18.9
	e. USDA Grading	e. sizes 1 thru 9	e. 6
	f. description	f. large medium small	f. medium
3. Shape of apples	Description	regular lopsided tapered pear-shaped flat, stem-to-blossom round	regular, tapered
4. Color	a. Description	a. red burgundy burnished red green yellow yellow with pink cheek	a. burgundy, overall
	b. USDA Scale	b. numbers 1 thru 24	b. #7
5. Quality	a. texture	a. crisp mealy woody	a. crisp
	b. moisture	b. dry juicy medium juicy	b. juicy
	c. taste	c. tart sweet sour Nyeh!	c. sweet
	d. USDA Scale	d. superior 4 good 3 average 2 poor 1	d. good—3

Unit Observed (Measured) for Obtaining Single Datum

The first category level is, of course, the variable (apple crop) concerning which observations are to be made. Since the variable relates equally to each item in the schema, it may be placed in the heading, and it need not have a column space. The listing of potential levels for identifying the data needed illustrates the usefulness of making explicit each of the five category levels for some types of data. It illustrates, too, that, for some types of observations, only the three category levels identified in a three-part definition are needed. In addition, the listing indicates that where the individual observation is to be made with a scaled measure, there is sometimes need to identify explicitly the unit to be measured. For example, where the scale of pounds is to be used, it is necessary to identify the unit to be weighed. Actually, whatever the nature of an individual observation, the unit to be measured (observed) must be known, but in many instances its identity can be readily inferred from the general context of the plan. This may be true even for some observations where scaled measurements are done. In the example of observations pertinent to the apple crop, it would be assumed that, where the specific measurement scale is centimeters, the unit to be measured will be a single apple. On the other hand, where the scale is bushels, there is need to identify the unit. Comparisons could appropriately be made of number of bushels per tree, per 10 trees, per acre of trees, or per orchard.

Data: Quantitative Qualitative, Descriptive

This example illustrates the extensive variety of data that may be gathered in any one investigation. It also serves to illustrate the three major classifications of research data and to point out that data within each classification may appropriately be sought in a single investigation. The three major classifications of data are: quantitative, qualitative, and descriptive. In order to evaluate the effects of the fertilizer, observations would be made of many attributes of the apple crop. There would be *quantitative* data of two types: (1) scale measurements, such as the number of pounds, the number of ounces, the number of inches, the number of bushels; and (2) frequencies, such as the number of apples, the number of trees, the number of plots of land, and so forth. There would be *qualitative* data: large, medium, small, superior, average, and so forth. And there would be *descriptive* data: regular shape, red overall, mealy with thick skin.

Qualitative and descriptive data have some commonalities, in that each relies on adjectives to identify the measurement of the attribute and each relies on a degree of subjective judgment by the observer. In contrast, quantitative data are obtained through use of established scales, and measurements are identified by fairly precise numbers, with need for little or no judgment on the observer's part. Qualitative data are usually expressed in terms of degrees of the attribute, whereas descriptive data are usually expressed in absolute terms. That is, a qualitative observation about the crispness of an apple might be "very crisp" or "somewhat crisp"; while a descriptive observation about the shape might be "symmetrical, squat, round with flattening on stem and blossom ends." Qualitative data are used for ranking subjects, although the "units" of the scales lack the precision of scales used for quantitative data. The rankings are used to compare subjects on several degrees of possession of the attribute. Descriptive data are not used to rank subjects and, where they are used to make comparisons, there are but two levels of comparison: the subjects either possess the descriptive attribute or they do not. Subjects being compared are either alike or different.

Both qualitative and descriptive data admit varying degrees of subjectivity. Data from either one of these classes may be useful in research: observations that may be reported only in descriptive terms, and observations that, while relying on descriptive terms, may be distinguished from others of like category by gross measures of degree. The definition of research noted that "quantitative" and "quantifiable" data will be analyzed, using appropriate statistical tests. Many data will be recorded in descriptive terms only, while some criterion measures will have two or more quantitative scale measurements appropriate for recording pertinent observations. For example, the size of apples might be measured by various scales applied to various diameters and circumferences. And the size might be "measured" in descriptive terms, such as large, medium, small; or the size might be in descriptive symbols, such as 1, 2, and 3; or A, B, and C. The symbols 1, 2, and 3, though they are numbers, would be considered descriptive and not quantitative, since they do not refer to a precise scale measure and are not, in such usage, additive. On the other hand, descriptive or qualitative data may be quantified, as is illustrated by the specific measurements 5. d. for quality of apples (page 143). There, scores were ascribed to qualitative terms, with the intent that scores for a group might be added and averaged to establish a group score. These scores, however, retain the limitation of subjective judgment of the person doing the "measuring." It is in such instances that experts are used to do the measuring, so that reliance on precision of measurement may be enhanced.

Transpositions of Data: Descriptive to Quantitative

In some instances, quantifying the data may serve little purpose, since the only meaningful measurements are descriptions as, for example, some of the measurements of quality. It would be possible to ascribe number symbols to the texture measurements of the apples, but they would have little meaning until converted to the descriptive terms of crisp, mealy, woody, and so on. The qualification of descriptive data implies that there are varying degrees of the same attribute, whereas crisp, mealy, and woody all are "measurements" of texture, but they are not degrees of the same texture.

Godfrey's study is a good example of process of quantifying data, since her data, as collected (as the measurements were made and recorded),

Example: Quantifying the Data

were in descriptive form. It will be remembered that students made process recordings describing their interactions with the children and the children's behaviors. Godfrey then developed a qualitative scale, using the following adjectives, with degree-modifying adverbs, as measurements:

| Very secure | Secure | Somewhat secure and Somewhat anxious | Anxious | Very anxious |

The raw data (the process recordings) were submitted to a panel of experts, who were asked to decide independently the qualitative description on the scale that was the best "measure" of each item of data (each process recording). Following this, Godfrey ascribed a numerical value to each qualitative description, as follows:

Very secure	2
Secure	1
Somewhat secure and somewhat anxious	0
Anxious	−1
Very anxious	−2

Thus, Godfrey's data moved through the three steps, from detailed descriptive, to the generalized qualitative, to the precise quantitative. Frequently, essentially descriptive data are collected in qualitative form, where a judgment of degree is made by the observer at the time of observation and recording. When this is done the process of quantifying the data requires but one step, that of applying the numerical scale to the qualitative measures.

Frequencies as Quantitative Data

Using frequencies is one other means of quantifying data, and this quantification can be applied to any type of datum. Often it is the only quantification that is reasonably applied: (1) where no valid scale of measurement has been established to measure a particular quality; (2) where development of a scale would entail a procedure so complex as to be impractical, either in itself or in light of the need for it; or (3) where scaled measurements are not required for the purposes of the study.

Sometimes frequencies are not even needed or may be undesirable when the purpose is to describe a situation or situations, with no intent to make comparisons or to ascribe values of any sort. An example of this type of datum and the rationale for so handling the data are well illustrated in Lesser and Keane's study, *Nurse-Patient Relationships in a Hospital Maternity Service.*[2] They wished to describe how mothers viewed the care they received and what they expected in the way of care, as well as what nurses thought mothers expected of nursing care and how they

Identification of Data Needed

viewed mothers' acceptance of the care provided. They wished to avoid all implications of good and bad, so they used no statistics, not even frequencies of various types of expressions.

Essentially, then, there are three types or general categories of data. They may be viewed as on a continuum from the broadly descriptive, through the ranked qualitative, to the precise quantitative. The amount of judgment required of the observer follows the same continuum: ranging from extensive reliance on observer judgment for grossly descriptive data, to little or no judgment being required of quantitative data that can be collected through use of established, validated measuring instruments. Quite obviously, it is advantageous to collect quantitative data from the outset. Wherever there is a choice among varied relevant data, the researcher would choose those data for which measurement scales had been developed. The key here, of course, is relevance. The researcher must identify the facts that are germane to his purpose and are relevant attributes of the variables about which he seeks information. For example, among measurements of the attributes of the variable "communicates" may be listed: (1) words per minute and (2) listens attentively. Words per minute would permit direct collection of quantitative data, which might well be relevant in a study of the skills of telegraphers or signal corpsmen. Such data would hardly be relevant in a study of skills of nurses teaching patients about postoperative ambulation.

Continuum: Descriptive to Qualitative to Quantitative— Movement From Subjective to Objective

Let it be said again: all data are collected one at a time! Whether it is counting apples, measuring their circumference, or determining their texture; be it observing the anxiety displayed by a child, or identifying the posture of a patient walking after surgery—there is only one observation and one recording of one study subject at any one time.

The data identified by 3B as she planned her design illustrate two points: (1) the efficacy of using a category level between a criterion measure and individual representatives of it; (2) the smooth flow of the planning from the hypothesis, to the definition of the dependent variable (wherein the criterion measures were identified), and to the identification of the data needed. The three-part definition of the dependent variable included for-instances excerpted from the definition of problem. These served to identify representative occurrences of a particular attribute of the variable. The listing of the planned data illustrates the logical evolvement of the identity of individual data from the three phases of the definition of the variable.

Example: 3B

Data needed to measure the dependent variable supported: (See hypothesis and definition of supported, pages 125 to 126).

Step 5: Kinds of Data Needed

CRITERION MEASURES	SPECIFIC CATEGORY	APPEARANCE OF ONE DATUM (Observations)
Anxiety (worry, fear, doubts, suspicions)	Physical manifestations: (example, overt signs which can be observed)	Thumb sucking, not talking, bed wetting, not sleeping nor resting.
	Verbal manifestations: (example, expressing in words fears and anxieties)	"Why am I not getting better?" Asking, "Am I going to die?" Stating, "Don't leave me!" Asking, "Why isn't the pain going away?"
Comfort	Physical (example, position, breathing, pain)	Stating that he is in a great deal of pain, complaining that his position is not comfortable.
	Mental and emotional	Putting his light on frequently, asking for same thing repeatedly. Exhibiting restlessness or suspecting behavior. Fingering his bedspread continually; watching every move of each person in room.
Needs met	Physical (example, personal care which he cannot perform for himself)	Expressing relief of pain following medication. Commenting that it feels good to be clean after his bath or mouth care. Remarks about easier breathing after being placed in O_2 tent.
	Emotional (recognition of his worries and fears, attempts made to alleviate them)	Someone on staff available to talk to after parents have left. Assistance to write letter to school friend.
	Mental	Playing games with nurse or other children on ward; games are mentally stimulating.
	Spiritual	Saying night prayers with nurse.
Loneliness and isolation (being left alone or isolated)		Stating, "I feel lonesome." Putting his light on frequently, making numerous requests that obviously only seek companionship.
Trusting relationship	Parents	Stating, "I know my mom and dad will come to see me whenever they can." "I love my mom and dad." Appearing contented when his parents are with him. Indicating apprehension as visiting hours approach, "I hope my parents come today."
	Staff	States, "The nurse always tells me when something is going to hurt." "I don't have to call the nurse, she comes to see me.

Identification of Data Needed

		Mostly she knows when I need her." Appearing comfortable and at ease with staff members. Asking to have nurse with him during treatments. Commenting that he'll wait for nurse to return, knows where she is.
Confidence	In staff	Accepts comforting from nurse at time parents leave. Comments, "My nurse knows when it hurts. She says it is all right if I cry. She tries to make it so it won't hurt."
	In self	Amuses self. Does not show apprehension when left alone for short periods.
Courage		"I'm not afraid. My nurse will stay with me when I need her." "It's all right for you to leave, now. I'll be all right till the nurse comes." "The nurse said it will not take as long as last time, and I'm not afraid."

(From here on, only the criterion measures and specific categories will be listed, though 3B developed all three levels.)

Outlook toward illness	Positive
	Negative
Goals set by patient	Realistic
	Unrealistic
Independence (ability to help self and feel satisfaction in accomplishments)	
Developing new interests	
Feeling of being "cared for": (example, having likes and dislikes considered, feels nurse is interested in him).	
Feeling secure and safe	
Freedom of expression	Verbally
	Through behavior
Comprehension of explanations given him by nurses	
Knowledge of what to expect or what might occur	
Reassurance	

IDENTIFYING CRITERION MEASURES

Judgment and Decision

Although many potentially useful criterion measures are introduced in the definition of problem, the selection of those most valid and reliable for measuring the dependent variable is not a simple or automatic process. The definition of problem will provide leads and, once decisions have been made about the measures to be used, it will provide descriptions of the measures. But not all potentially useful measures mentioned in the definition of problem will be used. The investigator will have some ideas about measures to use and should define them and describe the exact measurements of each, so that decisions can be made about each one's feasibility. In general, where needed facts are not measurements for which standard scales have been established (pounds, inches, degrees of temperature, and others), the more criterion measures used, the greater the confidence in the findings in relation to their test of the hypothesis. This, of course, presumes the validity, reliability, and relevance of the criterion measures (discussed below, pp. 151 to 155).

Suggestion From Nursing Service Personnel

The researcher would do well to seek recommendations for pertinent criterion measures from persons knowledgeable in his own and intimately related fields. The nurse researcher would discuss her planning with nursing service personnel, physicians, and paramedical personnel. Nursing service personnel are in daily contact with patients. Each day they make untold numbers of observations of patients' conditions, many of which are related to response to treatments. These persons can be a remarkably prolific source of suggestions for criterion measures. Few, however, will view themselves as such, and few will propose potential "criterion measures." But if the investigator asks them to suggest responses of patients that may be outcomes of particular kinds of treatment and care, most will be able to identify numerous relevant measures. Further, they will be able to describe them in detail and explain why they believe that the responses are related to the particular treatment or nursing care activity.

From Physicians

Because any single patient receives many kinds of care and treatment, it is usually difficult to identify particular responses to a particular treatment. Nurses have been especially reluctant to identify any response as resulting from nursing care. Physicians can be of marked assistance in this matter. The physician knows in detail all elements of the treatment that he provides or orders for the patient, and what results he expects from each. He also knows what changes he expects to occur in a patient as a result of care that he assumes the nurses will provide as independent actions. While nurses may be reluctant to relate some of these responses or changes to nurse action, the physician will not have this reluctance. For example, most surgeons will propose that lung reexpansion and prevention of pneumonia following thoracic surgery can be mainly attributable to nurse actions, rather than to anything done by the surgeon himself. Prevention of contractures, restoration of affected muscles in stroke patients, and prevention of thrombi, urinary calculi, and decubiti in many patients may be identified as resulting from nurse actions. These outcomes for patients that may be attributable to nursing care will depend on various factors: the cause of the potential conditions, other treatments, patients' general conditions, and others. The physician can be helpful in determining whether the outcomes can be ascribed to nurse action. He will suggest or confirm the appropriateness of using a particular type of patient response as a criterion measure in the dependent variable, where the independent variable is a form of nursing care.

Frequently, occupational and physical therapists can be of help, especially where the nurse researcher is interested in testing nursing care expected to affect skeletomuscular structures. Indeed, in many studies, the therapist cannot only suggest criterion measures but will have at hand the necessary measuring instruments and scales. Frequently, she will offer to make the necessary measurements. *From Therapists*

As with all phases of planning research, the investigator should not attempt to complete the identification of criterion measures without seeking suggestions from others. For the nurse researcher, the likely others are persons who contribute their own special care for the patient.

Criterion measures, as has been pointed out, are not arbitrarily chosen; they must be relevant to the dependent variable and to the stated purpose of the study. This was the qualification considered in the discussion of the operational definition of the dependent variable. It was there proposed that nursing care or patient response to nursing care or both may be dependent variables in many varieties of studies, as for example, one concerned with premature infants and another concerned with geriatric patients. Although the variable may be identified in the same terms (nursing care and patient response to care), the definitions of the terms would be rather different for the two studies. The general identification of the attribute to be observed (the criterion measure) might be "nutrient intake" for both studies. Yet some of the specific categories in the criterion measure would be different. In the study of geriatric patients, there would be the matter of roughage in the diet. This specific category of nutrient would not be relevant or, at least, would be less important in the study of premature infants. Here, again, the definition of problem can help in determining relevance. But the definition of problem explores a broad area and includes some speculative materials, so any suggestion drawn from it must be evaluated as to its relevance for the particular facet of the problem chosen as the focus of the study. *Relevance of Criterion Measures*

STEP 5: KINDS OF DATA NEEDED

Establishment of relevance, essentially, is establishment of face validity. That is, on the basis of gross examination and known relationship of attributes of concern, the criterion measure is indeed a measure of the dependent variable. 1A, in her definition of problem, described the physiological changes in a patient due to surgery and the limited movement that is a "natural" sequela of surgery. She described the effects of particular early ambulation activities on the changes in physiology, including descriptions of fluid accumulation in the lungs, the effects of deep-breathing, coughing, turning, and exercise on lung physiology, as well as the stases of blood in the lower extremities, and the effects of exercises, turning, and walking on the blood flow. In addition, she identified the crux of her problem as the postoperative behavior of the patients. As the focus of her study, she proposed a relationship between patients' being informed about early ambulatory activities and their performances of the activities. Since the activities could be expected to influence blood flow in the extremities and accumulation of fluids in the lungs, representative observations of these phenomena might reasonably have been selected as criterion measures. Yet, in addition to being more complex processes and requiring a much larger population from which to secure measurements, these variables would not have been directly relevant to the stated purpose of the study. They could not be identified as attributes of the dependent variable, performance of early ambulation activities. On the other hand, coughing, turning, sitting out of bed, and walking *are* logically attributes of such activities. Furthermore, these phenomena could reasonably be expected to be influenced by the independent variable, and were therefore directly relevant to the focus of the study.

It may be proposed, however, that 1A's ultimate concern was blood flow and accumulation of lung secretions. She might have proposed a relationship between early ambulation activities, on the one hand, and blood flow and fluid accumulation in the lungs, on the other. Had she done so, her dependent variable would have become the independent variable, and the variables that provided a rationale for justifying her investigation would have become dependent variables. The guide for deciding between these two paths lies in the very early phases of defining the problem: in recording early observations of the irritation. 1A's early concern was that postoperative patients were afraid to move, to get out of bed, to stand erect. This concerned her, of course, because of the potential harm to the patient in terms of blood stases and pulmonary secretions. Nonetheless, the actual observed conditions about which she decided something should be done were patients' manifestations of not ambulating and of fear as an element in the situation. Her observations were not that patients were displaying the ill effects of not ambulating, although knowledge of these potential ill effects was the basis for her initial irritation. Therefore, the reasonable facet of the problem for her study was the one selected. When a problem is well defined, decision may sometimes be made to select a facet for study other than the one most directly related to the original irritation. The use of the original irritation, however, is usually a good base for choosing the facet of the study and for judgments about the relevance of criterion measures selected.

Face validity is frequently the only validity the student researcher will establish for the criterion measures to be used in his study. This is especially true for the undergraduate or masters student. His primary purpose in doing an investigation is to learn the rudiments of the research process. He lacks the time to execute all of the details necessary in a full scientific inquiry. Validation of one or more criterion measures can be and usually is a long-term research project in itself. Some believe, however, that students should not be encouraged to proceed on the basis of face validity alone. They suggest that if no validated measures are available to students, they should be encouraged to test the validity of the proposed measures rather than pursue the original purpose of the study. It would seem preferable, however, to help students to understand what they are doing, rather than to have them redirect their study. They should understand that their study, at best, will be a pilot study, and that interpretations of their findings must be in light of various limitations, including those related to validation of criterion measures. Such a policy permits the students to proceed through the mechanics of a completed scientific investigation and gain an overview of what research is about. Along the way, they can be helped to recognize other types of limiting conditions that are very likely to be encountered in any investigation. Furthermore, even if students did devote their time and effort to testing the validity of criterion measures, it would still not overcome the matter of their proceeding under "false pretenses," so to speak, since it is not likely that the validation task, either, could be completed within the scope of the masters program or the masters student's competence.

Validity and Relevance

The matters of limited time in the educational program and how much a student can be expected to learn about research are a continuing plaguing concern for educators and students alike. Essentially, undergraduate and masters students will not test the validity of criterion measures as a prerequisite for using them in investigations. Nor will they, in most instances, collect sufficient data to test validity even at the completion of their studies, or as part of their data analysis. But they can be helped to understand the meaning of validity and the necessity for validation of measures before conclusive statements can be made; and they can learn to recognize that the work they do can serve as valuable initial steps to full-fledged scientific inquiries. Indeed, some students have designed studies that could be preliminaries to lifelong projects. The senior paper or masters thesis

How Encompassing: the Introduction to Research?

could be a first step, with outline of the doctoral thesis clearly visible in it, and the direction for continued investigation obviously implied.

Validation

Since validation of measures is an extensive study in itself, details of the process will not be presented here. Suffice it to remind the student that validity means that the measurements are measuring what they purport to measure. A test for validity of a criterion measure is the degree to which measurements of it agree with measurements of other criterion measures, known to be valid, of the same variable. For example, if Godfrey had (1) had available a valid test for anxiety in children, (2) had tested her children with it, and then (3) had obtained the measurements she did obtain, she might have tested the validity of her criterion measure. She could have done so by determining the degree to which her scores correlated with scores from the "known" (hypothetically known) valid measurement. Without an established valid measurement against which to evaluate a new criterion measure, it is still possible to validate a measure by examining observations made with the measure in terms of the face validity and of the amount of discrimination achieved. A criterion measure that yields measurements that discriminate among individuals measured, and with which those who make the observations (measurements) discriminate among individuals, may be said to be a valid measure. That is, the scores of the dependent variable derived through its use are valid measures of the effects of the independent variable. This delineation of validation is grossly oversimplified and represents only an introduction to the concept of validation. The statements made here about validity of measurements presume reliability and relevance of the criterion measure. The validity of the scores in the dependent variable can be increased through an increase in the number of criterion measures used to determine the score. For example, 1A may have used any one of her criterion measures: coughing, turning, deep-breathing, or walking. Using all of them, however, provided greater confidence in the validity of her measurements of her dependent variable. Of course, increased numbers alone will not increase nor assure validity. The added criterion measures must meet all qualifications of relevance, face validity, discriminating capability, and so on.

Reliability

The third attribute essential to criterion measures is reliability: that is, the measure must yield the same scores in repeated or multiple measurements of the same thing. Reliability is not as difficult to establish as validity but, for validity to be meaningful, reliability must be known. The process will not be described in detail, but reliability should be established in terms of repeated measurements of the same thing by one individual, and of several measurements of the same thing by several individuals. As with validity, the undergraduate or masters student will perhaps not test his criterion measures for reliability. He should, nonetheless, be aware of the limitation the omission imposes on the confidence he can have in his

DESCRIPTIVE DATA IN ALL STUDIES

Regardless of the purpose of the study, it is recommended that descriptive data be collected, even where the purpose is to test a hypothesis. This recommendation may seem to contradict an earlier recommendation that collection of unnecessary data be avoided. But this aspect of an investigation, along with many others, is one that requires judgment. Either too many or too few data in terms of quantity and variety can be inappropriate. The quantitative data needed for testing a hypothesis can frequently be gathered by merely recording figures in suitably labeled cells of a record form. The figures can be submitted to appropriate statistical analyses, and conclusions drawn about the substantiation of the hypothesis. On the basis of these figures alone, however, little else could be said about the subjects studied, let alone about the population they represent. Nor would these quantitative data furnish any information about facets of the problem other than the one selected for study.

More Data Than Needed to Test Hypothesis

Furthermore, should the hypothesis not be substantiated, there would be no information on which to examine findings in an effort to determine the possible reason for failure to substantiate the hypothesis. Two examples from the Uninterrupted Patient Care study[3] can illustrate the logic and ease of collecting descriptive data, and the invaluable purposes they can serve. Three criterion measures were: (1) activities of care performed by nursing personnel; (2) the time, in minutes, spent by nursing personnel in performing the activities; and (3) the number of requests for care made by patients. The observations were made by full-time, nonparticipant, nurse observers. Quite obviously, the data could have been recorded on a form divided into three sections: activities, time, requests. Each observation of an activity or request could have been recorded as a single hashmark in the appropriate section. The time spent in performance of each activity could have been similarly recorded. These were the only data required to measure one dependent variable, nursing requirements. With planning, however, it was possible to obtain a great deal more information, with no more effort on the part of the observers. The recording tool, instead of being divided into three sections, was sectioned according to types of care likely to be provided, such as personal hygiene, nourishment, medications, change of position, out of bed, and so on. When an activity was observed, the time it was begun and the time completed were recorded in one cell in the appropriate section. If the activity had resulted from a request made by the patient, an "R" was placed beside the recorded time. This plan

Example: Logic and Value of Collecting Descriptive Data

provided information about types of care most frequently provided, the amount of time spent performing particular types of care, and the types of care which the patient requested, as well the quantitative data needed to test the hypothesis. Thus, with only a modicum of planning, extensive additional information was obtained at no extra cost in time, money, or effort.

Example: Descriptive Data Invaluable

The second illustration from the study concerns another set of data that was collected. The nurse observers were asked to estimate the number of nursing care activities that would be required to provide comprehensive care to the patients. Securing these data required that the nurse observers develop what amounted to a detailed nursing care plan. As a part of this planning, the nurses developed a list of commonly performed activities of nursing care. This master list contained 83 activities arranged under headings that corresponded roughly to the 21 nursing problems identified by Abdellah, Martin, Beland, and Metheney.[4] As a nurse observer planned the care of a patient, she itemized the various activities of care that he would need and the number of times each activity would have to be performed in a 24-hour day. Estimates of the numbers of activities were made each day for nine successive days, with two nurse observers, independently, planning for each patient studied. Nurse observer A planned for seven of the days, and Nurse observer B planned for the other two days. There were four nurse observers. They were paired randomly for each two patients studied, with no two nurse observers being paired more than 18 times. So that the nurses would not have to write a detailed plan each day, each used the one individual plan she had developed for daily planning, but she recorded her estimates of numbers of activities on separate sheets, one for each day for which estimates were done. Modifications, of course, were made on the planning sheets as changes for patient care were indicated. On the recording sheets, it was necessary only to identify the activities by number and then to record the estimated frequency.

When the data for these estimates were examined, it was found that the nurse observers agreed only 40 percent to 68 percent of the time about the nursing activities needed to provide the patients with comprehensive care. With so little agreement, quite obviously these data could not be used to test the hypothesis. When considered only in relation to their quantitative values, the data were quite useless for the purposes of the study and might therefore have been dismissed as merely a "nice try"—except for the very disturbing fact of the meaning behind the lack of agreement among the nurses. What was the meaning of this for patient care? The nurse observers had been chosen on the basis of known competency. They had worked together to develop the guides for planning nursing care. Using data from the pilot study, they had shared development of the Master List of Activities. They had more time than nurses usually have to know the patients and to plan for them. If these nurses could not agree, what about other nurses who plan care of patients? What about an instructor agreeing with a student's nursing care plan? What of a supervisor evaluating a staff nurse's plan for patient care? What about care of patients from personnel, shift to shift?

Because of these questions, the data were examined in relation to their content. For example, on Day 1, nurse observer A may have estimated that activity #5 would have to be performed for the patient three times, but did not include activity #4. On Day 2, nurse observer B might have estimated that activity #4 should be performed three times, but she did not list activity #5. Statistically, these represent 100 percent disagreement on the two activities. When the activities were identified, however, it was found that activity #5 was "Feed patient," and activity #4 was "Assist to eat." Here, quite obviously, these two nurses did not disagree either in relation to the needs of the patient and the particular activity required to meet the needs, or in relation to the frequency of the performance of the activities. As one further illustration: on Day 1, nurse observer A listed activity #9, with an estimate of one performance required; on Day 2, nurse observer B did not list activity #9. Again, statistically, there is 100 percent disagreement. Activity #9 is "Irrigate catheter." But the catheter had been removed on the evening of Day 1, so there was no disagreement, after all. After all data were examined, it was found that there was 78 percent to 90 percent agreement among the nurse observers, with 85 percent or better agreement for most patients.

There are several lessons to be learned from this experience. First is the value of descriptive data even where quantitative data are all that seem needed for the immediate purpose of the study. Further illustrated are the admonitions often repeated by statisticians, and frequently ignored by those who seek the help of statisticians: (1) Statistics are only as useful as the observations they represent. (2) Statistics will tell only that variables are or are not related or that subjects are or are not from a common population. (3) Statistics will not identify the variables, nor will they tell why or how populations are different. Goshen suggests that there is need to "show more attention to the source from which data is [sic] derived and less attention to the language of its expression."[5]

Statistics Only as Useful as Observations They Represent

The importance of knowing the identity of the observation represented by the statistic, as described in the example above, suggests another matter of importance to the investigator: the need for research to be conducted by persons knowledgeable about the problem of concern. Nursing research should be conducted by nurses, psychological research by psychologists, and so forth. This is not to say that members from other disciplines cannot be of help to nurses or nurses to them in their research. It does say that, where nursing research is to be done, nurses must be

Nursing Research By Nurses

intimately involved in all aspects of the study. Only a nurse could have been aware of the far-reaching meaning and implications of the limited agreement found among the nurse observers. Members of other disciplines might have merely reported the finding as fact and dismissed the matter with note that there was one less set of data than anticipated by which to test the hypothesis. A member of another discipline could not have made the judgments necessary to determine whether two activities were sufficiently similar as to indicate the same patient need and similar provision of care.

Essentially, then, descriptive data can frequently be collected with very little additional expenditure after the planning is done. Such data should not be collected merely because they will not be difficult to secure. But, if good judgment indicates that there may be value in having these particular data, though they are not immediately needed to meet the stated purpose of the study, their collection should be planned for. Suggestions to guide decisions and identification of particular data that might be of value will come from the definition of problem, where speculations about many closely related facets of the problem have been delineated. Besides this, there will always be interested persons who will suggest kinds of data the investigator might wish to collect.

An Investigator Must Say "No"

The investigator will do well to listen to these persons. Nonetheless, a warning should be interposed here: depending on the focus of their interests, watch out for them! If their interest is purely to help a fellow being, they may help. If their interest is a pet concern of their own, no matter how subtly demonstrated, the data that they propose collecting might very well be tangential to the investigator's purpose. This is not to say that the two can never be compatible, but the investigator's problem is to make sound judgments. He must say "NO" to collecting data that cannot add information to the problem as he has defined it and to the focal area he has selected for study.

Other considerations that must enter into decisions about types and quantities of data to be gathered are potential availability of the data and the means for making the necessary observations. There is also the matter of the time available, not only for collecting the data but, perhaps even more important, for analyzing them. A general idea about the potential complexity of this problem can be estimated at the time specific observations are identified as potentially useful data. As with other aspects of planning, the competence of the investigator will be an important consideration. By now the student will have recognized that each identifiable entity in the planning for research, no matter how simple it may seem on first thought, has many elements composing it and must be considered in the light of many impinging factors. Identifying potentially useful data and deciding which to collect or not to collect, require extensive planning with many interacting considerations. Once this planning has been completed and each type of datum precisely described, the investigator is really on his way. There are many complex steps to be planned but, once the data are known, all items needing planning become concrete. Thinking and planning will be in terms of individual, one at a time, observable phenomena.

REFERENCES

1. Godfrey, A. E. A study of nursing care designed to assist hospitalized children and their parents in their separation. Nurs. Res., 4:52, 1955.
2. Lesser, M. S., and Keane, V. R. Nurse-Patient Relationships in a Hospital Maternity Service. St. Louis, Mo., The C. V. Mosby Co., 1956.
3. Wandelt, M. A. Uninterrupted Patient Care and Nursing Requirements. Detroit, College of Nursing, Wayne State University, 1963, pp. 121-126.
4. Abdellah, F. G., Beland, I., Martin, A., and Metheney, R. Patient-centered Approaches to Nursing. New York, The Macmillan Company, 1960.
5. Goshen, C. E. The tyranny of words. Saturday Review, February 6, 1960, p. 57.

STEP 6
METHOD OF STUDY AND SOURCES OF DATA

TERMS DEFINED

Method: Method is "a way of doing anything; mode; process; especially, a regular, orderly, definitive procedure or way of teaching, investigating, etc."

Technique: Technique is "the method of procedure (with reference to practical and formal details) in rendering an artistic work or carrying out a scientific or mechanical operation."

Method of Study: Method of study is the general pattern (the blueprint) for organizing the procedures for gathering all the data for the investigation.

Technique of Data Gathering: Technique of data gathering is the process of making individual observations of phenomena or entities. A technique is a process by which data are collected, one datum at a time. All accumulated observations will compose the data for the investigation.

Type of Research: Type of research refers to the general purpose for doing a particular investigation, such as pursuing a study for the purpose of describing, demonstrating, applying, testing. For example, as a type of research, descriptive research is done for the purpose of revealing new knowledge by describing situations or conditions. Applied research is done for the purpose of learning how to utilize knowledge. General purpose is not to be confused with the definitive statement of purpose, which makes specific the focus of the study.

Population: Population is the general group or category of entities under study; individual entities in the population may be animate or inanimate; animal, vegetable, or mineral. The population is represented in the study by selected subjects (the study sample) from whom the facts needed as data derive.

Study Subject: Study subject is an entity from which the facts needed for study derive: the object of study that manifests the qualities and actions to be observed.

Source of Data: Source of data is an entity from which facts needed for study are obtained by the investigator. A source may be the study subject from which the facts are obtained by direct observation. A source may also be an object or person from which the needed facts, as observed and recorded or reported by others, are obtained. By way of example, the datum, age, may be available to the investigator from various sources. One source may be the study subject: the investigator may ask the patient his age. Another source may be a person who knows the patient: the investigator may ask the patient's relative, his nurse, or his physician. Still another source may be a record: the investigator may obtain the datum, age, from the patient's clinical record. Essentially, then, the study subject is the ultimate source from which the facts needed for study derive, and from which the facts needed for study may be directly or indirectly obtained. The study subject may be thought of as a direct or indirect source of the data, but not all direct sources are study subjects. The study subject is the entity which possesses and manifests the observable phenomena of concern (the data sought). The data may be obtained either directly, by observation of the study subject as the source, or indirectly, from other sources, by excerpting or eliciting observations recorded or reported about the study subject.

Setting for Study: Setting for study is the general locale in which the sources of the data are expected to be located and in which the data collection procedures will be carried out.

CONCEPTS PERTINENT TO DEFINED TERMS

Distinct Meanings: Method, Technique

The terms "method" and "technique" are used interchangeably by most researchers. It is difficult to understand why they persist in this practice, since it is quite simple to ascribe a precise and distinguishing meaning to each term as it is used in reference to research. The distinct meanings could encompass the generally accepted concepts of each, but could be devised in such a way as to eliminate the fuzziness about distinctions in their meanings. Distinct meanings could allow each to refer to a specific set of concepts and, in turn, not allow either to refer to the set of concepts "belonging" to the other. One possible explanation for the persistence of the practice of interchanging the terms is that "method," as a word standing alone, has not been defined in terms of its particular meaning or connotation in research.

Most authors "define" method by identifying various "methods" and then launch into a discussion and description of the individual "methods." None defines the term as an entity in itself, one that can stand alone. Instead, they presume that identification of several examples of the generalized concept will serve to define it. Here is a converse from the usual difficulty with definitions. Usually, definitions are limited to broad generalizations expressed in very abstract terms, without concrete illustration to promote common understanding. In contrast, most researchers, in defining method, omit a generalization that would encompass all methods, and limit the definition to describing several individual methods. Similarly, entities frequently are defined by identifying their actions, without describing the entity itself. For example, an automobile may be defined as a vehicle used for transportation, either as a luxury or a necessity; it may be a sports car used for pleasure or a taxi used as a necessary commodity. This definition identifies some attributes of an automobile, but does not identify the entity itself. No matter how extensive the listing of illustrative examples, it cannot be exhaustive, whereas a definition of the entity itself encompasses all examples of the phenomena of its class. A definition of the entity itself permits common understanding of the concept denoted by the term.

Method of Study

The common understanding derives from knowledge of the qualifying properties of the general class that would be possessed by all particular members of the class. It is entirely possible to define the general class of *method* by identifying usually understood properties of the word, along with those peculiar to a general concept meaningful in research connotations. Such a definition would promote understanding and serve as a base for clarifying distinctions among, and understanding of, particular methods. A distinctive definition of the term "method" is needed, not only because it is interchanged with other terms which may well have distinguishing definitions of their own, but also because researchers rarely agree as to the precise meanings of particular methods. This lack of consensus means that a listing of particular methods, with detailed descriptions of several, still does not provide for identifying concepts of sufficient commonality to permit intelligent, succinct communication.

The dictionary definitions reveal that, in general context, the meanings of the two words, method and technique, are indeed similar. Procedure and process are given as synonyms of method. Method of procedure and carrying out a scientific operation are used to define technique. Yet it is entirely possible, for the purposes of communication about research, to ascribe meanings that would provide distinct meanings for each term and thus facilitate communication and thinking. This would seem necessary because of the confusion resulting from the fact that researchers so often use the word "method" as a term with specific research connotation, referring to one step in the total process of investigation, and then, later on, use the word interchangeably with technique, when they are referring to another entity in the investigation process.

Distinct Steps: Method, Technique

The definitions for the two terms, as presented at the beginning of this chapter, do identify specific, distinct meanings for each term. Each can be reserved for reference to the set of concepts identified in its definition. Each should and does refer broadly to an individual step in the process of research. Both definitions—method (of study) and technique (of data collection)—encompass the concept, orderly procedure, used in the general (dictionary) definitions of the terms. In each the procedure is one designed for securing the facts needed, but the procedures are of quite different scope.

Method "of Research" Technique "of Data Gathering"

The concept "organizing the procedures" encompasses the planning for and execution of the activities of persons, the accomplishment of tasks, and the scheduling needed to carry out the data collection portion of the investigation. The activities of persons, of course, means the activities of the study subjects, the observers (data collectors), and those who will introduce the independent variable, as well as activities of others who may be involved. The *method* is the blueprint for obtaining all of the data for the investigation, whereas the *technique* is the blueprint for securing one single datum.

The definitions proposed here for the two terms do not differ from the meanings ascribed to the terms by other researchers. The difference lies in the recommendation that *method* be used to encompass a procedure of broad scope, with *technique* referring to a procedure of limited scope. The terms should not be used interchangeably.

Analogies: Diagnosis, Method, Treatment, Technique

A help in remembering these specific meanings is to attach to each the phrase proposed in its definition: method "of study," and techniques "of data gathering." Conceiving of method as analogous to diagnosis, and of technique as analogous to treatment, provides some rationale for the distinction of meanings. Diagnosis is defined as "a careful investigation of the facts to determine the nature of a thing; the decision or opinion resulting from such an examination or investigation." Further analogy between method and diagnosis may be seen in the relationship of the sources of data to the determination of the method of study. Essentially, the diagnostician examines the subject or situation and, on the basis of all facts observed, combined with related knowledge, he "makes a diagnosis."

Concepts Pertinent to Defined Terms 165

The examination reveals the immediate facts about the patient, the physician relates these to knowledge he possesses, and he identifies the set of facts and concepts so derived with a single word or brief phrase: a diagnosis. In research, the investigator determines the facts he must secure as data, he relates these to knowledge he possesses about potential sources of data and the setting in which the sources may be expected to be located. He then identifies the set of facts and concepts so derived with a single phrase: the method of study. In both instances, the particular word or phrase alludes to a generalization that all persons knowledgeable in the area would understand. Given the same sets of facts, all would agree to the ascribed title of the diagnosis or the ascribed title of the method. The analogy holds even further. The concepts denoted by a particular diagnosis give rise to proposals for particular actions and so do the concepts denoted by a particular method. For example, the diagnosis lobar pneumonia would identify for a physician a general set of signs and symptoms that exist in the individual patient and that he readily associates with specific knowledge. These, in turn, suggest to him a particular set of actions to be taken for treatment. The method experimental would identify for the researcher potential sources of data, the setting for location of the sources, and a general set of plans for the data-securing procedure. It would also suggest a particular set of actions to be taken for securing the data.

Parenthetically, it may be noted that, in relation to nursing care of patients, nurses use the term "diagnosis" to refer only to the general concept of the examination process. They do not delineate any individual diagnoses nor ascribe identifying titles, nor do they identify particular sets of facts and principles with identifying words or phrases to serve as generalizations referring to a particular diagnosis. They do not declare a particular "diagnosis," in a single word or brief phrase, that represents to them and to others a commonly understood set of facts and concepts, along with an appropriate course of action.

Nursing Diagnosis

Many nurses have thought extensively about the concept, nursing diagnosis, and have delineated the applicability of the concept to nursing actions. They describe the process of developing a nursing diagnosis: the nurse observes the facts about (symptoms of) the patient; she relates these to her background of scientific knowledge; she prescribes a course of action; and she plans the evaluation of outcomes to be followed, as indicated, by modifications of actions. All this follows the pattern and process of the physician as he makes a diagnosis. But nurses have not delineated an array of generally understood patterns of symptoms, interrelated science facts, and pertinent principles to guide courses of actions. They have not ascribed names to individual patterns that would provide generalizations for succinct communication of ideas commonly understood by all knowledgeable in the field. The analogy between a nursing diagnosis and a medical diagnosis holds for the detailed process of arrival at the needs of the patient and plan for his care. It falls short in relation to one-word or brief-phrase generalizations that permit succinct communication of the outcomes of the process.

Common Understanding: Exists for Method, Lacking for Technique

Another cause for wonder at the persistence of the practice of interchanging the terms "method" and "technique" is that, when a particular method is identified by its generalized term—"experimental," for instance—most researchers have a common understanding of the pattern or set of facts and concepts that is under consideration. Whereas, although technique is generally perceived as referring to a narrower "set of facts and concepts" than method, there is much less common understanding of any particular set of facts and circumstances identified by the name of a particular technique. The analogy of method to diagnosis may be extended to elaborate an analogy of technique to treatment. The analogies may serve to explain the differences in degree of common understanding associated with titles of individual methods and those associated with the titles of individual techniques. Any particular, individual diagnosis communicates a commonly understood pattern of symptoms and interrelated science facts. Similarly, any particular, individual method communicates to a researcher a commonly understood pattern of potential sources of data and settings in which sources may be located. A diagnosis communicates a commonly understood course of action (treatment), but the implied treatment is not nearly so narrowly definitive as is the pattern of symptoms and related science facts. For example, the diagnosis lobar pneumonia clearly identifies the symptoms manifested by the patient and the related pathophysiological facts. It suggests, too, a general course of action—physical rest and antimicrobial drug therapy—but the total treatment must be described in more complete detail in order to communicate common understanding of it. So it is with method: a particular method communicates a commonly understood course of actions for data collection (techniques). The implied techniques, however, are not nearly so definitively identified by the title of the particular method as is the pattern of sources and settings. Experimental method communicates the concepts that two groups of similar subjects, in comparable controlled settings, will be sources of data. It also suggests that the data will be gathered through use of some general observation technique: some form of direct observation of the study subjects. But only a detailed description of the technique will communicate common understanding of the total process planned for use in the particular experimental investigation.

In summary: (1) There are many more techniques than there are methods of research. The number of methods may be set at four (philosophical, historical, survey, and experimental). The number of techniques continues to grow, as new ones are developed. (2) The sets of facts and concepts identified by any particular method are accepted in common by most researchers. (3) Few techniques have been identified with a fairly circumscribed set of facts and concepts commonly understood by all researchers. (4) Most techniques used are combinations of several identified techniques. Communication about them must be done with detailed description and qualifying statements, rather than with a generalized term used to identify the set of facts and concepts mutually understood and accepted by the researcher and knowledgeable peers. (5) Most investigations will utilize more than one technique, whereas, essentially, only one method will be used in any one investigation.

Returning to the analogies, a particular diagnosis is a generalization that communicates a commonly understood pattern of observations and known facts and the general direction of treatment. But, for complete understanding of the treatment to be used in any one case, a detailed description of the treatment is necessary. The details of treatment individualize the physician's plan for the individual patient. So, in research, the particular method communicates a commonly understood pattern of sources and their settings and indicates the general process for collecting the data. But for complete understanding of the technique (the process) to be used for securing the data, a detailed description of each technique is necessary. The details about the techniques will individualize the techniques and will fit them to the particular data to be derived from particular sources in a particular setting or settings.

SOURCE DICTATES METHOD

Since the sources of data must be considered before the method of study can be identified, the position of the two concepts might be reversed in the title of Step 6. The designation, as given, is in deference to general thinking about elements in the research process. Many writers discuss only briefly the planning for sources of data, while most devote entire chapters to a single method. The fact remains, though, that thinking about sources of data actually initiates the thinking about method. The latter is dictated by the sources the investigator decides to use. Furthermore, the details of planning the method need not be and usually are not completed until Step 9. Although these two phases, determining method and determining source in the planning of research, are usually treated as though they were distinct steps, there is no logical reason for so designating them. As the investigator elaborates the rationale for selecting the particular source from which he will seek data, he is elaborating the rationale for the method of his study. Indeed, the sources of the data rigidly dictate the method to be pursued for establishing conditions pertinent to data collection. This concept is self-evident from the definitions to follow of the four methods of study. The terms (titles) identifying the various methods offer general indications of the sources from which data will be secured.

Data: Derived From Subject, Obtained From Source

The population to be studied will have been identified in the statement of purpose, and the exact representatives, the study subjects, will have been made specific in the definitions of terms. The sources of the data, however, cannot and should not be determined until the planning for the types and precise descriptions of the data has been completed. At first thought, "population to be studied" and "sources of data" may seem synonymous. But, although it is possible for the subjects representing the population to be the sources of data, they are not necessarily and always the immediate sources from which the investigator directly obtains the data. In order to proceed with planning, it is necessary to distinguish between study subjects and sources of data. In turn, it is necessary to distinguish each from the persons who will collect the data. It is possible for one individual to serve in all three of these roles but, when this is so, it should be made explicit; it should not be left implied.

To identify the sources of data, it is helpful to remember that data are gathered by making one observation of a phenomenon at a time and that all observed phenomena used as data in scientific inquiry will ultimately be recorded in some form. After the data have been precisely described, it is possible to begin planning about various stiuations and places where the phenomena occur or observations of them are recorded. It is possible, also, to envision the potential forms in which they may be observed and recorded. Only rarely is there but one possible source from which to obtain the necessary observations. After several possible sources for needed data have been identified, the feasibility of using each can be evaluated. Among the factors influencing the final selection will be the availability of subjects and of persons to make and record the observations, the length of time required to make observations in various settings and conditions, and the time required for the anticipated effects of the independent variable to become measureable.

Example: Uninterrupted Patient Care

In the Uninterrupted Patient Care study, for instance, the hypothesis was:

> If a chronically ill patient receives care for an uninterrupted period of time from a professional nurse, his care requirements, implied or expressed, will be modified and the attitudes of the nursing personnel responsible for his care will be modified—modifications will trend in directions judged desirable by those responsible for his nursing care.[1]

The study subjects were randomly selected, chronically ill, hospitalized adults. The data sought were observations of activities performed by nursing personnel to meet nursing needs of the patients, the time required to perform the activities, requests made by the patients, the attitudes of personnel toward the patients, and estimates of the nursing care activities needed to provide optimum nursing care. Pertinent terms were defined (here abbreviated):

Nursing care requirements are the activities which must be performed by nurses to fulfill patient's nursing care needs. Nursing care activities change as the patient's nursing needs change.

Activities are those tasks performed by the hospital nursing personnel to provide nursing care for the patient.

Time is the amount of time (in minutes) spent by members of the hospital nursing staff in performing the nursing care activities for one patient during any specified period of a day.

Requests are overt signs made by the patient to indicate a need, or wish, for assistance from members of the nursing staff. Requests might be verbal, body motion, or mechanical signal, such as a bell or light.

Attitudes are expressions of the way persons feel about patients. The concept of an attitude as a "set for some kind of action" was basic to the development of the tool to measure the attitudes of personnel and to the inclusion of this variable in the hypothesis.

Chronically ill adults were the population being studied; randomly selected patients, the study subjects. Yet, except for the number of requests made for care, the patients were only indirectly sources for any of the many types of data collected. The nursing service personnel were the sources for the activities performed and the time required to perform the activities. The activities and time were two criterion measures of nursing care requirements. The data were observations of personnel as they interacted with patients, but the personnel were the sources of the data. The criterion measures and the individual measurements (individual observations) influenced the selection of the "entities" to be observed—the sources of the data.

Nursing service personnel, in addition, were asked to fill out a checklist, Patient Rating Scale, which measured their attitudes toward individual patients. For these data, the personnel were the subjects being studied, the sources of the data, and the collectors as well, since they recorded the "observations" of their attitudes. When the nurse observers estimated the nursing care requirements, they were sources as well as data collectors. In this instance, however, unlike that for measuring personnel attitudes, the subjects were the patients. The data were intended to measure changes in the patient, not the nurses' ability to make the estimates.

It would have been possible, in the course of this investigation, to ask patients to indicate the attitudes that personnel displayed toward them, or to ask head nurses to estimate the attitudes of personnel toward individual patients. Had this been done, the subjects would have remained the personnel, as they were when they filled out the Patient Rating Scale, but the sources of data, in distinction, would have been the patients or the head nurses or both. This illustrates how the distinction between source, subject, and observer (data collector) can become sticky. When head nurses estimate attitudes of personnel, are they reporting observations of the subjects, with the latter being the study subjects? Or are they reporting observations of phenomena that stem from themselves, which would make them the study subjects *and* the sources of the data? Since their "observations" would not be single, individual, identifiable phenomena manifested by the individual whose attitudes they were reporting, it could be said that the head nurses were the sources of the individual observations, though the subjects of study would be the personnel. The data considered in these examples more or less required using the subjects of study or persons in communication with them as sources.

Time and Cost Influence Selection of Source

Time and cost are frequently inextricably related to each other as they influence the selection of sources of data. They, in turn, are dependent on the techniques selected for making the observations. The sources of data used by 3B (pages 148–149) illustrate how time and cost influenced the selection. A quick consideration of the nature of the phenomena to be observed would indicate that hospitalized, fatally ill children, the subjects of the investigation, would be the sources of data. Further consideration, however, indicates that finding even 20 such subjects who might be directly observed, even if for only a few days each, would require a considerable period of time. It was therefore determined that parents of the subjects might serve as sources of data. They would have observed and could report the various actions, responses, and comments of their children. From the parents it would also be possible to obtain items of data (phenomena) occurring over an extended period of time, while only brief periods could feasibly be involved were the children themselves to serve as sources and direct observations used for securing the data. The decision made by 3B exemplifies how consideration of potential sources, other than the study subjects themselves, can lead not only to identification of other sources, but also to a source that might be expected to yield more extensive and more complete data than might be expected from direct observation of the study subjects.

Considerations Beyond the Obvious

The example of 3B also emphasizes the fact that the researcher must do his planning with an open and searching mind. The source from which any one type of datum will be sought should not be selected until all possible sources have been considered. The illustration from the Uninterrupted Care study and the comment about any one type of datum, of course, remind the student that sources must be selected for each type of datum sought. Although many types of data may be secured from a single source, sometimes several sources will be needed for the various data. Occasionally, data of a single type will be secured from more than one source. An example of two different sources for a single type of datum might be the study subject and the clinical record as sources for observations of the patient's vital signs. This is not the same thing as when patients, nurses, and physicians, for example, are all asked questions about the routine of strict bedrest for a cardiac patient. In this instance, the three groups would not be three different sources for the same type of datum, as in the previous example. Rather, they would be three different sources for three different types of data about three different study subject groups.

Perhaps the first thing an investigator should think of when considering sources of data is whether the needed data already exist in recorded form. He needs to be sure of this, however, before he goes any further in his planning. Frequently, it seems so obvious that the data would exist that no check is made until all planning has been completed and the time to collect data has arrived. Only then is it discovered that the data that "naturally" would be on record are not. It is remarkable that observations made and recorded for one purpose, although seemingly the exact observations needed for another purpose, can be so unlike those needed for the second purpose. This is true to such an extent and with such frequency, that an investigator should not presume that even recordings of age made for some prior purpose will serve his purpose. For instance, he may need data on age to the nearest month, or to the last birthday, or to the coming birthday. Or he may want to categorize age to the nearest birthday. The source to which he might go may record age only in years with no indication of birthdate or relationship of stated years to time of birthday. Or suppose a nurse researcher is concerned with patients' fluid intake and output. There are few observations more frequently recorded by nurses than patient's intake and output, yet no nurse would plan to use existing charts as sources for these data for her planned research. This is because the usual recordings of these phenomena are notoriously imprecise and could not serve research purposes. Though existing recorded data may be limited in usability, because of the potential economy, this source should always be considered as a possibility.

Existing Records as Source of Data

Another precaution in relation to using already recorded data is that such sources should not be prematurely identified. In other words, investigators should not begin to plan their research on the basis of knowing of a set of recorded observations and believing that something should be done with them. Such a procedure is almost certain to lead to frustration. On the other hand, some investigators reject what might well be the most meaningful data they could secure for their study. They believe it would be impossible to find a source from which the data might be obtained. They reject the idea of searching for the most meaningful data and plan to seek data more conspicuously obtainable. Either extreme, whether planning research around existing data or deciding to seek less meaningful data

Influence of Ready Availability of Data

on the basis of potential difficulty in finding a source of more meaningful data, may be in error. Each should be given fair examination before completion of Steps 5 and 6.

The investigator should always attempt to determine the most likely source of data and give consideration to the setting in which the source is likely to yield the data sought. This may not always be the most obvious place or the most convenient, as illustrated by the story of the intoxicated man who was diligently searching the ground around a lightpost. When asked, he said that he had dropped his keys. The solicitous person joined in the search. After a few minutes of no success, he asked the man where, exactly, he thought he had dropped them. The reply: Oh, I dropped them over by my car, but I'm looking here, because the light is much better.

As the investigator thinks through the many considerations pertinent to selecting sources of data, he will concomitantly be considering the methods by which data are collected. The rationalizations that underlie the decisions made about the sources of data will also apply to the selection of the particular method chosen for obtaining the data. The intricate interrelationships of the two phases will be further delineated, below, in the discussion of concepts about method and particular methods for organizing the data-collecting tasks of the investigation. The complete pattern of the data-collecting phase of the investigation will be described in Step 9.

Other Labels for Concepts of Method

The method of study will be dictated, primarily, by sources of the data and the settings in which the sources are expected to be located. How many possible research methods are there? This is a matter on which research authorities rarely agree. Furthermore, as any text on elements of research will indicate, there are various conceptions of "method." Some writers, rather than identifying method as a step in the research process, speak of it in terms of "types of research" and "categories of research." Still others use words, such as "experimental" and "survey," as adjectives to modify the words "research" or "study," although most researchers use these words to identify specific methods. They then use the resulting phrases as though they referred to the complete process of a particular investigation, rather than to the plan for organizing its data collection phase. For example, they may discuss "experimental research" or "descriptive research" as though either phrase identified all facts and concepts of the entire investigational process. Or they use them as though the researcher could decide first the method of research to be used and then proceed to define his problem, decide on his data and their sources, and develop the plans for collecting the data. In all probability, the titles of the methods for data collection are used as titles for the entire investigations because the data-collecting portion of the investigation is the one in which the most people are involved and is the most concrete and visible portion of the study. Furthermore, since each method title implies the sources of the data, it also implies,

Four Methods

grossly, the nature of the data to be used. From these broad hints of the nature of the study, the overall nature of the study is inferred.

The four methods to be described may make the rationale for the above concept a little clearer. It is, indeed, true that certain broad aspects of the findings may be anticipated from the identity of the sources of data implied by the title of the method. But imputing the implications of all of these entities to the concept of the method of investigation will produce one of two undesirable results: (1) planning in relation to the many entities will be left in broad outline; (2) the large concept of method will have to be analyzed into multiple smaller concepts and detailed plans developed in relation to each one. The first result will permit gaps in planning and unnecessary flaws in the completed investigation. The latter will result in a cannot-see-the-forest-for-the-trees situation: the method will be lost in the maze of details about its many purported components.

Limitations When Method Connotes Total Research Process

Kaplan proposes: "Methods include such procedures as forming concepts and hypotheses, making observations and measurements, performing experiments, building models and theories, providing explanations, and making predictions."[2] The only purpose that such a conglomerate sentence can serve is to alert the student to the fact that he may anticipate finding the term "method" ascribed to any entity or any conception of entities composing the research process. Perhaps the term should be retained only as a catch-all word, with no definitive meaning. But it would seem that ascribing a definitive meaning to the term—one that can serve as a reasonable generalization and that can hold constant in its meaning in relation to other terms—can provide the student with a definitive concept to use in thinking and developing his own conceptualizations of relationships among the entities of the research process.

FOUR METHODS

Four distinct methods of research can be identified to account for all patterns for organizing procedures used to accomplish the collection of data in scientific inquiries. The four methods are: (1) philosophical, (2) historical, (3) survey, and (4) experimental.

Philosophical method refers to the general pattern for organizing procedures for collecting facts that derive from the minds of men, where the phenomena, the observations of which will make up the data, are thoughts of men from the past, present, and future.

Historical method refers to the general pattern for organizing procedures for collecting facts derived from study subjects from the past, where the phenomena, the observations of which will make up the data, are no longer available for direct observation, but must be excerpted or inferred from "records."

174 STEP 6: METHOD OF STUDY AND SOURCES OF DATA

Survey method refers to the general pattern for organizing procedures for collecting facts that are derived from study subjects of the present, where the phenomena, the observations of which will make up the data, are currently occurring and observable.

Experimental method refers to the general pattern for organizing procedures for collecting facts that derive from study subjects of the future, where the phenomena, the observations of which will make up the data, will occur and be observable only in the future.

Method and Degree of Concreteness of Data

Essentially, these four terms describe the ultimate source from which the data derive and the sources from which they will be secured. The nature of the types of data pertinent to specific methods of study may be thought of as moving from very abstract along a continuum to the very concrete. Some facts collected for a study are ideas about nonobservable concepts. Others are ideas about observable phenomena, and still others are clearly measurable (observable) entities. Thus, facts collected as data range from (1) those that exist only in mental conceptualizations with no concrete referents, to (2) mental conceptualizations with concrete referents, to (3) observable objects with mass, form, and texture.

Nurses and Changes in Philosophy

The philosophical method will be chosen where the facet of the problem selected for study is one involving moral and/or ethical issues, and the facts needed are ideas pertinent to the issues. The source of data will, ultimately, be the minds of men. Nurses have engaged in little philosophical research and perhaps will do very little in this area for some years. Yet they should be aware that society must address itself to study of philosophical problems and that nursing practice will be greatly influenced by findings from such studies. Nurses should feel a responsibility for contributing in this area of exploration. Just as they are beginning to recognize responsibility for sharing in the provision of better physical and mental health care for people, so, too, they must share in shaping changes in philosophies that dictate the nature of the care provided. Nurses should not wait to be told of philosophical changes and of the consequent changes in care; they should share in making those philosophical changes. Indeed, there is no reason that nurses should not lead in this important area.

Methods Related to Era

The definitions of each method indicate that the method for organizing data collection procedures is determined by the period in time at which the phenomena to be observed occur: (1) If the phenomena occurred in the past and the facts to be collected as data were observations of the phenomena recorded at the time of the occurrence or were observations of objects from the past that may be interpreted as facts about past phenomena, the method of study will be historical. (2) If the phenomena exist or are occurring in the present, if the facts to be used are observations of what is, of phenomena as they exist and may be observed today, the method will be survey. (3) If the phenomena have yet to occur, if the facts to be collected as data will occur only in the future, with the investigator manipulating conditions in a manner calculated to effect their occurrence, the method will be experimental.

The lines dividing these methods may sometimes be fuzzy, with some mingling of methods in any one investigation. For example, in a retrospective study of hospital infections occurring during the past three years, but including patients currently hospitalized, the direct or immediate sources of the data would be patients' clinical records; some of the phenomena would have occurred and been recorded in the past, and some in the present. Or the situation may be one where measurements will be made of phenomena in the dependent variable, followed by introduction of the independent variable, and subsequent measurements made of the dependent variable. It may be argued that the first measurements of the dependent variable are observations of phenomena that exist in the present, and those taken following the introduction of the independent variable would be observations of phenomena occurring at a future time. In the first example, is the method for collecting the facts historical or survey? In the second, is it survey or experimental, or are two methods used in each study? This impasse may possibly be handled by considering the definition of method of study as an overall pattern for organizing procedures for collecting data, with particular methods referring to commonly understood patterns.

Historical Method

The commonly understood pattern for historical method is one where the researcher seeks data about phenomena no longer available for direct observation, due either to extinction of the study population or to extinction of particular settings or situations involving the population of study. For example, a sociologist may wish to trace changes in family relationships in three-generation families, with all family members residing in the same community, from families in colonial New York to present-day families in New York State. Study subjects of the three-generation families are available for direct observation today, but many of the phenomena involving study subjects of three-generation families of colonial New York are not. The general pattern for collecting the needed data would involve seeking recordings and other evidences of phenomena that occurred in the past.

Survey Method

The general pattern for organizing procedures for collecting data denoted by survey method is one where the facts sought are observations of phenomena involving study subjects existing today and available for direct observation. This does not mean that all observations will be directly from the study subjects since, in some instances, they may have been made in the recent past, but the subjects are available and the observations could be made directly. It would be possible to make the observations today, though it may not always be feasible to do so. In the example cited in the discussion of definition of sources of data (page 162) about the

176 STEP 6: METHOD OF STUDY AND SOURCES OF DATA

age of a patient, the datum needed might be obtained from a previous recording of the fact or directly from the patient. The study subject is available or potentially available so that a direct observation can be made; the phenomenon and its ultimate source, the study subject, exist today.

Experimental Method

Experimental method refers to a pattern for organizing procedures for collecting data, or a study process, wherein the phenomena to be observed will be expected to occur as a result of controlled circumstances. The phenomena to be observed will be available only in the future. The investigator will have determined that the conditions under which he expects the phenomena to occur do not now exist or do not exist in a place available to him for observation. He will plan to establish the conditions by controlling the variable he believes will have predictable influence on the study subjects, thereby making the phenomena available for observation.

Method and Data Analysis

Before detailed plans for the collection of data are developed (Step 9), it is necessary to decide on the techniques to be used for making the observations and the tools for recording them (Steps 7 and 8). First, however, let us consider some other elements in the research process that some have identified as "method." Some writers perceive method as implying patterns for analyzing the data as well as the pattern for collecting them. This, however, does not seem consistent with the components of other steps in the research process. The patterns for analyzing data are dictated more by the stated purpose of the study and the nature of the data than by the sources from which the data are collected. The relation of data analysis to focus of study and nature of data will be discussed in detail in Step 11.

METHOD, TYPE, GENERAL PURPOSE

Perhaps the most confusing interchange of the term "method" to mean something other than the general organizing pattern for collecting the data is its interchange with the term "technique" to mean the process by which observations are made. Next to this is the interchange of the term "method" with the term "type" when it is viewed as meaning the general purpose for doing the research. Yet those who use the word in the latter context describe the various "types" of research as though the term referred to a generalized description of the presentation of the findings. On the premise that all research is done for the purpose of revealing new knowledge, identifying specific types of research can help to clarify this point. (1) Descriptive research is done for the purpose of revealing new knowledge by describing situations and conditions, the entities and phenomena composing them, the interrelationships of phenomena, and so on. (2) Philosophical research is done to reveal new knowledge through the study of philosophical issues as they are conceptualized by various thinkers. (3) Epidemiological research is done for the purpose of revealing new knowledge by studying all factors (and their interdependence) that affect the occurrence and course of health and disease in a population. (4) Basic or pure research is done for the purpose of revealing knowledge about phenomena where interrelationships with other phenomena are unknown and hypotheses about them are nebulous. (5) Practical or applied research is undertaken for the purpose of learning how to utilize existing knowledge to improve the welfare of society. (6) Demonstration research is done for the purpose of demonstrating processes of interrelationships of phenomena, with close observation to identify sequence and effects of occurrences of phenomena under study.

These and many more *types* of research have been referred to as *methods* of research. In terms of meaning "a regular, orderly, definite procedure or way of . . . investigating," and meaning "an overall pattern," method may be considered an appropriate term to use in reference to these various types of research. Where it is so used, it does not cause as much confusion as when it is used interchangeably with technique. This may be because, in such usage, the general context of the materials in which it is found identifies the concept to which it refers. From the context, its meaning is readily distinguished from the meaning "pattern for collecting data." Whereas, in contexts where method and technique are used interchangeably, the precise referents for each may be difficult to identify. The interchange of the term "method" with the term "type" to refer to a broad description of the presentation of the findings (which, in turn, is identified by the users of the term "type" as meaning the definitive or general purpose for doing the study) is not overly confusing and will not frequently be misunderstood. Nonetheless, it does seem an unnecessary interchange of terms.

All of the above is intended to give the student researcher an awareness of the fact that the term "method" is used with a variety of connotations and to help him understand these connotations. He will then have bases for determining the particular connotation intended whenever he finds the term in research writings.

Guides and Relationships

It is anticipated that, through the concepts and guides presented in this text, the student will better visualize elements of the research process as distinct entities. As he learns to think about and to formulate his own conceptualizations of these various elements, he will proceed with greater understanding and clarity if he: (1) identifies precise meanings for various frequently used terms, (2) learns to use each to refer to its own definitive concept, and (3) avoids using terms interchangeably. These guides should also enable him to identify the relationship of one step to another and to the entire process.

SUMMARY

To recapitulate, then, the term "method" is used by others to refer to many elements in the research process and it is most frequently interchanged with the terms "technique" and "type." It has been proposed that precise and distinct meanings be ascribed to each of these terms and that they not be used interchangeably. The method of study may be thought of as the overall pattern for organizing and scheduling tasks and procedures for collecting the data, with the specific method being dictated by the sources from which the data will be sought. Essentially, there are four methods of study: (1) philosophical, where sources of data are the minds of men—past, present, and future; (2) historical, where the sources of data are records and remnants from past events, where study populations and pertinent phenomena are no longer extant and no longer available for direct observation; (3) survey, where the sources of data exist and are available for observation, though all data may not be collected by direct observation, but may be obtained from records or reports; (4) experimental, where sources of data lie in the future, and where the plan is to use sources from situations in which conditions are controlled by the researcher. Decisions about sources of data require extensive planning in relation to the nature of the data to be sought, the availability of the sources, the costs and time involved in utilizing the various sources, the time required for the independent variable to produce a measurable effect, and other factors.

Method is most frequently used interchangeably with the term "technique" to refer to the processes for making the individual observations of the phenomena that are the facts or data for the study. It is interchanged next most frequently with the term "type" to refer to the descriptions of the findings from the particular investigation. Such interchanging of terms leads to confusion both in communicating and in thinking. Restricting the use of each term to refer to its precise meaning places no restriction on communicating or thinking about concepts to which each refers nor about the relationship of these concepts to other elements in the total research process.

Essentially, Step 6 involves planning for and selecting the sources from which the various data will be sought. The sources will dictate the method of study, the overall pattern for organizing the tasks and procedures for collecting the data.

REFERENCES

1. Wandelt, M. A. Uninterrupted Patient Care and Nursing Requirements. Detroit, College of Nursing, Wayne State University, 1963, p. 1.
2. Kaplan, A. The Conduct of Inquiry. San Francisco, Chandler Publishing Company, 1964, p. 23.

STEP 7
TECHNIQUES

TERMS DEFINED

Technique: A technique is a process for making or obtaining individual observations of phenomena or entities. It is the process by which data are collected, one datum at a time.

CONCEPTS PERTINENT TO TERM DEFINED

The previous step differentiated between method and technique, identifying method as the general pattern for organizing the procedures for gathering the data needed for the investigation. The particular method is dictated by the sources from which data will be sought. Technique is identified as the data-collecting process by which observations are made a single datum at a time. Selection of techniques is dependent on the nature and sources of the needed data.

A second differentiation is needed to establish the concept of technique as a distinct entity not to be confused with other elements in the research process: a technique may be identified by describing the process of obtaining a single datum. The process of making a single observation of a single occurrence of a phenomenon is in contrast to the concept im-

Collecting One Datum

plied for Step 9, Collection of Data. Step 9 elaborates details of the method wherein plans are made for executing the many and varied activities necessary for collecting all needed data. Step 9 involves planning for securing permissions and cooperation from all persons to be involved in data collection; introducing the independent variable; scheduling time, place, and activities of data collectors; application of techniques and utilization of tools; and many other tasks.

Technique, Tool; Observation, Record

It is difficult to think about techniques without thinking about tools. Yet, the student should distinguish between them and be careful not to move on to Step 8 before he has completed Step 7. This is a temptation because the tool is concrete and easier to think about and plan than the technique. The student, as he is planning techniques, may move ahead to thinking about tools, not only because this is an easier task but also because one type of tool that may be needed is one required for making some of the observations. For some studies it will be necessary to develop tools for making, as well as for recording, the observations. But even when such tools are needed, the process for making the observation can and should be planned before the observation-making tool is developed. It is possible that the needed tool may be one already developed, such as a thermometer or a stopwatch. Or the needed tool may be one where a general idea about its nature is all that is needed to plan the process for using it. An example is an open-end questionnaire.

Many students, unfortunately, try to develop their tool long before they have decided, definitively, how the observations are to be made. Such practice usually gives rise to great frustration. Frequently, the student gives up, with the protest that he "just can't" figure out a tool that will be usable. He is usually right: he cannot develop a workable tool for recording his data when he has not yet determined the manner in which individual data, possibly of varying types, will be observed. It is hoped that before he reaches the point of complete frustration, he will recognize the cause of his difficulty and back up to complete work on Step 7.

Need for Caution About Thinking Ahead

Some thinking about tools, of course, will take place legitimately when techniques are being planned. Indeed, as each successive step in the planning is undertaken, there is increasingly greater involvement with other steps. Planning for the earlier steps can be done with attention focused on the single step. Beginning with Step 6, however, thinking ahead to other steps becomes necessary for making some of the decisions pertinent to planning the step of current concern. So it will be with all remaining steps. The student should be alert, nonetheless, to the purpose for which he allows himself to think of later steps as he plans for any particular step. That is, when planning for techniques, the student will think about tools, but he should think about them only to the extent that is essential to planning the technique. If a student who purportedly is addressing himself to planning for techniques finds himself picking up a ruler to facilitate precision in spacing for the tool he is thinking about, he has gone too far! He is now developing a tool and not merely thinking about it in terms of its relationship to the technique.

PLANNING TECHNIQUES

The plural, techniques, is used advisedly. Most investigations will involve utilization of more than one of the many techniques that have been developed for observing phenomena. Occasionally, a technique, as developed for one study, may be *adopted* without change for use in another study. More frequently, however, it is necessary to *adapt* previously developed techniques; sometimes, entirely new techniques must be developed. Considerable evidence of the proliferation of techniques may be found by thumbing through the journal *Nursing Research*. Not only does almost every report of research describe a specific, distinct technique, but the main purpose of many of the articles is to report the development and testing of a single technique.

For Every Study— One, Two, or More Techniques

Prior to beginning to plan the techniques he will use, the student should return to the library to learn about various existing techniques. Most detailed reports of investigations will fully describe the techniques used for making observations. Briefer reports published in journals will provide sufficient information about techniques to enable an investigator to decide about their potential usefulness for his own study. These reports will usually identify sources of more information about the techniques. Most introductory texts on research describe a number of techniques. Indeed, there are entire books devoted to describing techniques; some to describing a single technique. The student should develop a file of references of descriptions of techniques, making out a bibliography card for each new technique that he notes in his readings from the very beginning. He need not necessarily make notes of sufficient detail for his purposes, should he later decide to use the technique, but he should include enough information to identify the nature of the technique and to ensure finding the report again.

After becoming familiar with some of the techniques, the student should consider again the precise nature of each type of datum he plans to collect. He will think of these in relation to the sources from which the data are available and the particular ones from which he has decided to obtain the various data. He then will consider the total process needed to make the observation of one occurrence of one phenomenon. He will consider several elements in the process: (1) the entity to be observed (the object or subject selected to be the source of the data); (2) the immediate

Multifaceted Process

setting in which the source will be found at the time the observation is to be made; (3) the identity of the individual making the observation; (4) the process of making the observation (visual, auditory, tactile, and so forth); (5) whether a scaled measuring device is to be used to make the observation (thermometer, ruler, stethoscope, or others); (6) the relationship, in time and space, of the observed to the observer; and (7) other pertinent considerations. This planning must be done for each type of datum to be gathered. The development of planning about techniques can be made clearer by describing some techniques as they have been used.

Techniques in Behavioral Sciences

The techniques discussed here are mostly those developed for use in behavorial science research since, to date, most research done by nurses utilizes these techniques. (In general, before most nurses can undertake investigations where techniques from the physical and biological sciences would be used, they would have to enlarge their basic knowledge in the field of concern.) In the course of acquiring her background information, the student will learn many of the techniques appropriate for making observations in her chosen field. Many of these have been given names that are more or less descriptive of the process involved. A few of them will be listed and briefly described, with the reference list at the end of this chapter identifying sources for more detailed descriptions of the many techniques of particular usefulness to nurses.

ADOPT, ADAPT, COMBINE TECHNIQUES OF OTHERS

For most investigations, techniques will not be adopted for use; rather, they will be adapted or new ones will be developed. Furthermore, most studies will not involve a single technique as developed for another study, but rather a combination of "techniques." For example, Godfrey combined participant observation and process recording as the technique for securing the observations of the children studied. She used a questionnaire to secure the observations on the parents. And, in Example 2J (page 94), the investigator decided that observations of fear and anxiety experienced by nurses as they cared for tracheostomized patients could best be obtained by having nurses report critical incidents. The subject was asked to describe in detail a situation in which she experienced fear or anxiety as she provided care that involved suctioning or changing the tube. The investigator planned to interview nurses and have them tell her of their experiences. This represented a modification of the critical incident technique, as well as the interview technique for securing "observations" of phenomena. It is obvious that combinations of several other techniques might have served to secure observations needed as data in 2J's study. She could have used process recording and questionnaire; a projective technique, utilizing photographs and tape recordings; or others.

Adopt, Adapt, Combine Techniques of Others

Because "pure" techniques are seldom used and because the processes used to make needed observations for any one investigation or even for any one type of datum are usually hybrids of two or more techniques, the student frequently has difficulty in deciding on the *right* name for the technique he plans to use. This is the reversal of Col. Pickering's observation in *My Fair Lady*: "The French don't mind what they do particularly, so long as they pronounce it properly." It does not really matter what a technique is named, so long as the process is described adequately.

A title that applies to the primary elements in the technique might be used, but even this does not always help; sometimes more than one technique has major import. Another solution might be hyphenated titles, which could serve two purposes: (1) to be more definitive of the process than any single-concept title could be; (2) to alert the reader to the fact that the process is not a "pure" adopted technique, but rather an adaptation of two or more techniques.

The critical incident technique is an example of how infrequently techniques are adopted and how frequently they are adapted. Critical incident has potential for extensive use in nursing studies in adapted form, but only limited use in pure adopted form. This technique was developed by John C. Flanagan for studying behaviors of men in the United States Air Force.[1,2] He developed a rather precise process, which utilized nonparticipant observation and included a specific scaling for the observations. The technique, as he detailed it, is usable only for collection of data very similar to those in the studies for which he developed the technique. He conceived of the critical incident as an episode wherein the behavior of the subject would make a difference in the situation, either for the subject or for others involved. In addition, enough of the episode must be observed so that a decision may be made about the direction the result would take; that is, whether the behavior would have a positive or negative effect. Many studies of concern to nurses will require data about nurses' or patients' behavior or about processes such as nurses' responses to patients' questions, changes in patients being treated for shock, or changes in patients receiving oxygen therapy. In such instances the concept of the critical incident is very useful to nurse researchers. Another illustration of the usefulness of the critical incident concept is delineated as it is contrasted to process recording, pages 193–194, below. It should be noted, however, that utilization of the *concept* of the technique implies the adapting rather than the adopting of the technique. Several techniques useful for nurses will be briefly discussed here to demonstrate the usual pattern for utilizing techniques developed for other studies. The pattern is to utilize the general concept of the technique with adaptation for delineating many components of a process suitable for making observations requisite to the planned study, and to the specific data and sources pertinent to it.

What's in a Name

Adaptation: Using the Concept Rather Than the Original Process

Participant Observation

Participant observation is a technique wherein the individual making the observations becomes, or already is, a member of the study subjects' group. Or the observer may assume the role of an individual commonly associated with the study subjects. Godfrey, to a degree, used a dual aspect of this concept when she had her students record observations of the children's reactions and behaviors.[3] The students were nurses who usually provided care for the children; yet, for the experimental group, they extended their care to assume somewhat the role of the parents. (One of the classical examples of the use of participant observation is the study reported by Margaret Meade, in her *Coming of Age in Samoa*.) Information about the technique, participant observation, has been widely reported as it has been used in studies of street gangs. Originally, in these studies, college students sought to be accepted by the gangs and they lived with them. Recently, youngsters of the same ages as members of the gangs have been trained to be observers. They have been youths selected from specific gangs, or youths who have ostensibly "moved" into the neighborhood and become members of the gangs. Participant observation is useful for gathering data in many nurse-patient situations. For the nurse who wishes to consider this as a potential technique for her purposes, Marion Pearsall's "Participant Observation as Role and Method in Behavioral Research," is perhaps the best first reference.[4]

Two major factors influence the decision to use participant observation. First, it may be the only technique whereby needed data can be obtained, as in situations where the presence of an individual in any other role would change the character of the phenomena about which observations are wanted—for example, in studies of people of primitive cultures on an isolated island or of street gangs in a large city. Either the presence of an outsider would result in changed behavior, or the outsider would not be allowed to witness usual behavior. Nurses will find participant observation a useful technique when seeking observations of behaviors of mentally disturbed patients, whose behaviors might be modified if they were aware of an outsider in their presence. Perhaps even more important for the mentally disturbed might be the untoward effect on the course of their treatment that would be imposed by an outsider making observations.

The second major reason for using participant observation is that it may be the least expensive means for securing observations. It not only eliminates costs of salaries for persons who serve as observers but, frequently, the cost of orienting observers to the setting. Involved would be only the lesser costs of training persons already in the setting to make and record the specific observations needed.

Example: Godfrey

Since one of Godfrey's objectives was to determine whether an instructor carrying on a full-time job could complete a scientific investigation, it may be assumed that one of the reasons she chose participant observation was the cost of salaries for observers. Cost, however, would not necessarily have been the sole basis for her selection. She may well have viewed the experience as a particularly valuable learning one for the students. Further, her primary concern may have been the children, who would have known the nursing students. Their serving as participant observers precluded the need to introduce additional strangers. In relation to purely research concerns, however, the cost of hiring observers would have been pertinent.

Although the use of persons already in the setting as participant observers sounds like a built-in boon for the researcher, this lovely situation can have its drawbacks. (1) The researcher must not ask too much of individuals. In many nursing studies, it would be most convenient to ask the head nurse to make the needed observations—not only because she is in the setting, but because, in many instances, she is the person best qualified to make the observations. The head nurse knows nursing care; she knows patient reactions; she has had extensive experience in observing both. Nonetheless, the investigator should be cautious about the amount of involvement he requests of head nurses. Indeed, he should ask them to serve as participant observers only when there is absolutely no other person who could make the needed observations. In some instances, he might even forego obtaining some it-would-be-nice-to-have data, with the view to obtaining the most needed data. He would do this, rather than risk overextending the involvement of the head nurse to the point where she may refuse to participate at all. The investigator should avoid requesting head nurse involvement where participation would be a grave burden and might require that she neglect some of her primary responsibilities. (2) Individuals in the setting may be too close to it to be objective and unbiased in relation to observations needed. (3) Some persons in the setting may not really be competent to make the observations needed. The fictitious example used to illustrate the potential validity of assumptions can serve here: the necessary observations are manifestations of anxiety by patients; nursing students providing care for the patients may be considered for their potential as participant observers; yet, if they are in their first clinical experiences, they may not be competent to make needed observations.

Caution: Do Not Ask Too Much of People

Nonparticipant observation is a technique wherein the individual making the observations is in the environment of the study subjects, but remains as unobtrusive as possible to the doings of all persons making up the normal environment. Pearsall's article on participant observation identifies this opposite end of the continuum. Just as the name "participant observation" is rather descriptive of the technique, so the name "nonparticipant observation" indicates the general process of the technique. Pearsall comments that there are perhaps few situations in which either complete

Non-Participant Observation

188   STEP 7: TECHNIQUES

participation or nonparticipation is possible. The researcher planning to use nonparticipation must examine the total situation to determine the interplay of many factors and identify the degree of nonparticipation that is possible.

Degrees of Nonparticipation

The nature of the phenomena to be observed will determine the extent of the precautions necessary to ensure that the observer is indeed not participating in the group's activities. Many devices have been used to ensure nonparticipation, including one-way screens, hidden mirrors, tape recordings, and the very controversial wire tapping. These devices are necessary for making some observations where known presence of an observer would cause subjects to modify their behavior as, for example, in situations where study subjects are known to be suspicious of outsiders and indeed have reason not to want outsiders to know of their actions, plans, or thoughts, such as some prisoners or members of crime syndicates. Similarly, members of fraternal organizations like to keep some beliefs and rituals esoteric. Certain information is imparted only to those who become one of them. Under these circumstances, participant observation or secretive nonparticipant observation would be the only way to secure data about actions and rituals of the organization or its members. There are few, if any, types of observations needed in nursing studies where the subjects entertain such suspicions of outsiders. In most instances, where the data needed can best be obtained through nonparticipant observation, the process can be planned whereby the observer remains as inconspicuous as possible, yet within the subject's realm of awareness. Repeated studies have demonstrated that, in situations where subjects have no reason to be suspicious of outsiders, the subjects and others in their immediate environment soon get used to having the observer in his appointed place. They go about their usual activities, paying little or no attention to the outsider.

Questionnaire

Questionnaire is a technique wherein study subjects record observations about themselves, their knowledge, or their opinions. It is the one technique whose name is the same as that of the tool used to record the observations and it is perhaps the most widely used of all techniques in behavorial science investigations. On the surface, it appears to be simple to use. Yet, if judged by the errors committed in its use, it might well be classed as the most complex of all techniques. An investigator who contemplates using the questionnaire as the technique for obtaining his data should recognize that, for even the simplest kinds of data, the questionnaire has many intricacies. Many complete books have been written about development and use of questionnaires, including Paine's *The Art of Asking Questions*,[5] and the reader is referred to these sources for more detailed information about developing questionnaires.

One admonition is in order: *All* questionnaires should be pretested—every one! This practice is perhaps the most flagrantly neglected of all practices involved in data collection by behavorial scientists or others studying human behavior. There are several reasons for the pretesting. (1) No matter how brief or simple the questionnaire, there is no way of being sure that it will yield the needed data without putting it into use and actually having respondents answer the questions. (2) Pretesting can provide the investigator with information about the length of time needed to respond to the questionnaire, so that he may be specific about this factor when he asks subjects to give of their time. (3) An investigator can justify his asking subjects to give of their time only on the basis that they will be contributing to science in addition to giving of themselves. Therefore, he cannot justify his request if he has not done everything possible to ensure that the contribution he asks will result in information that will improve the lot of other men.

Admonition: Pre-test the Tool

Preliminary prestesting may be begun by asking colleagues to imagine themselves in the role of a study subject and to respond to the questionnaire. Such a test will usually provide suggestions about terminology, sequence, and relevance. Following revisions resulting from the first testing, the investigator will want to ask persons meeting the criteria for the eventual population sample to respond to the questionnaire. The pretesting may be done in the setting where the data for the study will be collected or in a similar but different setting. To illustrate, if the purpose of the questionnaire is to obtain information, from patients having general surgery for nonchronic conditions, about what they plan to do during their first week after leaving the hospital, and if the pretest is to be completed two months before the beginning of collection of data for the study, it would be advantageous to do the pretest in the setting of the study. The patients who would be the actual study subjects would be admitted to the hospital long after the test period and would not be influenced by the testing. Other advantages would be orientation of the data collectors to the program and setting, and familiarization of the staff with the work of the study. On the other hand, if the data sought were opinions of nurses about supervisory policies and practices in their hospital, pretesting in the study setting would involve the very persons who would be needed as subjects for the study itself. Testing in the setting would influence the study data to a degree where they would be useless. These two examples are extremes, but they illustrate factors that must be considered by the investigator as he plans details for collecting the data needed for his study.

It may seem that the above discussion of testing the questionnaire belongs to the next step, planning and developing tools, and that including it here is jumping ahead in sequential planning. In a way, this is true. On the other hand, the discussion should be viewed as proposals about testing the technique, not about testing the tool. The obligation to test is so intimately related to the thinking about using the questionnaire and asking people to give of themselves that discussion of it is appropriately part of planning the technique. Elements related to testing tools that do not have the moral connotations so conspicuously inherent in the questionnaire are elaborated in discussion of Step 8, Tools.

Interview

Interview is a technique wherein observations are obtained by the observer's asking questions of study subjects and recording the answers on an interview schedule. It is like the questionnaire technique in that subjects are asked to verbalize observations, knowledge, and opinions. In fact, the tools—the questionnaire and the interview schedule—may be indistinguishable from each other in form and format. The admonition about pretesting is equally applicable to both, and, for some kinds of data, either the interview or questionnaire will serve equally well. Where there is a matter of social acceptability, the respondent may possibly respond as he thinks the interviewer would expect him to, rather than as he really believes or thinks. In such instances, a questionnaire may be preferable. But even the latter must be screened for social acceptability of its items. The questionnaire would not become the automatic choice of technique if the data sought involved problems of valid responses and social acceptability. Where the response to any one question is expected to be lengthy, the interview may serve better, since persons will elaborate in speech when they will not undertake the chore of lengthy writing.

These are but a few elements that must be considered when deciding between questionnaire and interview. Besides learning the intricacies of developing a useful questionnaire or interview schedule, the student should read publications about both techniques to learn of the many factors needing consideration in planning the application of the techniques.[6, 7]

Content Analysis

Content analysis is a technique wherein observations are excerpted from records of facts that have been recorded for some purpose other than providing data for the current study and usually prior to it. This definition of content analysis will seem very strange to those who first developed the technique. It is defined in this way, however, because content analysis, as a technique for obtaining data in most behavorial science investigations, resembles the critical incident technique in that it is used only in a form much modified from the original. Essentially, the concept of content analysis, rather than the technique as originally developed, serves as a base for planning techniques useful in nursing studies. A further analogue to the critical incident technique lies in the fact that the description of the original process of the technique outlines the pattern for analyzing the data as well as the process for making the observations. Though he did not originate the idea of content analysis, Bernard Berelson, in his *Content Analysis in Communication Research,* delineates perhaps the best description of the technique in relation to the purpose for which it was developed.[8]

Adopt, Adapt, Combine Techniques of Others

The technique, as indicated by the title of the book, was developed for the purpose of studying, in detail, various elements in written communications. It has been extensively used to examine the contents of elementary school texts, with the texts serving as subjects of study. Essentially, the technique was used to study content of written materials to permit understanding of the sources themselves: the written documents being studied. The concern of the behavorial scientist's research, however, is behavior of persons. He obtains facts from records, not to gain understanding about the records, but to further his understanding of human behavior. Although written records may be the immediate sources of his data, his study subjects are human beings, not written records.

Books, the Study Subjects

Therefore, the behavorial scientist adapts the underlying concept of content analysis. He uses the gathering-of-facts and the immediate source-of-the-facts aspects of the technique, without the data-analysis aspect, to devise a plan for securing data he needs for his study. The rationale for the proposed definition is another instance of possible interchanging of two techniques. Content analysis may be considered a part of the processes of several techniques, such as process recordings, critical incident, and others. In utilization of each of these techniques, the observations are recorded in detailed narratives and the narratives must be analyzed to identify specifically the observation that represents a single datum. Although the "content" of "process recordings" must be "analyzed" to identify the "critical incident" that composes a single datum, it is proposed that the term "content analysis" not be used to refer to a part of the process of analyzing the data secured from their sources by other techniques. Rather, it should be reserved to identify the technique used by the researcher when the sources of data are records of facts made for purposes antedating the plan for study and for purposes other than recording facts needed in his particular study. For example, in a study to determine the frequency of elevated morning temperatures among patients who had elevated temperatures the preceding or following evening, or at both times, the researcher might use a content analysis technique. Patients' body temperatures are usually recorded at these times. The investigator could therefore plan to use, as sources of data for his study, these temperature records, which may have been made months or even years before. To gather the data, the collector would extract the facts from the contents of the records and record them in the tool prepared for the data collection. This process is a modified content analysis technique.

Using the Concept of the Technique

Since the observer (data collector) must identify only items pertinent to the needed data, it may seem that, in the above example, there are elements of the critical incident technique. This is true, but it is suggested that the title of the preponent technique be used to identify the technique being used. The preponent technique may be identified by

The Preponent Technique Provides Title

considering the actions required of the observer as he obtains the observations from their sources. In either the process recording or critical incident techniques, the data collector will make direct observations of the study subjects themselves as sources of data, or he will use individuals who have observed the study subjects as sources of data and obtain reports of observations from them. The observations will have been recorded specifically to provide data for the investigation. Whereas, in content analysis, the observer will search recorded materials for recordings of observations made by others for some purpose not related to the study at hand. This, it would seem, identifies specifically when the process used for obtaining the data may be termed "content analysis."

Record Analysis

Record analysis, as a technique used by the behavorial scientist to obtain observations, is essentially the same as content analysis. The observer peruses records of observations recorded for some purpose other than the current investigation and extracts observations contained in the records. As with content analysis, the technique of record analysis was originally developed to learn something about the nature of the records; the latter were the subjects of study. But, when the behavorial scientist uses the concept of record analysis as a base for devising a technique for obtaining data for *his* study, his subjects are human beings about whom the records contain observations. His purpose in excerpting observations from the records is to learn about his human subjects; it is not to learn about the records themselves. Actually, for the modified techniques usually identified by the names "content analysis" or "record analysis," the behavioral scientist might use the terms interchangeably. For greater precision, he might use the title "content analysis" to indicate that his data will be obtained from general-type recordings, such as texts, histories, and others; the term "record analysis" would indicate that the sources of data will be records of observations about particular individuals, such as students' school records, patients' clinical records, and motorists' driving records.

Nursing Audit

Examples of the use of record analysis are currently prominent in nursing literature, under titles including the term "nursing audit." [9] In the nursing audit, the record analysis technique, in its original intent, is more strictly used than is true for most uses of the technique in nursing studies. Records are examined on the premise that their contents reflect the nursing care provided the patients. Thus, the nursing audit is essentially a modification of the technique record analysis. Maria Phaneuf has described details of the process of nursing audit in several publications.[9-12]

Least Costly of Time and Money

As in decisions on sources of data, recordings of observations made for a prior purpose and possibly unrelated to the current investigation should always be given early consideration. Obviously, these sources would be the least costly in time and money of any sources from which to secure needed data. In addition, for many types of data, a less skilled observer would be able to excerpt the data from the records. Still another reason for looking first to previous recordings is that it is perhaps the most efficient means for determining the potential of the source for yielding the type or types of data needed. All that is required to know the exact nature of the data obtainable is for the investigator to examine a small sampling of the recordings. With these he can know whether the observations he needs are recorded and whether they are recorded in sufficient detail, form, and specificity to meet his requirements.

If the purpose of the study is to test a hypothesis and consideration is being given to using observations recorded for some other purpose, great care will have to be taken to determine all circumstances in the situations or conditions under which the observations were made and recorded. Only rarely will circumstances be found that provide confidence that control and experimental situations were entirely similar. And only rarely can there be certainty about the precise nature of the existence of the independent variable in the experimental situation. The needed assurances about these conditions are difficult enough to obtain when survey of existing conditions is used for collecting data, wherein observations are made specifically for the purpose of the study. Being able to establish that required conditions of control existed when observations were made for some other purpose, with no attention having been given to the requirements of a scientific study, may be too much to hope for.

Caution: Improbability of Conditions Satisfying Control Requirements

Process recording is a technique wherein the observer records, by writing or dictating, a detailed description of all behavior occurring during a specified period of time. Usually, the number of individuals involved in the setting is very limited. The focus is on a single subject, and reporting about other persons in the setting is limited to the interaction of the study subject with them or to their influence on the study subject's behavior. Frequently the observations are interactions between the observer and a single study subject. The recordings may be limited to objective reporting or may include interpretations of the behavorial phenomena observed. The process recording technique is usually combined with participant observation. Nonparticipant or self-observation may sometimes be used. The element that differentiates it from the direct observations techniques is not the manner in which observations are made, but rather in the character of the recording of the observations. The title of the technique is descriptive of the raw data that may be expected. The data will be recordings of sequential actions, interactions, and reactions.

Process Recording

An essential difference between process recording and critical incident is the way in which the boundaries of individual observations are determined. In the process recording, the observations are bound by a preset duration of time: one hour, three hours, 20 minutes. In the critical incident, the boundary is determined by the nature of an episode of behavior.

Boundaries: Starting and Closing Times

The process of the behavior is described or recorded from the beginning to the end of an action-reaction—from the start to the close of the incident, the start and close being determined by the judgment of the observer. He will describe as much of the setting and of the study subject's behavior as he believes is necessary to recount a meaningful behavior and to identify clearly the nature of the result, or effect, or meaning of the behavior. In other words, the two techniques may utilize the same observation techniques (processes), but the observers will be attuned to slightly different emphases on observations to be noted and recorded. Through the modest differences, the techniques will yield data of two quite different natures. Should the investigator be interested in observations of only one or two well-defined types of behavior, the critical incident will yield the data. Should he require observations of behavorial sequence (which, incidentally, need no less specificity of definition) to learn relationships of various "critical" behaviors to other behaviors, then the process recording would be needed.

Differences in Focuses of Attention

It may seem that the process recording would yield critical incident data, but that the critical incident technique would not yield process recording data. To a degree, this is true. Yet there are several excellent reasons for not using process recording when a critical incident is the type of datum needed. (1) Process recordings yield volumes of written words, and the task of excerpting the needed data would be unnecessarily enlarged. (2) Persons grow weary of writing, and it is not logical to request that they report more than is needed. (3) The focus of attention of the observer is different in the two situations. Where process recordings are to be done, the observer is alert to transitions between behavorial episodes for their potential meaning in adjacent or remote episodes. He would be less alert to the identification of beginning and end boundaries of definitive episodes. There seems to be sound base for proposing that the two techniques serve distinct purposes in data collection and should not be used interchangeably. On the other hand, there may be the infrequent situation where process recordings have been made for one purpose and will contain critical incidents adequately described to provide data for a study of another purpose. Researchers should be alert to this possibility and should examine potentially useful process records as they plan for sources of needed data. Should the process recordings contain usable, relevant incidents, the technique, of course, would be a content analysis-critical incident process for collecting the data.

Diary

The diary is a technique whose name identifies the process for obtaining observations. Just as with any other technique, diary keeping must be described in terms pertinent to the specific observations to be made and to the stated purpose of the investigation. Data will not be collected merely through the maintaining of a diary. Rather, they will be collected through the maintaining of a diary recounting specified types of episodes and previously characterized surrounding circumstances and commentary about the episodes. Many of the comments pertinent to the process recording and critical incident techniques are applicable to the diary technique. The researcher would do well to review the concepts and processes of those techniques as he plans the use of the diary for his data gathering.

Activity analysis, work sampling, time sampling, and others with similar titles are techniques originally developed for study of workers in industry. In their original uses they were distinct techniques, each with a well-delineated process. Behavorial scientists have since adapted those processes to fit requirements of particular investigations. Furthermore, the titles have been applied to new processes, so that the once definitive titles no longer identify the process the investigator has in mind. Indeed, most of these terms originally were more descriptive of the purpose for which data were collected than of the process for collecting them; they identified the nature of the use to which the data would be put, rather than the process by which the observations would be made. This may have been because the studies for which they were developed were more of a problem-solving than of a research nature. Employers wanted to know how a worker used his time: how much time was spent in each category of activities (time sampling). Unions wanted to know the amount of work that constitutes a fair day's work (work sampling). Employers wanted to know what activities various categories of workers were engaged in (activity analysis).

Activity Analysis Work Sampling, Time Sampling

As nurses began doing research, they were interested in what nurses do. With guidance from behavorial scientists, they addressed themselves to studying nurses. Most of what is called nursing research prior to 1955 is behavorial research. In their early research efforts, nurses seem to have been more "irritated" by problems of nurse behaviors than by problems of patient care needs. This is probably because the interests and directions taken by early nurse researchers were dictated by circumstances and expediency. They turned to behavorial scientists for assistance, and the concerns and interests and knowledge of these scientists had just recently turned to the whole fruitful field of studying employees in work situations. Assisting nurses to study nurses represented to them the opening of a new area in that field. Since learning the process and skills of research through the early studies, nurses have more and more addressed themselves to nursing research: that is, they are now testing theories about relationships between nurse actions and outcomes for patients. They study the applicability of hypothesized and established theories of the basic sciences to the improvement of nursing care outcomes.

Nurse Researchers and Nursing Research

In our materialistic world, a prime justification for doing research is possibility of securing knowledge needed to improve a product. Nursing's product is nursing care of patients. Nurse researchers' efforts, it seems reasonable to suggest, should be directed to learning ways and means for improving nursing care of patients. This is not to say that studies of nurses and nurse behaviors are not proper subjects for research by nurses, but, rather, to help the student to identify various types of investigations and to distinguish between what a study is purported to be and what it actually is.

As the nurse researcher looks to these techniques developed for industry, she will find much that will be helpful for planning the processes to be used for obtaining observations needed for her investigation. This will be so whether the problem be nurse-employee related or patient-care related. But she should be prepared to find various components of the techniques under various titles in different references. Although the nurse researcher will seldom find it feasible to adopt one of these techniques in its pure, original form, this need not pose a problem. She may take pertinent concepts from whatever source and use them in any combination for planning the processes that will facilitate securing needed facts. As to what she will call her technique, she may adopt or adapt a title that seems descriptive of her process, or she may coin a new name.

Pertinent Concepts

If the student keeps in mind that the technique is the process by which a single observation is made, he will perhaps identify his technique in terms connoting some action of the observer, based on a previously described technique. He may find concepts from work and time sampling "techniques" more useful for planning for Step 9, Collection of Data, than for planning Step 7. Briefly, the concepts composing some of the pertinent techniques from industrial studies are:

1. *Activity analysis* involves recording a large number of activities performed by one or more categories of worker over a period of days. Observers may be participants or nonparticipants. Activities may represent all activities performed during the stated period of time or they may be samples of activities, with observations made at predetermined, randomly selected times.

2. *Work sampling* involves timing the worker as he performs particular activities, the purpose being to determine the length of time required to perform any particular activity or job. As the title implies, planning for collecting the data involves developing a schedule designating the activities that will be timed and when each will be done.[13]

3. *Time sampling* involves recording large numbers of activities, wherein each observation recorded identifies whatever a worker is doing at a predetermined time.[14] Observations are recorded every 10 to 15 minutes for 8-hour periods (the work day), over a series of days. Through calculations of the percentage of the total number of activities that fall into each category, it is possible to determine the percentage of time spent in each

of the various categories of tasks. The most extensive use that nurse researchers are likely to make of the work sampling techniques is to use ideas from the general concept in planning a hybrid technique and to schedule times for making multiple observations.

4. *Time study* is a technique wherein observations of difficulty, complexity, and time of production line tasks are obtained, with the view to determining what production may be expected of an individual in a one-day work period. The full implications of such studies are concepts rather foreign to nurses, and the technique in its pure, original form is not likely to be used for nursing studies. It is mentioned here, however, because the title is sometimes used to refer to other techniques and because nurses should know that time study has a specific denotation and is not merely another term for time sampling or work study.

A projective technique is one where the subject is provided with a stimulus—most frequently visual, sometimes auditory, and, least often, other sensory—and asked to tell what comes to mind, or to rate or categorize items.[15] One objective is to secure spontaneous, uninhibited responses. In some situations, where conveying requisite ideas in words would be difficult if not impossible, the use of pictures makes it possible to focus the respondent's attention on the subject of concern and to communicate intended meaning to him. This is particularly true when the investigator is seeking expressions about feelings or ideas from persons who have limited experience and facility in perceiving abstract concepts expressed in language. For instance, it has been demonstrated that persons with limited education understand little of the concepts of rest and exercise in relation to treatment for a heart attack, when instructions are given verbally or in writing. But when explanations are accompanied by and related to a series of pictures, the individuals are able to grasp the concepts and to follow prescriptions for treatment. Another purpose served by using pictures to elicit responses is that it eliminates putting answers into the mouths of respondents; this is sometimes almost impossible to avoid when using verbalizations to inform subjects about the concept to which a response is sought. The use of pictures provides assurance that all subjects are exposed to identical stimuli. If the accompanying technique is interview, however, with verbal description used, the stimuli may be varied from subject to subject: by tone of voice, by altering words or sequence of words, and by additional explanation for some subjects.

Projective Technique

The projective technique has merit, but development and validation of the set of stimuli to be used are time-consuming and require considerable competence and knowledge in the development of psychological measuring tools. The student researcher should probably use this technique only if his particular study requires data obtainable through use of a projective tool already developed. Another prerequisite would be that the tool have clearly defined guides for interpretations of the responses to it. The student researcher may also use a projective technique where the purpose of his study is to explore and describe and where the precise measurements required to compare various groups or situations are not essential.

Q-sort

Q-sort is a technique wherein the study subject is asked to sort a pack of cards, each of which identifies a task or opinion pertinent to the focus of the study.[16] The technique has been used most frequently to study jobs. The subject is asked to arrange the cards in an order that indicates what he considers most important to least important in relation to his expectations about the job—his own or someone else's. The development of the cards is an extensive undertaking and the student researcher should perhaps not attempt it. Whiting developed and tested a 100-card pack that is usable for studying opinions about the composition and meaning of the "job" of nursing.[17] His pack has been adopted or adapted for several studies of nurses' jobs, another demonstration of the influence of the behavioral scientists' concerns. Q-sort is considered extremely useful by some, and extremely limited by others. A major limitation is that it permits only the study of six or seven of the extremes, either the most important or the least important tasks, and tells little or nothing about the many tasks in between. Data gathered with the Q-sort itself seem to have limited value. The technique has potential, nevertheless, for studies where interest is in determining the relationship between kinds of performance and opinions about importance of various tasks.

Miscellaneous Comments

In most reports of nursing research, the student will find one or more of these technique titles, but in very few will he find indication that a technique was adopted for use in its pure, original form. The student researcher is apt to believe that he must utilize a previously described technique or at least that he must attach one or more of their titles to the process he plans for making his observations. Neither of these practices is mandatory. The researcher's primary responsibility is to describe precisely the process he will use to secure the observations he seeks. He is responsible for ensuring that the process will, indeed, yield the facts he has identified as being needed, from the sources he has designated. He may give his process a title or not, as he chooses. Indeed, the beginning researcher should resist trying to fit a title to every type of observational process he will use—for example, the process of collecting background data about study subjects from their clinical records. The researcher should identify the items of background data he will collect and simply state that these data will be obtained from the clinical record. There is no need to elaborate the process for this commonly used task.

The researcher must consider many and varied factors as he determines the techniques he will use. Some may seem unrelated to the process of the research. An example of an unexpected, yet entirely necessary, consideration may be illustrated by a fictitious study of behaviors of hippies. The researcher determined that the needed data could be secured only through participant observations. As part of his plan he had to allow time for his observers, before they could become participants, to become *that* dirty.

SUMMARY

A technique is the process by which observations are made. Essentially, it is a description of the process required to obtain a single datum—to make the observation of one phenomenon that has been identified as representative of a type of datum needed. Deciding on the technique requires consideration of (1) specific identity of each type of datum, (2) sources of data, (3) activities required of the persons making the observations, and (4) the setting in which the observations are to be made. The researcher should examine the potential usefulness of several techniques before selecting the one best suited for his purposes. Although some thinking about them will enter into the planning of Step 7, detailed development of tools for recording the data or of the institutional setting in which the observations will be made are not essential to the decisions about techniques.

Many techniques have been developed for obtaining observations pertinent to nursing studies, but few of these can be adopted in pure, original form for use in other studies. More often, concepts from established techniques serve as bases for planning a modified technique or for developing a wholly new technique suited to making the observations sought. New techniques are being developed rapidly; for many studies only a new technique will do. Nonetheless, the researcher should think first about adopting or adapting a technique already developed and tried by others. Many suggestions have been made about ascribing a title to the technique used, and various rationales have been proposed in support of factors influencing title selection. Yet the researcher's main responsibility is precise description of his technique in terms of securing a single datum. Of remote second concern should be the titling of the technique.

REFERENCES

1. Flanagan, J. C. The critical incident technique. Psychol. Bull., 51:327-358, 1954.
2. Fivars, G., and Gosnell, D. Nursing Evaluation: The Problem and Process. New York, The Macmillan Company, 1966.
3. Godfrey, A. E. See reference 4, Step 1, page 62.

4. Pearsall, M. Participant observation as role and method in behavorial research. Nurs. Res., 14:37-42, 1965.
5. Payne, S. The Art of Asking Questions. Princeton, New Jersey, Princeton University Press, 1951.
6. Kahn, R. L., and Cannell, C. F. The Dynamics of Interviewing—Theory, Technique, and Cases. New York, John Wiley & Sons, Inc., 1957.
7. Richardson, S., Dohrenwend, B., and Klein, D. Interviewing: Its Forms and Functions. New York, Basic Books, Inc., Publishers, 1965.
8. Berelson, B. Content Analysis in Communications Research. New York, American Book-Stratford Press, Inc., 1952.
9. Phaneuf, M. C. A nursing audit method. Nurs. Outlook, 12:42-45, 1964.
10. ——— The nursing audit for evaluation of patient care. Nurs. Outlook, 14:51-54, 1966.
11. ——— Analysis of a nursing audit. Nurs. Outlook, 16:57-60, 1968.
12. Donabedian, A., and Phaneuf, M. C. Evaluating the quality of medical care. *In* Selected Papers: Institute on Planning and Administration of Nursing Service in Medical Care Programs. Ann Arbor, Continuing Education Service, School of Public Health, University of Michigan, 1968, pp. 169-189.
13. Barnes, R. M. Work Sampling. New York, John Wiley & Sons, Inc., 1957.
14. How to Study Nursing Activities in a Patient Unit. Washington, D.C., Government Printing Office, 1954, #370.
15. Meyer, G. Tenderness and Technique. Los Angeles, University of California Press, 1960.
16. Stephenson, W. The Study of Behavior: Q-Technique and Its Methodology. Chicago, The University of Chicago Press, 1955.
17. Whiting, J. F. Q-sort: A technique for evaluating perceptions of interpersonal relationships. Nurs. Res., 4:70-73, 1955.

STEP 8
TOOLS

TERMS DEFINED

Tools for Obtaining Facts: A tool for obtaining facts (an observation-making tool) is a tool or instrument used in the process of securing observations that are to compose the data for the study; examples are a thermometer, a yardstick, an electrocardiograph, a rating scale, a true-false test, an interview schedule, and many others.

Tools for Recording Facts: A tool for recording facts (an observation-recording tool) is a form on which observations are recorded; examples are a temperature graph sheet, an electrocardiogram tape, a video tape, a checklist, a bibliography card, a diary, and many, many others.

CONCEPTS PERTINENT TO DEFINED TERMS

In many instances the observation tool and the recording tool are one and the same. For example, in most instances where a true-false test is used, the respondent indicates his responses on a form that contains the answers. Thus, the measuring instrument and the recording instrument are one and the same tool. On the other hand, if the test questions were on a separate sheet or flashed on a screen and the respondent were to write or check his responses on an answer sheet, the two tools would be different. Thus, the identification of a tool by name alone does not reveal much about its nature or intended use. This is especially true if the name is one of the many generalized terms used to refer to research tools. For example, the term "checklist" can refer to innumerable types of instruments: a ballot, an employee time card, or a multiple-choice test, which usually has a checklist format. Any form on which the individual is asked to "check the answer that best expresses your thoughts" is a checklist. It may be a single-item form, or it may run to several hundred questions. Many forms that are given slightly more definitive names may be checklists, too. A questionnaire, a job satisfaction rating scale, or a hobby-avocational interests inventory may all be in the form of a checklist.

Many of the comments made about techniques are applicable to tools. For almost all tools, a generalized title is applicable, but the exact nature of the tool can only be identified through a detailed description of it. Indeed, looking at the tool itself will not always give full understanding of it. In many instances, the tool itself, along with instructions for its use, will be sufficient for an understanding of its nature. Sometimes, however, the rationale underlying its development and the description of its intended application are necessary for complete understanding. Phaneuf's Nursing Audit and the Slater Nursing Competencies Rating Scale are examples of the latter.[1,2]

Observation-making Tools

Tools for making observations are of three types:

1. Sensory-enhancing tools, sometimes referred to as the hardware. The sensory enhancers enable an observer to identify phenomena that could not be "sensed" or identified by the unaided senses (without the tools). Among the sensory enhancers are the stethoscope, the microscope, the electrocardiograph.

2. Standard-scales tools. These permit relatively precise measurements of amounts of the variable, or the phenomenon, to be observed at any one point in time. Among these are the thermometer, the sphygmomanometer, the yardstick, the Wexler-Bellevue IQ test, the stopwatch.

3. Nonscaled tools. These make it possible to obtain nonscaled descriptive observations of phenomena or entities. Among them are the open-ended questionnaire, an essay type test, a Q-sort card pack.

Observation-recording Tools

Among the tools for recording observations (facts) are types that correspond, in some characteristics, to the three types of observation-making tools:

1. The "hardware," or mechanical tools, that require a special machine for recording and displaying the recordings of the observations, such as dictaphones, tape recorders, films, video tape, and others.

2. Prescaled recording tools, with printed scales on which the observer records or checks a precise measurement at the time the observation is made. This type of tool may be further divided into two categories:

a. A tool on which observations made with the aid of the standard scales tools, such as graphs and sectioned forms, are recorded: for instance, scaled measurements of individual observations of time, weight, length, blood pressure, and many others.

b. A tool on which the observer would record a judgmental evaluation score, having made the judgment against a defined scale that may be reproduced on the tool itself, or that may be described in a guide to the use of the tool, such as the Slater Nursing Compentencies Rating Scale, and the qualitative scale used by Godfrey (page 146).[2, 3]

3. Nonscaled recording tools used for recording essentially descriptive, nonscaled observations, where the actual recording may be a check alongside a descriptive word, phrase, or sentence; a written word, phrase, or sentence; or a process recording or an entire diary.

The materials of the first type of recording tools are usually tapes, films, phonograph records, and others. The materials of most of the tools in the second two categories are paper-and-pencil type. Some recording tools may fall into either the first or second type. Among them are electrograms, or time-o-gram recordings of temperatures or pressures in machinery on an around-the-clock basis. Since these recordings employ paper-and-pencil material and do not require a machine to display the recordings, they perhaps more appropriately belong in the second type or prescaled category.

Tools Developed for Other Investigations

To a larger degree than for techniques, the investigator should use observation-making or measurement tools developed and used for other investigations. This is because development and scaling of measurement tools frequently require more time and work than are needed for all the rest of the investigation for which they are developed. This fact has become so well recognized that many researchers now devote their full attention to development of tools. And sophisticated researchers modify plans for investigations when they find that they will have to develop a new tool to make required measurements. Either they markedly extend their time schedule, or they select other criterion measures. The beginning researcher is less likely to be aware of the considerable work involved in developing a new measuring tool. He will frequently plan to develop a tool and complete the planned investigation, only to meet with frustration from one of two sources. Either the tool will be incompletely developed and tested, so that little confidence can be had in the data secured with it, or so much time is devoted to the development of the tool that little is left for completing the investigation. In turn, the stepped-up schedule for completing the study usually allows little time for thorough analysis of the data.

Students Developing Measurement Tools

The beginning researcher is frequently a student planning an investigation to be conducted as part of his educational program: a senior project, a masters thesis, or a doctoral dissertation. Faculty advisors have an obligation to assist these students to develop a plan wherein the required data may be collected through use of tools developed for other investigations. Should the plan not so develop, but the needed tool can be developed as a logical and limited modification of an existing tool, it may be feasible for the student to persist in his original plan. Should the needed data require measurements for which no tool has been developed, the student should be guided to pursue some alternative aspect of his problem. Otherwise, he can unwittingly get into a situation where he must greatly extend the time required to complete his educational program. Or, he may encounter the frustration of having to wind up his investigation knowing that his data are not valid.

Students may be disappointed when advised against developing their own tools; they may believe that instructors are placing restrictions on student prerogatives to pursue studies of their own interests. Despite these concerns of students, the instructor concerned for students will continue to guide them along paths that can lead to satisfying outcomes and help them avoid paths that can lead only to multiple frustrations. It is hoped that these comments will help a student to understand an instructor's reasons for suggesting that he revise his planning and pursue an alternate course in the study he plans to do.

Example: Slater Scale

To illustrate this point, during one year I received communications from five graduate students, all in different schools, two in doctoral programs and three in masters programs. Most of them were far enough along in planning their studies to know that the tool they needed was a scale to measure nurse performance in the clinical setting, and each was planning to develop such a tool. They wrote to me for information about the Slater Nursing Competencies Rating Scale, whose testing I had guided. The Slater Scale had been in the process of development for over five years. By rough estimate, 100 nurses have used the scale; over 5,000 evaluations have been done in some 40 varied settings; the evaluations have been of nurses ranging from sophomore students to graduate nurses. Two masters students shared the testing of the scale's reliability for their masters thesis. All tests produced high levels of anticipated results. At the time of the correspondence, it was expected that the final testings of the scale would be completed during the ensuing year. Despite information about the extensive amount of work involved in development of a valid and reliable tool, two of the students seeking information reported that they wished to use the Slater Scale only as a source of ideas. Each planned to develop her own tool to measure nurse performance in the clinical setting. Unfortunately, many students, despite presumed guidance from their instruc-

Concepts Pertinent to Defined Terms 205

tors, seem to insist on learning by personal trial and frustration, rather than from experiences of others. It is therefore repeated: the researcher should search for tools that he may adopt or adapt for making the observations that will compose the data for his investigation.

The search for such tools will take the same path as the search for techniques: *Search for Tools*

1. Searching indexes to discover books and articles about tools.
2. Skimming research reports to identify tools that have been used in other investigations.
3. Thumbing journals for articles describing new tools and for reports of investigations where tools used might be appropriate for collecting the data needed in the current investigation. When searching for observation-making tools, the student should also take note of observation-recording tools. The latter, more frequently than not, will have been developed specifically for the investigation in which they were used.

The researcher may glean many ideas about tool development and format from tools developed by others but, essentially, he will have to think through the design for his own recording tools "from scratch." This does not mean, however, that he will begin with materials or ideas picked at random. Rather, if his prior planning has been thorough, he will know specifically the character of the observations to be recorded and the exact form that each recording will take. He will know the various types of data needed and the identity of each variation of individual observations to be made in each type. He will know the sequence and the setting in which observations will be made and he will know precisely what the observer will be doing as he makes the observations. He will know whether machines will be required to make observations and whether the machines will record the observations as well as facilitate making them. He will know many other things about the observations he needs to make and record. He will use all of this information, along with ideas from tools developed by others, in planning the recording tools for his investigation. *Tool Developed From Scratch*

The general appearance of a tool can be best conceptualized when it is thought of in terms of the material, form, and construction necessary to make possible the observation and/or recording of a single phenomenon. The researcher, when planning for techniques, will visualize the observer in the setting where the observations will be made, along with the observer's actions as he observes a single phenomenon. Similarly, as he plans the design of the tool for recording the observation, he will visualize the observer recording the single datum. The thinking about techniques and tools may well occur simultaneously. Yet the admonition to complete the planning for techniques before planning for tools still holds. Once the planning for techniques is completed, the researcher can mentally review *Recording One Datum at a Time*

Example: 1A

what the observer will be doing as he makes the observation. He can then plan to insert the activity of doing the recording into the pattern of the activities composing the making of the observation.

1A needed observations of patients' deep-breathing and coughing, turning in bed, sitting out of bed, and walking. She had determined that the technique for making the observations would be nonparticipant observation. Since her data were to be in the form of enumerations or frequencies of each type of action by patients, a single datum might have been recorded as a hash mark, as the number 1, or as a time of occurrence. Since the recording of each datum would require little space, she could visualize a form on which might be listed the names of each type of observation about which she wished information.

After this point in planning tool design is reached, it is necessary to think ahead to Step 9, Collection of the Data. Decision must be made as to the approximate number of observations that might be recorded on each copy of the tool. Since, for 1A, the types of phenomena to be observed would probably occur only sporadically and since it would have been costly to observe one patient on a full-time basis, she decided to use a modified time sampling plan. She made 15 observations of a study subject, during a 3-hour period, on each of four successive days. A copy of her tool is displayed in Exhibit 1.[4] It may be seen that she was able to visualize the appearance of a single datum recorded for any one of the patient activities to be observed. In addition, the completed tool provided for organization of her data as successive observations were recorded. This data organization was made possible by the column in which were listed the times at which observations began. It was planned that, at any one observation time, the observation of a single phenomenon would be recorded. That is, if a patient were sitting out of bed and deep-breathing and coughing, only one of these activities would be counted. This would be the one considered to be representative of greatest patient progress: in this instance, the sitting out of bed. Such detailed and specific planning was required in order to ensure equal opportunity for early ambulation activities to be observed and recorded in both the control and experimental groups of patients. This situation is the reverse of thinking ahead to a later step and its influence on planning. Here, thinking about the process for making and recording a single observation made it necessary to return to an earlier step in planning. It is unlikely that the planner would have made explicit, in the identification of data needed, the specification about which phenomenon should be recorded when two pertinent phenomena were observed simultaneously. This is an instance where later thinking will result in a return to more detailed and precise planning for an essentially completed step.

1A's tool illustrates several important points about tool construction—among them, the value of securing descriptive as well as quantitative data.

EXHIBIT 1

OBSERVATION RECORD

Page _____ of _____ pages

Patient _____ Date _____ Postoperative Day _____

Room _____ Type _____ Age _____ Sex _____ Marital Status _____

Date of Admission _____ Previous Major Surgery _____

Type of Surgery _____ Date _____

Complications _____

Time	Activity							Code
	Coughing		Turning		Out of Bed				
	S	A	S	A	1	2	3	4	
									S = self
									A = assistance
									1 = sitting in chair
									2 = walking back very bent
									3 = walking, back slightly bent
									4 = walking, back straight
Sub-Totals									— = no activity
GRAND TOTALS									

COMMENTS: Group _____

Instructions _____ Reinforcement _____ Visual Aid _____

Provide for Descriptive Data

Descriptive data should be collected where: (1) they have potential meaning for understanding findings; (2) they can be obtained with little or no additional time or effort for the observer; and (3) extensive additional time will not be required to utilize the added findings in analyses of the data.

1A's hypothesis required only a count of the frequencies of early ambulation activities. Essentially, a tool to record these might have been a form with a place for the date and a column with the heading, Patient name. The names of the patients to be observed might have been listed, and a hashmark placed on the line to the right of a patient's name each time he was observed performing an activity. This would have provided the quantitative data needed to test the hypothesis. But the more extensive planning and the resultant tool yielded not only the required quantitative data but also information about kinds of activities performed. For example, 1A found patients deep-breathing and coughing only seven times in 1,200 observations of 20 abdominal and thoracic surgery patients during their first four postoperative days. She found that the 10 patients in the control group were out of bed, sitting or walking, only 50 times; while during a comparable time, the experimental patients were out of bed, sitting or walking, 169 times. She found that the frequencies for turning were essentially the same for the two groups. Each of these descriptive identifications of the nature of the activities has meaning for nurses. Yet the additional information required no additional work or time for the observer, and comparatively little more time for data analyses. In this, as in most similar instances, the secret to the collection of meaningful descriptive data, where rather simple quantitative data are all that are strictly required, lies in the planning for the recording tool. The construction of 1A's tool, Exhibit 1, and that of Exhibit 2, illustrate the point without need for elaboration.

1A's tool also made provision for background data. These of course, would not have to be recorded each day. Provision for them appeared on each copy, however, since this eliminated the need to have two essentially-the-same tools. The calendar date is not always needed. Yet, since it frequently serves identifying purposes, it is recommended that the date be a part of every recording tool. 1A's tool consisted of but one page, so numbering of successive pages was not necessary. When a tool is multi-paged, however, numbering is helpful—particularly for tools several pages in length, where the study subjects will fill in the recordings or where several observers will use the tools. It precludes omission of pages during the use of the tool.

The display of the code for identifying particular observations on the face of 1A's tool is another useful feature. Sometimes space limitations make it impossible to provide this feature; the codes should not be included if they will result in a cluttered form. The student researcher may

EXHIBIT 2

Form O

OBSERVATION FORM

Patient _____ Nurse Observer _____

Date _____ Day of Study _____

Activity		Time and Duration				Total		
						Time	Act.	R.

Personal Hygiene
  Wash hands and face
  Shave
  Teeth
  Hair
  Backrub
  Environment
  Elimination
	D*
	
	B
	
	H
		9:20
		25'37"
		7:05
		
		R3'12"
		11:52
		
		6'20"
			10:10
			13'42"
			
			12:05
			– –
			3'0"
				
				12:10
				
				20'18"				

Meals, Fluids and Nourishment	A F	7:35 14'23" 11:01 R						
Medications	J	10:12 30"						
Change Position	G I	11:10 R 1:01 6'05"	 1:01** 5'50"	**In red on original				
Out of Bed	E	9:32 B 3'07	***	***In green on original				
Observation of Condition	C	9:15 1'15"						

*These letters and the times recorded did not appear on the forms used to record observations. They are used here as adjuncts to the Form O-G, Guide to Use of Observation Form, Part I.

EXHIBIT 2 (Cont'd)

Form 0, page 2

Activity		Time and Duration				Total		
						Time	Act.	R.
Nursing Procedures	C'	9:16						
Answer Questions	G	11:10 "21"						
Diversion								
Teaching Patient and/or Family								
Recording and Reporting								
"Just Checking"								

not always consider including the codes, since he usually thinks in terms of his being his own data collector. He reasons that, by the time he is ready to make and record his observations, he will be thoroughly familiar with his own plans and will need no guiding code. True though this may be, he should, nonetheless, develop appropriate codes for several reasons. (1) A distinguishing attribute of research is that the design is made sufficiently explicit that the investigation could be replicated. (2) Though the student may anticipate doing his own data collection, plans may later change and involve other observers. (3) The best way to clarify ideas is to put them on paper. (4) The concepts will never be more vivid for the investigator than at the time he is developing his tool.

Explicit Codes and Instructions for Use

These same comments apply to the need for writing detailed instructions for the use of each tool developed. There are excellent illustrations of guides and instructions for use of tools in the report of the Uninterrupted Patient Care study.[5] Exhibits 2 and 3 provide one example.

Another important feature of 1A's tool is the provision for recording "no activity." For any tool that provides for a specific number of recordings, provision should be made for noting when no observation is made. That is, wherever there is occasion for recording a datum, some recording should be made. A blank is not sufficient. A blank may mean either that there was no observation or that the recording of an observation was overlooked. But when "no activity" is recorded, there is no doubt about the meaning.

Accommodation for No Observation

Finally, the provision of spaces for entries of totals, in 1A's tool, facilitated organizing the data for analysis. This feature is desirable when it can be done without cluttering the tool.

For recording most data, a separate form should be used for each observation period for each study subject. Where observations may be influenced, even in minor degree or even on an unconscious level, by subjective judgment of the observer, the separate tools are imperative. This is true whether the observer be the same person from one observation period to the next or there be different observers. For example, in the Uninterrupted Patient Care study, the nurse observers were asked to estimate, each day, the number of nursing care activities that would be required by the patient. Since estimates of previous days may have influenced those made on any one day, it was imperative to provide for blank recording forms for each day. In the same study, personnel were asked to respond to the Patient Rating Scale (a simple one-page checklist) on the first and final days of study. The tool could have been so designed that the two recordings could have been made on the same copy. Yet each respondent was provided with a second copy for his second rating, so that he might not be influenced by seeing his previous opinions. This practice also facilitates the organization of data.

Separate Copy for Separate Collection Periods

EXHIBIT 3

PART I. GUIDE TO USE OF OBSERVATION FORM

1. The purpose is to record the number of nursing activities performed, the time required by <u>nursing personnel</u>, and the number of requests for care made by the patient. Categories of nursing activities are listed on the left. Record the time of onset of a particular activity and the duration of the activity in the space designated for each activity. See A on sample. When recording duration of time, use the following symbols: 0-hour; '-minute; ''-second.

2. The onset of an activity is the time of arrival of nursing personnel at the patient's side.

3. The termination of an activity is either the time the nurse leaves the bedside or when a task, such as aftercare of equipment, is completed. Since it may be impractical to follow nursing personnel in order to time the preparation or aftercare of equipment, estimates of time required to perform these functions may be used.

4. Simultaneous or contiguous activities, such as observation of the patient and discontinuing an I-V, are to be treated as two activities during one period of time. Record the time duration in the space devoted to the activity for which the patient contact was initiated. Record the second activity with a check mark and the time of occurrence in the appropriate square. See C and C'. A second activity is defined as one which would be carried out without the initiation of the primary activity. On the other hand, if the person who feeds a patient makes him comfortable again after the meal, the change of position is considered part of the meal activity; no check mark is necessary. See A. The onset of some activities (socialization, for example) will be difficult to identify. The time of occurrence need only show a relationship to the primary activity.

5. If additional activities are carried out by a second nurse, record the time of onset and duration, so that the total nursing time is accounted for when two nurses are at the patient's side. See E. Indicate the presence of more than one person at the patient's side by entering (in green) a "B" to denote one additional person, a "C" to denote two additional persons, etc.

6. If additional personnel approach the patient's side to engage in a simultaneous, but unrelated, activity, treat this as a separate activity by charting time of occurrence and duration in an appropriate square. See J and D.

7. If activities are carried out by members of the patient's family, record time of occurrence and duration in red.

8. If an activity is carried out by nursing personnel and family simultaneously, show the time of occurrence and duration (family) in adjacent square. See I.

9. If an activity such as personal hygiene is administered and not carried out over a continuous period of time, but the intent to return is obvious, enter the time of onset of the activity and the duration of time in a square; record the time of resumption of the activity and the duration of time required for completing the activity in adjacent square; indicate the resumption of activity by connecting the two squares with an arrow. See D. (This is to be tabulated as one activity.)

10. When portions of an activity, such as shaving, combing hair, placing a paper bag, or leaving part of a meal at the bedside, are carried out at a later time, the continuations can be treated as separate activities. The nurse observer will notice the intent to sever the patient contact.

EXHIBIT 3 (Cont'd)

11. If a second activity occurs during an interruption of an activity, indicate the resumption of the first activity with a dotted arrow through the square denoting the second activity. See H.

12. If a patient has requested care, enter "R" in the same space in addition to the onset of the patient contact and duration of the activity. See B. (Each time a patient puts on his light, chart as "R" under the appropriate heading. Record in margin until the nature of the request can be identified.)

13. In the event that a patient requests care and there is not time involved on the part of the personnel and the request is not granted, chart under activity heading the time the event occurred and "R". See F.

14. If a patient requests care and the person moves to the bedside to hear the request, but the request is not granted, chart the time of occurrence and time involved under "answering questions." Place an "R" and time of occurrence under the heading that applies, (e.g., fluids). See G.

15. If the nature of an unanswered request is not identified, record time of occurrence and "R" in answering questions.

16. The category, "Answering Questions," refers to isolated incidents, rather than questions answered during a conversation, and each entry will include an "R" unless "R" is recorded in relation to the activity to which the request relates.

17. When medications and nursing procedures are administered by the functional method of assignment, record an estimate of the proportion of time required for preparation, aftercare of equipment and recording for the observed patient.

Exceptions

There are, of course, exceptions to the usefulness of individual copies of the tool for individual data collection periods. For some types of data, such as repeated standard-scales measurements of body temperatures, a single copy of a form may be used to record observations for an entire week or month for one patient. Also, with this type of datum, a single copy might be used to record data for several subjects. This would pertain where recordings are of a relatively brief nature and are objective observations, such as repeated standard-scales measurements. Although there are some notable exceptions, tools, like Topsy, "just grow." The exceptions, of course, derive from the fact that the format of a tool will grow in relation to the appearance of the recording of a single datum.

Further Elements Influencing Format

The nature of the recording will have been determined in relation to the phenomena to be recorded. Planning for ease in handling the symbols when the data are to be organized for analysis will also influence the format of the tool, as will the numbers of observations to be recorded and the period of time in which any set of observations will be made. So, too, will the pattern of activities of the observer as he makes and records the observations. The researcher should be imaginative in designing his tools and should try several forms and types of materials. Bibliography cards of various sizes are frequently convenient for recording the data and particularly convenient for its later organization. Different colors for different forms are a good idea. As with observation-making tools, the researcher should adopt and adapt recording tools wherever possible. Where tools are adopted, the researcher should make certain that he has permission to use copyrighted tools. Where adaptations are made, credit should be given to the original source of the idea; if extensive use is made of the original, permission should be obtained.

Pretest the Tool

Where adaptations are made or new tools designed, the researcher should try several formats until he finds the most useful one. For both observation-making and -recording tools, pretesting is imperative. The first pretest should be "recording" hypothetical data—not just any hypothetical data, but recordings as they may be expected to appear in the actual data collection situations. The researcher should imagine himself actually making observations. He should then record, in appropriate form in the planned spaces on the tool, what he expects to observe in his imagined situation. If prior steps in the planning have been thoroughly done, this will not be difficult. IF (1) the investigator's problem was thoroughly defined; (2) the definitions of terms were pulled from the problem-defined; (3) the terms were operationally defined; (4) the types of data to be sought were precisely identified; (5) individual data of each type were identified, each at a ground-ham-on-rye level; (6) the sources of data and the process for obtaining the observations to compose the data were reasonably planned; and (7) these steps led smoothly one to the other and all were completed, THEN the items that must appear on the recording tool have all been identified. To pretest the tool, the planner needs only to insert the previously identified data recordings into the spaces he has designed in his tool. It is easy to visualize the ease with which 3B was able to develop designs for potentially usable tools. The thoroughness of her plan for Step 5 (pages 147–149) provided her with concretes with which to work in planning Step 8. If there has been a gap in the continuity of the planning of prior steps, that gap (or gaps) will have to be filled in before the recording tool is developed, or as it is being developed. Step 8, the student is again reminded, is the culminating point. Movement may be made to succeeding steps on the basis of incomplete prior steps—until Step 8. What has not been done before Step 8, now will have to be done.

Identify Gaps in Prior Steps

The student will readily recognize gaps in his previous planning if he: (1) imagines himself in the setting that he has planned for collecting his data, (2) pictures himself performing the activities needed for making a single observation, and then (3) writes down the notation that he has envisioned as a recording of a single datum. The notation may be a hashmark beside a descriptive term or phrase, the record of a scaled measurement, such as a blood pressure reading, a written word or phrase such as "turned without assistance," or a full-paragraph description of a critical incident. If data have been identified on ground-ham-on-rye levels, there will be illustrations from Step 5 that can be placed in the developing tool, to try them for size. The detailed listings of potential data by 3B (pages 147–149) demonstrate this point. In some instances, the student will have identified in Step 5 only a few illustrative examples of his anticipated data; this does not constitute a gap in planning. In Step 8, the student will, as he develops and tests his recording tool, identify an additional number and variety of data illustrative of observations to be made. How completely the tool will be developed during the planning of the entire design for the investigation will depend on the number of varieties of data that must be identified. If there is a limited number, the tool or tools may be completely designed as Step 8 is being planned. If there are a great many varied types of data, only a portion of each tool will be developed at the time of design development. Completion will await evaluation of the total design and decision to move forward with data collection and execution of the total investigation.

Degree of Completion of Tool

A further example from 1A's study (Exhibit 4 [4]) can illustrate this latter point. She planned to seek information from patients about what they had been taught about early ambulation and how they felt about performing the activities, and decided to use an interview as the technique for collecting these data. She identified five major areas about which she wished to question the patients. For each major section, she identified three to eight main questions, each with one to nine subquestions. As she planned Step 8, she made explicit the five major areas. She developed the main questions for two of the areas and the subquestions for all main questions in one area. The rationale for this procedure was that, having identified the five major areas of concern, she knew the scope of the data she would be seeking and could be confident that she would explore all areas of her concern. By developing all main questions for two major areas, she could know the nature of the questions to be asked and the number of questions needed to elicit all information required. By developing all subquestions for all main questions in one area, she could anticipate various responses that patients might make and ensure that she had questions that would elicit all needed information from all patients about the particular area. This planning also allowed her to visualize the pattern that the recording of each response would take, and she could estimate the approximate length of time that would be required to conduct the interview. In addition, it provided for planning for spacing on the tool.

The device of listing an extensive number of subquestions serves two important purposes. When descriptive, explanatory data are sought, the subquestions ensure that areas are completely explored and that no facets

EXHIBIT 4

PART I:

    <u>Comment to Patient:</u>   First I would like to ask you about some of the things you did <u>after</u> your operation.

1. Approximately how soon after your operation were you asked to cough deeply.

    1.1 Did you know you would be asked to cough?

    1.2 What is your understanding of the reason you were asked to cough?

    1.3 Did you have help with coughing?

    1.4 Tell me how you felt about coughing deeply?

    1.5 What made you feel that way?

2. Approximately how soon after your operation were you asked to turn in bed?

    2.1 Did you expect to do this?

    2.2 Did you have help with turning?

    2.3 What is your understanding of the reason you were asked to turn in bed?

    2.4 Tell me how you felt about turning in bed?

    2.5 What made you feel that way?

3. Approximately how soon after your operation were you asked to get out of bed?

    * * * * * *

    3.7 Did you have any medicine for pain?

    If no to 3.7 ask:

    3.8 Did you know you could ask for pain medication?

    3.9 Approximately how many times did you get up to walk during <u>each</u> of the first three days after your opera<u>tion</u>?

PART II:

    <u>Comment to Patient:</u>   I would now like to ask you about some of the information you may have had <u>before</u> coming to the hospital.

There were 6 major questions, with subquestions.

PART III:

    <u>Comment to Patient:</u>   Now I would like to ask you about information you received after you came to the hospital.

    <u>Experimental Group:</u>   When you are answering these questions try to recall the instructions you received from other persons, rather than the instructions that I gave you.

Concepts Pertinent to Defined Terms 217

EXHIBIT 4 (Cont'd)

PART III (Cont'd)

1. Did you wonder about what you would be expected to do <u>after</u> your operation?

    1.1 What particular things did you want to know?

2. After you came to the hospital did you receive definite instructions about the things you would be asked to do after your operation?

    2.1 Experimental Group only: Did persons other than myself offer to give you instructions?

3. Did the nurse give you any definite instructions about:

    a. coughing deeply?
    b. turning in bed?
    c. walking?

    * * * * * * * *

PART IV:

<u>Comment to Patient:</u> The next questions will be about your opinion of instructions for patients.
There were 8 questions, with subquestions.

PART V:
<u>Give copy of visual aid leaflet to all patients</u>

<u>Comment to Control Group:</u> I would like you to look over this leaflet. This is sometimes given to patients before their operation.
<u>Comment to Experimental Group:</u> Do you remember the leaflet I gave you before your operation? Here is another copy; I would like you to look it over again.
There were 6 questions, with subquestions.

---

will be overlooked. Where data for testing a hypothesis are being sought, they ensure that similar questions will be asked of all subjects. For both types of data, the division into key and subquestions permits some free-association responses from the subject. That is, he is asked to respond to the encompassing key question. The subquestions are used only if he does not include answers to them in his response to the key question. The device eliminates many stilted, short-answer questions. If needed, it provides for probing with them. The latter is particularly helpful with subjects inclined to laconic responses or those unused to expansive verbal communications where some degree of abstractness is involved. The student is cautioned, however, about probing when seeking data for testing a hypothesis. Depending on the plan for quantifying the data and on other matters, decisions

EXHIBIT 5

SLATER NURSING COMPETENCIES RATING SCALE

Page _____ of _____ pages

Date _____

Nurse being rated: _____ Rater (name or No.): _____

Column headings (diagonal): Best Nurse | Between | Average Nurse | Between | Poorest Nurse | Not Applicable | Not Observed

PSYCHO-SOCIAL: INDIVIDUAL
Actions directed toward meeting psycho-social needs of individual patients.

1. Gives full attention to patients. ( ) ____ ( ) ____ ( ) ____ ____
2. Is a receptive listener ( ) ____ ( ) ____ ( ) ____ ____
3. Approaches patient in a kind, gentle and friendly manner ( ) ____ ( ) ____ ( ) ____ ____
4. Responds in a therapeutic manner to patient's behavior ( ) ____ ( ) ____ ( ) ____ ____
5. Recognizes anxiety in patient and takes appropriate action ( ) ____ ( ) ____ ( ) ____ ____
6. Gives explanation and verbal reassurance when needed ( ) ____ ( ) ____ ( ) ____ ____
7. Offers companionship to patient without becoming involved in a non-therapeutic way ( ) ____ ( ) ____ ( ) ____ ____
8. Considers patient as a member of a family and of a society ( ) ____ ( ) ____ ( ) ____ ____
9. Is alert to patient's spiritual needs ( ) ____ ( ) ____ ( ) ____ ____
10. Identifies individual needs expressed through behavior and initiates actions to meet them ( ) ____ ( ) ____ ( ) ____ ____
11. Accepts rejection or ridicule and continues effort to meet needs ( ) ____ ( ) ____ ( ) ____ ____
12. Communicates belief in the worth and dignity of man ( ) ____ ( ) ____ ( ) ____ ____
13. Utilizes healthy aspects of patient's personality ( ) ____ ( ) ____ ( ) ____ ____

NOTE: To facilitate identification, Best, Average, and Poorest Nurse columns are those with the parens marking spaces.

*Copyright © 1967 College of Nursing, Wayne State University.

about the nature and amount of probing permissible will vary with each investigation. The device of the key and subquestions is useful, but it must be used with discretion.

The reason for developing the entire set of main questions for two areas and the entire set of subquestions for one area is that it ensures that the tool will enable the securing of usable data. It also provides a pattern for doing the remainder of the tool at a later time. If only scattered questions and subquestions are done, there is no basis for judging that the final tool will secure all data that will be required. If the investigator does one or two sections completely and identifies the nature of all main sections, he will know the exact character of his tool and he will have assurance that what he "has in mind" will indeed be executed and will serve his purpose. Furthermore, it is only with a completed section that he can pretest his tool for spacing needed to make the recordings.

Rationale for Details for Few Areas

For detailed planning for only two or three major areas, planning need not be limited to the first areas in the projected sequence. It may very well be advantageous to select areas out of sequence. With such selection, the investigator is apt to explore more varied areas than if he planned in logical sequence. As illustration, 3B would have thought of a variety of concerns in her study as she completely developed subquestions for her key questions #3 (What does he ask about his brothers and sisters, and about school friends?) and #8 (What physical discomfort does your child complain of?) Whereas, had she planned in relation to question #3 and question #4 (How does your child like the other children on the ward?) she would have planned for only a limited facet of her concern.

The same planning may be done where the nature of the anticipated data is such that the tool would take the form of a lengthy list of items with adjacent spaces for the appropriate notations. For example, the Slater Nursing Competencies Rating Scale is composed of 84 nursing actions divided into six major categories of activities.[2] As that tool was developed during the planning of a research design, the six categories would have been identified and all activities for one category would have been delineated. The format of the tool would have been drawn for the first page of the tool (Exhibit 5).

Example: Slater Nursing Competencies Rating Scale

Materials from 3B's work illustrate one more aspect of tool construction and format: overly detailed planning. 3B followed a pattern similar to that of 1A for planning her interview schedule. She looked to the criterion measures and specific categories of data (pages 147–149) that she had identified as areas about which she would need facts to test her hypothesis. She identified and constructed 30 key questions and 3 to 5 subquestions for each. Actually, 3B developed plans in far greater detail than was necessary. Such extensive planning, on the part of 3B and others like her, may stem from the following reasons: (1) eagerness on the part of

Admonition: Details Beyond Need

the student, (2) anticipation of completing the study, and (3) once involved in planning any particular facet, it is difficult to stop before completing it. A deluge of ideas demanding to be recorded pours forth. Here, again, there is need for guidance on the part of the instructor and self-discipline on the part of the student. Occasionally there is justification for excessively detailed planning in the design for individual facets of the study. One may be anticipation of completing the study. Yet, even in this instance, the student should be mindful that there are still other steps to be planned. It may seem as though it will take only a short time to complete detailed plans, while warmed up to the work and while ideas are proliferating. Yet several of these short periods can cut deeply into the total time available for developing the entire design. The student should resist planning beyond the details necessary to understand the precise nature of the materials being planned and to establish the pattern for the complete planning of the particular facet. He must move on to next steps.

There may be one further justification for the student's planning details beyond those needed for the design itself. The student is thinking broadly and deeply about his problem as he elaborates details. He is learning something. All reasons justifying excessive detail are worthy. The pros and cons of the discussion lead to a platitude applicable to many other facets of planning: there is not a right and a wrong. The researcher must plan in detail suited to the many factors inherent in his individual investigation.

SUMMARY

Tools are needed for two purposes: to make the necessary observations and to record them. Wherever possible, tools developed for other investigations should be adopted or adapted. This is particularly true for the observation-making tools, since these require a great deal of time and know-how for development and testing. The researcher should adopt whenever possible, adapt when no tool can be found to fit precisely the requirements of his data needs, and start from scratch only as a last resort.

When planning for tools, the investigator will think first of the identities of his data, the sources of the data, the activities of the observer in observing and recording the phenomena, and the form that the recording of the data will take. The most helpful procedure is for the investigator to visualize himself as the observer in the planned setting as he observes and records a single phenomenon. The recording should be exactly as he expects it will be in the actual collection of the data: a hashmark, a number of pounds, a narrative description of a critical incident, or any other. Where observations are limited in variety, complete tools can be designed. Where there are a large number of varied observations, the major areas should be identified and one or two major sections completely developed.

All tools should be pretested for the purposes of assuring: that (1) anticipated data will be obtained through their use; (2) spacing for recording is appropriately planned; (3) the amount of time required for gathering the data can be estimated; and (4) there will be base for planning the final four steps of the design. As for numerous other aspects of the design, planning for tools should be as simple as possible and as complex as necessary.

The first testing of the tool should be done by the investigator, imagining himself as the observer collecting data during one planned observation period and filling in a complete copy of each tool. For tools only partially planned, he would fill out the part that has been completed. He will visualize each phenomenon as it might be expected to occur, and he will record a hypothetical datum illustrative of a recording as he anticipates it will appear in the actual situation.

REFERENCES

1. Phaneuf, M. C. The nursing audit for evaluation of patient care. Nurs. Outlook, 14:51-54, 1966.
2. Slater, D. The Slater Nursing Competencies Rating Scale. Detroit, College of Nursing, Wayne State University, 1967.
3. Godfrey, A. E. A study of nursing care designed to assist hospitalized children and their parents in their separation. Nurs. Res., 4:52, 1955.
4. Couture, N. A. Planned Pre-operative Teaching of Early Ambulation for Patients Having Major Abdominal Surgery. Unpublished masters thesis, Detroit, College of Nursing, Wayne State University, 1961, pp. 85-94.
5. Wandelt, M. A. Uninterrupted Patient Care and Nursing Requirements. Detroit, College of Nursing, Wayne State University, 1963, pp. 121-152.
6. Murphey, H. M. Greater support of the dying child. Unpublished research design, Detroit, College of Nursing, Wayne State University, 1967.

STEP 9
COLLECTION OF DATA

Collection of data is what all that has gone before has been about. All the planning described in the earlier steps will now be tied together in this step. The student may feel that he is now ready to do what he has labored so long to prepare to do. Indeed, some persons refer to Step 9 in such terms as "doing the study" and "the actual study." It seems quite erroneous, however, to refer to one aspect of the study as "the actual study" —particularly when the aspect may, in many ways, be considered the least important of the entire investigation. But attempting to place a level of importance on any one aspect of a scientific inquiry is like attempting to establish the relative importance of one blade of a scissors or one wheel of an automobile. The analogies also contradict the idea of any one step of a study referred to as the actual study. One wheel does not make an automobile; nor one blade, a scissors; nor collecting data, a study. In this chapter, plans will be developed for coordinating all of the elements that, to this point, have been so carefully planned. Briefly, Step 9 is the plan for *who* will do *what,* with *whom, when,* and *where.* Many of the elements of this planning will have been considered previously, and rightly so. But the actual detailed, specific, and precise planning has not been required until this particular point.

Misnomer: Actual Study

One of the early decisions to be made in relation to the collection of data is the number of data to be collected. Where a hypothesis is to be tested, a statistician will have been consulted early in the planning and

Number of Data Needed

will have assisted in determining the number of subjects required and the numbers of various data needed. The statistics-based guides for making such determinations are described in various statistics texts and in some guides to research planning. The details about them are beyond the needs of the beginning researcher, but he should understand that statistics is a fundamental tool in all hypothesis testing and that consultation with a statistician is practically always necessary. As he moves on to more sophisticated scientific investigations, he will learn more and more about the statistics needed for his purposes. But, as he is learning the process of research, he usually works under a marked time limitation and his first research effort will in all probability be a pilot study. For it, he will make an arbitrary decision about the numbers of subjects to be studied, depending on such factors as the time needed to introduce the independent variable, for its effects to become measurable, and to collect the data.

Introduce Independent Variable

Where a hypothesis is to be tested, the planning for the independent variable must be completed as part of Step 9. Frequently, in nursing investigations, the independent variable will be some form of instruction, of either patients or personnel, or of both. For the design, the investigator will develop the "course outline," which will indicate the general content and plan of instruction. Detailed plans may be completed after the entire design is completed and the plan for the investigation found to be feasible. Where the independent variable is a form of "treatment," its nature and the precise method and schedule for its application must be made explicit as a part of Step 9. Once this has been done, the planning moves to consideration of the introduction of the variable to the experimental subjects.

WHAT THE INVESTIGATOR WILL BE DOING

At this point, the investigator should think in detail about who will be doing what, with whom, when, and where. Some of the first considerations will be what the investigator himself will be doing.

Subjects and Sources

1. What will he be doing in relation to study subjects and sources of data? In some instances, the investigator himself will introduce the independent variable. For example, 1A gave preoperative and early postoperative instructions to the experimental patients in her investigation. On the other hand, Godfrey had her students introduce the "treatment." In the Uninterrupted Patient Care study, the nurse observers provided the care that was the independent variable, for most of the patients. Hospital staff provided the experimental care for some of the subjects. The investigator served as coordinator of much of the work and identified all potential study subjects, did the random selection of those to be studied each study period, and planned the nurse observers' schedules for their

work with the patients. Quite obviously, each of these approaches required different planning, including planning for the investigator's relationship with those who would introduce the independent variable to the experimental group of subjects.

2. From whom will the investigator request permission to use data sources? When the investigator is a student, his advisor should be involved in this procedure. The advisor can help the student to plan for the most likely sites for successful execution of his data collection, and can frequently gain entrée, where a student might be refused. This implies some control, so that particular agencies or individuals who are generous in their contributions to the school and its students will not be overtaxed with excessive requests. The original contact will be made by the advisor—usually by phone in the presence of the student. Frequently, a meeting between the individual whose permission is being sought and the student can be arranged at this time. After that, the student may make all other permission requests. The original request will usually be made to the director of the service of concern. For example, a nurse would communicate first with the director of nursing in the agency. In some instances there may be some question about the individual with whom first to communicate. For example, 1A had to have permission from the surgeons whose patients she would be studying as well as from the nursing service director. In such an instance, the appropriate approach is through the director of nursing; the study was a nursing care study, and a nurse would be "working" in the agency.

Permission to Use Data Sources: Strategy, Courtesy, Self-interest

Even where the study may involve few if any of the nursing staff, the investigator's first communication should still be with the director of nursing, as a matter of professional courtesy. Furthermore, of importance to the self-interest of the investigator, the director of nursing can open doors that would remain closed without her assistance. What usually happens is that, following the student investigator's introduction to the director of nursing service, the director or her assistant will set up appointments with other persons who must be involved—physicians, hospital administrators, social workers, research committee chairmen, nurse supervisors, and head nurses. In many instances, they will accompany the student investigator for her introductory interviews. It cannot be recommended too highly that the investigator seek entrée to the agency through the director of the service related to his own discipline.

Sometimes, quite inadvertently, the investigator may become extensively involved with planning an investigation with a member of another discipline before having communicated with the director of the service of his own discipline. This may happen when a nurse investigator has worked closely with a physician. For example, the nurse, while serving as a member of the nursing staff, may have begun thinking of study of a particular prob-

Inadvertent Involvement

lem and, at that time, discussed the problem with one or more physicians whose patients were involved. The physicians may have expressed interest, and planning may have continued without any notification to the director of nursing. The nurse investigator should be alert to this possibility and should request an interview with the director of nursing at the earliest possible point in the plan development. This is particularly important if the investigator's relationship with the agency is not a formal one involving an independent contract with the agency, but instead is one such as a former employee or instructor or student might have. This suggestion applies to investigators in any discipline. The director of that discipline within the institution can offer great varieties of assistance. In addition, he will be interested in the investigation and is one more individual with whom the investigator may discuss his plan, thereby further enlarging and clarifying his own thinking about it.

There are times when the student investigator may be acquainted with a member of the service of his own discipline in the agency where he plans to collect his data. In this circumstance, the student may prefer to make the initial communication with that individual. This presumes, of course, that the acquaintance is in a position to grant the required permission. But even where the student does know someone in an agency, the plan to seek permission to conduct the study in that agency should still be discussed with the advisor, and the request for permission should be addressed to the director of the service.

Information for All Participants

3. How will the investigator acquaint the persons to be involved, with the nature of the study and with their particular involvement? The desirable procedure is to bring these persons into the planning as early as possible. The "early as possible," however, is subject to great variation and is influenced by many factors. Essentially, a student investigator will have his design completed and approved by his faculty committee before members of the agency where the data will be collected are apprised of the study. Where the investigator is not a student, he will communicate with persons in the agency early in his planning—certainly, by the time he is deciding about the sources of his data. The first communication will be an exploratory one, to determine the agency's interest in becoming involved and cooperating in the study. The initial inquiry will include determination of potential availability of data in the agency and discussion, with persons knowledgeable in the field, of the evolving plans for the study. The first communication may be with the director of the service alone, or at his discretion, it may include one or more of his assistants. As plans develop and there is relative certainty that the investigation will be pursued, there will be further communication with the agency to include more of the persons to be involved. These communications will coincide with Step 9 in the planning, when one or more members of the agency

What the Investigator Will Be Doing

will be assigned to work with the investigator to assist in developing details for the data collection.

Orientation of Data Collectors

The investigator must plan details of the process through which he will instruct the observers (data collectors) and those who will introduce the independent variable. These instructions should include at least one practice session, during which these persons will perform each of the activities they will be expected to do in the actual data collection period. The degree of formality of the orientation and the amount of time spent on it will depend on the complexity of the tasks and the degree to which the tasks are new to the individuals. The practice session should be in the actual setting of the data collection or in a nearly exact replica and it should include use of exact copies of the recording tools. The practice session will take place within a day or two of beginning the actual data collection. At this time, ample supplies of all material will be ready for use. Supplies will include outlines of plans, along with guides and instructions, for use of all tools.

Advance Notice

The anticipated degree of involvement of various members of the agency will determine the amount of information supplied to each. Those responsible for agency functions and programs will be supplied with an outline of the total study plan. They will receive such details about the study as the problem of concern, the focus and timeliness of the study, and a description of the planned involvement of themselves and of persons for whom they are responsible. Study subjects are usually individually informed about the study and their part in it at the time they enter into the study. Advance notice in some form of a general group communication, however, can be helpful. For patients, a memo attached to their morning newspaper or placed on a breakfast tray, and a flash on the house radio are appropriate and effective means for such communication. For personnel who are to be study subjects, brief discussions during change-of-shift reports, locker room bulletin board flashes, or individual letters delivered either at work or sent to their home addresses are appropriate. How formal these communications should be will depend on the character of the participation requested. These communications would, of course, go only to those who might be involved: potential subjects of study and sources of data, and persons working in the setting.

The nature and amount of advance notice will depend on the number of persons to be involved and the nature of their involvement. Although advance information seems to favorably influence responses to requests for cooperation, there are situations when this procedure must be sacrificed. In the Uninterrupted Patient Care study, there was the potential of some 300 nursing service personnel and 70 physicians to be involved during the course of one year. General information meetings with these persons were not feasible, since the cost in time for them would have been large. Besides, there was the possibility that some might never be involved and some might not be involved until six months or more after the meetings would have been held. Therefore, two meetings were held with head nurses and supervisors: one, early in the planning to inform them about the study and to seek suggestions from them; and the second, later on, to plan detailed procedures and seek their ideas and cooperation. Individual letters were sent to each person who might possibly be asked to cooperate in the study. One letter was sent just prior to the beginning of data collection (during the three-week orientation of the nurse observers), explaining the study and informing the individuals of the types of assistance they might be asked to provide. A second letter was sent following the pilot study and prior to renewal of the data collection activities. At the beginning of study of each new set of patients (four patients were studied each two-week period), when patients had not been studied on the unit during the prior two-week study period, the general aspects of personnel involvement were explained during the change-of-shift reports. Essentially, the persons who may be involved in a study should be given prior information, with those selected for actual involvement given additional individual instructions. All should be offered opportunity to ask questions and, should they so desire, to refuse to participate.

The Truth

4. What should be told to persons who are to be involved in the study? First and foremost, all involved in the study should be told the truth. This includes the purpose of the study, the reason that they are being asked to participate, exactly what will be expected of them, and how much of their time they will be asked to give. They should be told whether they will be identified in any report of the findings from the study, and they should understand that they may refuse to take part in the study. All of these things should be explained fully and truthfully.

In some studies, however, if the study subjects, and sometimes even others, were to know the entire plan of the investigation, the findings would be influenced to the point that they would be biased or without meaning. In such instances, the individuals can be given some information about the study. Then they should be told that an explanation of the exact nature of the study would possibly affect their actions, behaviors, and responses. An appeal should be made to them to participate, with the assurance that they will remain anonymous and that results of the study will be made available to them if they so wish. They should be informed, *truthfully*—whether they be patients or personnel—that persons responsible for their care and welfare know the details of the study and the contribution they are being asked to make, and that these persons approve the conduct of the study and their participation in it. Very seldom will persons so informed refuse cooperation. Any that ask that they not be included in the study should have their wishes respected.

The investigator should plan what he is going to tell the individuals concerned. The best rule of thumb is to make the explanation as brief as possible without compromising the truth. (By and large, most persons are amazingly generous with their time. When studies are done in hospitals, the problem is not likely to be one of obtaining cooperation of patients and personnel but, rather, of reassuring and giving recognition to those who would like to participate, but will not be asked to do so.) The reason for keeping the explanation brief is that most persons do not feel that they understand much of what the study is about, anyway. A lengthy explanation seems to confuse rather than to clarify. Furthermore, a detailed explanation can indeed become complex, and it becomes more difficult to adhere to the truth and still not reveal facets about the study that would influence the subject's responses or behavior. Nonetheless, those who wish detailed information should be given an opportunity to request it.

"Barkus Is Willin'"

The desirability of a brief explanation may be illustrated by two real-life stories. A health worker when asked questions by one or all of his three preteenage children was frequently admonished by them, "Please, Daddy, don't tell us a whole long story; just answer the question."

How Much to Tell

The second story is of a public health nurse, who, with her husband, took two nieces, ages 7 and 8, for a leisurely drive one summer evening. They had not gone far when one of the children asked a question. The aunt, who had no children of her own, gulped a bit and thought, "This sort of question is their mother's responsibility; yet, children should have answers when they ask questions." Whereupon she launched into a detailed story of where babies come from. When she had finished her tale, she turned to look at the children in the back seat. The seven-year-old was sound asleep, and the eight-year-old said, "I don't believe a word of it."

Still another episode illustrates the small amount of explanation needed and the willingness of people to participate. An instructor approached a little old man with snappy black eyes, sitting up eating his breakfast. She checked his bed tag and greeted him by name. He said, "Good morning. Are you doing a study? Have you come to interview me"? and seemed disappointed when she gave a negative reply.

5. What will the investigator be doing in terms of the accumulating data? The student investigator is most likely to be the only data collector. Even if this is so, he should have a plan for orderly filing and for keeping track of the recorded observations. Depending on the number and variety of forms that will be involved, these plans may be simple or complex. They may involve a single manila folder or envelope, one folder each for the control and experimental groups, one folder for each study subject, a series of office files, or many other arrangements. Planning will also be necessary in relation to collection of the completed forms. The complexity of these plans will depend on the number and variety of forms, the

Chores Related to Accumulating Data

number of persons involved, and the work locations of the persons. Where data are collected within a single agency, housed on a single campus, the planning is not overly complex and members of the agency will usually assist. Where the observations composing the data are made in separate geographic locations, planning will be more complex and will require assistance from more liaison persons. To ensure against loss of data through errors in collection of forms, the investigator should prepare a written set of directions for handling the forms and should discuss these with each individual who will assist with any phase of their handling. Where others than the investigator handle data collection forms, the investigator will want to check during the first one or two runs of handling the forms to make certain that each understands what he is to do and to determine that all forms are getting to the point planned for their final pick-up. Where several varied forms are to be used, it is a good idea to plan to log forms out and in, each day or other appropriate time period.

Selection of Study Subjects

6. What is the investigator's role in the selection and scheduling for participation of study subjects? As mentioned earlier, a part of Step 9 is to decide on the number of data that will be needed. This will lead to determination of the number of subjects needed. These determinations are sometimes sequential and sometimes independent of each other; sometimes, the only determination is the number of subjects. As a part of planning for the data collection, the researcher will outline his plan for identifying the potential study subjects in the agency. He will decide on the particular formula and process he will use to randomize the selection of subjects and to assign them to control and experimental groups. Some of this planning will have been done during considerations about sources of data.

Sequence of Use of Study Subjects

Whether the study is to be of a before-and-after nature or if subjects in the control and experimental groups are to be studied at the same time will be influenced by choice of sources. Before-and-after can imply one of two major considerations: (a) The hypothesis proposes that individuals will change as a result of the experimental variable. (b) Subjects exposed to the experimental variable will be different from subjects not so exposed. In condition (a), the before-and-after plan is imperative; the study subjects must serve as their own controls. In condition (b), before-and-after is usually used to avoid contamination of the control group, though it is not essential to the testing of the hypothesis. Consideration must be given to the many factors involved in being sure that all variables will be the same for the two groups, except for the exposure of the experimental group to the independent variable. Where the independent variable is to be used in the same setting as that in which the control data will be collected, the control data should be collected before the independent variable is introduced. This will prevent its influence from spreading to the control group.

For example, if Godfrey had decided to have half of her students introduce the independent variable (sustaining care for the children and parents) while the other half were supposedly carrying on the established practice, it is entirely probable that there would have been communication among the students.[1] Some of the students providing care for the control children would have been providing—even if only in small degrees and unintentionally—some aspects of the care composing the independent variable. This would have tended to obliterate any difference between the treatments of the two groups. Furthermore, any differences found in outcomes of care could not have been attributed to differences in treatment. To prevent the influence of the independent variable from spreading to or contaminating the control group, it is comparatively simple to collect the control data in a situation known to be void of the independent variable, then to introduce the variable and collect the experimental data.

Example: Godfrey

Where studies are of a markedly "practical" nature, the before-and-after is perhaps a good plan, since, once a seemingly useful practice is introduced, it is difficult to withdraw it or to withhold it from persons who might be helped by it. This may not be a very scientific point of view, but it is a human and natural one. The researcher becomes so convinced of the value of his "treatment" that he cannot tolerate withholding it from potential candidates. Most testing of BCG vaccine in Europe, during the 1930's and 1940's, suffered from this fault. An example of resistance to this tendency, on the other hand, was the testing of the Salk vaccine under the guidance of Dr. Thomas Francis.

Giving and Withholding "Treatment"

Selecting study subjects and planning to introduce the independent variable can both be intricate; each investigation will encompass many unique factors that will influence the final details of the procedures. Abdellah and Levine have discussed the many influencing factors, using examples from nursing studies in Chapter Six of *Better Patient Care Through Nursing Research*.[2] The student will find their discussion helpful for guidance about particular planning and for ideas about best procedures in the light of his own particular influencing factors. An even more detailed discussion may be found in *Experimental and Quasi-Experimental Designs for Research*, by Campbell and Stanley.[3]

The desirable plan is to follow the classic pattern of experiment. That is, the sample of study subjects, who are representatives of the population being studied, should be divided into two equal groups. Both groups should be maintained in identical environments. The "treatment" (the independent variable) is introduced to the experimental group and simultaneously withheld from the control group. Observations are made of all subjects in both groups on the same basis at the same times. Such, briefly, is the desirable plan for obtaining data to test a hypothesis. Obviously, it is not always,

Classic Pattern of Experiment

nor even frequently, possible to achieve the desirable plan when studying human beings—and especially when the study subjects are individuals with health care needs. Frequently the investigator must choose between: (1) studying the control and experimental groups at the same time in two different settings, and (2) studying two groups in sequence in a single setting. Frequently, the less undesirable of these two less-than-desirable situations is the second approach. There are apt to be fewer variances of influencing environmental factors at two different time periods in a single setting than there would be in two different settings during a simultaneous time period. Of course, if the investigator could control all components of an environment where persons live and work and receive health care, there would be no reason for concern. But it is almost impossible to maintain complete control over all environmental factors, simply because of the magnitude of the tasks,—there are so many potentially influencing factors. In addition, and frequently more important, is the matter of the health care needs of the study subjects. They often need particular care and treatment, even though the requirements of the research make the care undesirable. In such circumstances, the investigator must modify his research plan to accommodate the prerogatives of the patients to receive care.

RIGHTS OF HUMAN SUBJECTS

Guidelines for Nurse Researchers

The question of rights of persons who are asked to participate as study subjects in research has had extensive attention in recent years. Most organizations that conduct studies involving human subjects and those that support and otherwise foster such research have published guidelines to assist researchers as they plan investigations that will involve human subjects. Investigators should provide the study subjects with information sufficient for them to know and understand the nature of their involvement and participation in all facets of the study. Guidelines developed for nurses, and titled *The Nurse in Research: ANA Guidelines on Ethical Practice,* were adopted by the board of directors of the American Nurses' Association, in January, 1968.[4] Obviously, such guidelines require interpretation to accommodate variations in individual investigations. The researcher will usually have available to him in his own agency or in the agency responsible to and for the study subjects, a committee on ethics. The members of this committee will assist him in his planning and approve the plan he develops in relation to the involvement he plans for his study subjects. They will also assist him to plan and evaluate the information given to the subjects as a basis for the latters' decision to participate or not.

Many of the details about the selection of study subjects apply only when a hypothesis is to be tested. Where no hypothesis is to be tested, there is no need for random selection or random distribution of subjects among groups. This is not to say that in exploratory studies there is no need for definitive identification of study subjects. In fact, for exploratory studies, the identity of the study subjects must be as definitive as in studies to test hypotheses. The process of identification will have begun in the definition of terms. In Step 9, however, the researcher will describe his population in greater detail, the degree of explicitness depending on the stated purpose of the study. The illustrative studies that have been used throughout this text indicate the degree and types of explicitness needed. Godfrey limited her population to ill children, between ages 2 and 6 years, hospitalized more than one day, whose parents visited them, and who were in contact and able to communicate. 1A identified her population as men and women, between ages 18 and 60, having nonemergency major, abdominal, or thoracic surgery, with no complications that would preclude out-of-bed ambulatory activities. For exploratory studies, similar definitions would be used to identify precisely the population from whom observations would be obtained and to whom findings would be generalizable. While random selection of individuals from the potential population pool would not be necessary, a degree of representativeness would be sought. The means for obtaining representativeness will depend on the nature of the characteristics which the investigator wishes to have represented. As with many facets of planning, the scope of representativeness and the means for its attainment require consideration of many relevant factors. The characteristics that would be controlled for and the distribution of various degrees of the characteristics necessary to assure the study subjects' being representative of the study population should be relevant to the problem and focus of the study. For example, 3N was concerned about techniques and support provided patients having nasal gastric tubes inserted.[5] It was important that she have patients who had experienced this procedure two or more times, as well as those who had had the tube inserted only one time. On the other hand, the subjects' occupations would not be expected to influence their expressions of their experiences related to the procedure and would not have been taken into consideration when planning for representativeness of the study population. In many but not all exploratory studies, geographic distribution is utilized as one of the variables in seeking representativeness. All relevant variables should be accommodated in the design; unnecessary ones should not be incorporated.

7. Who will introduce the independent variable? This question has already been considered in the discussion of some of the things the in-

Study Subjects Representative of the Population

Who Gives "Treatment"

vestigator will be doing in relation to data collection. The investigator himself may introduce the independent variable to the subjects of the experimental group; this is especially likely if the investigator is a student. Sometimes one or two persons may be responsible for introducing the independent variable, or many people may be involved. Under any of these circumstances, however, the investigator should outline, in writing, a plan and schedule for the activities required by this procedure. Similar planning must be done in relation to identification, orientation, and functioning of the individuals who will make and record the observations.

WHO DOES WHAT, WITH WHOM

Who will be doing what, with whom?

Plans must be outlined, in writing, for the type of interactions among persons involved in the data collection phase of the study. The investigator should imagine exactly what a person will do as he introduces the independent variable to a study subject. He should then consider what all persons will do as they introduce the independent variable to all subjects in the experimental group. This will provide the base for developing the time schedule for the data collection. The complete time schedule, of course, must include the collection of data from the control as well as the experimental subjects. The imagining should include interactions between those who introduce the independent variable and the study subjects; between observers and study subjects; and between all involved persons and other persons in the setting.

The thinking through of individual patterns for each category of persons will help the investigator to visualize precisely what may be expected. The four exhibits from the Uninterrupted Patient Care study (Exhibits 1 through 4) illustrate this type of planning.[6] Such guides can help the observers know where they are to be and what they are to be doing, at any one time, on any one day, and on each day of the period of study of any one subject. Such elaborate planning is not always necessary. Frequently, the study of a single subject is of short duration and involves only a few types of observations. Nonetheless, a plotted time schedule is comparatively simple to make and provides assurance against error.

WHEN?

Who will be doing what, with whom, and when?

The *when* must be planned in terms of the time of day, what days of the week, and how many days and weeks.

EXHIBIT 1

SCHEDULE AND OUTLINE OF ACTIVITIES OF NURSE OBSERVER A DURING ONE 11-DAY STUDY PERIOD

Time of Day	Activities of NURSE A on Days:									
	1	2	3	4	5	6	7	8 9	10	11
A.M.	Hear report Pt. A Read Hist.	Hear report Pt. B Read Hist. Pt. B Obs. Pt. B	Hear report Pt. A Exp. Care Pt. A	——————————→					Hear report Pt. A Obs. Pt. B	Hear report Pt. B Obs. Pt. B
P.M.	Obs. Pt. A Assmt. Pt. A Est. Ill. Pt. A	Obs. Pt. B Assmt. Pt. B Est. Ill. Pt. B.	Obs. Pt. B Assmt. Pt. A	——————————→					Obs. Pt. B Assmt. Pt. A Est. Ill. Pt. A.	Obs. Pt. B Assmt. Pt. B Est. Ill. Pt. B

EXHIBIT 2

SCHEDULE FOR NURSE OBSERVERS A AND B PERFORMING PATIENT-CENTERED ACTIVITIES FOR PATIENT A

Activity	Nurse Observers for Days:									
	1	2	3	4	5	6	7	8-9	10	11
Assessment	A	B	A	A	A	A	A		A	B
Observation	A	B	B	B	B	B	B		B	B
Estimate of Illness	A	B							A	B

WHERE?

Who will be doing what, with whom, when, and where?

The *where* must be planned in relation to the name of the agency,

Step 9: Collection of Data

EXHIBIT 3

SCHEDULE AND OUTLINE OF NURSE OBSERVERS' ACTIVITIES FOR STUDY OF TWO PATIENTS

Day of Week	Day of Study	Nurse	Functions of Nurse Observers
T	1	A	A.M. Patient A: Hear morning report. Become acquainted with patient through record, conferences with head nurse and physician as indicated to plan care. Record Observations of nursing care given by nursing staff. Meet patient when observations begun. Begin Background Information.
			P.M. Patient A: Record Observations for 11 a.m. to 3 p.m. period. Record Assessments for Day 1, 24-hour period, Tuesday, 7 a.m. to Wednesday, 7 a.m., and 4-hour period, 11 a.m. to 3 p.m. Record Estimate of Illness.
		B	Same activities, Patient B.
W	2	A	A.M. Patient B: Hear morning report. Become acquainted with patient through record, conferences with head nurse and physician as indicated to plan care. Record Observations. Meet patient when observations begun.
			P.M. Patient B: Record Observations. Record Assessments for Day 2. Record Estimate of Illness.
		B	Same activities, Patient A.
Th See Exhibit [4] Schedule for one day of experimental care	3	A	A.M. Patient A: Hear morning report. Give experimental care.
			P.M. Patient B: Record Observations. Patient A: Record Experimental Care given in A.M. Record Assessments for Day 3.
		B	A.M. Patient B: Same activities.
			P.M. Patient A: Record Observations. Patient B: Record Experimental Care. Record Assessments for Day 3.
F S S M	4 5 6 7	Same	Same
T & W	8 & 9	A & B	Days off. Patient receives routine care from hospital staff.
Th	10	A	Patient A: Hear morning report. Record Assessments. Record Estimate of Illness.
			Patient B: Record Observations A.M. and P.M.
		B	Patient B: Hear morning report. Record Assessments. Record Estimate of Illness.
			Patient A: Record Observations A.M. and P.M.
F	11	A	Patient B: Hear morning report. Record Assessments. Record Observations. Record Estimate of Illness.
		B	Patient A: Same activities.

Where?

EXHIBIT 4

SCHEDULE FOR ONE DAY WHEN EXPERIMENTAL CARE IS GIVEN

Time	Functions of Nurse Observers	Relationship of Nurse Observers A and B to Patients A and B	
		Patient A	Patient B
7:00 a.m.- 11:00 a.m.	Hear morning report Give experimental care	Nurse A	Nurse B
11:00 a.m.- 11:40 a.m.	Lunch. Change from uniform to street clothes and white coat.		
11:40 a.m. to 3:30 p.m.[1]	Record Observations of care given by hospital nursing staff.	Nurse B	Nurse A
	Charting Experimental Care given during the morning in special form.	Nurse A	Nurse B
	Making Assessments on special form.	Nurse A	Nurse B

[1] Although observations were made from 11:40 a.m. to 3:30 p.m., for brevity's sake, the period is referred to throughout the report as the 11 a.m. to 3 p.m. or the 11 to 3 period; and the duration, as a 4-hour period.

the addresses of the buildings where observations will be made, and of the appropriate areas in the buildings. This planning may range from the relatively simple to the very complex. In almost all situations, the investigator will want to do some of the planning with assistance from persons in the agency. The agency will usually have to provide some space in which the study personnel may work. Even if the observer does no more than copy items from clinical records, he will still need work space, a place to hang a coat, and cafeteria and restroom accommodations. For the Uninterrupted Patient Care study, the director of nurses provided a room with closet space, desk, and chairs for the full 15 months that it was needed. Again, the thinking through of one day's activities for one person will provide the concretes for the planning. Activities from the time the individual leaves home or his usual work area, through his arrival at the agency, to the observation setting, to his leaving the agency should be envisioned. Each activity should be plotted in outline in terms of time of beginning and exact site of action. These plottings will provide the general outline of who will be doing what, with whom, when, and where.

Step 9 may seem so obvious that one might think there would be little need for detailed planning. But it is just because of this apparent "obviousness" that the investigator needs to think it through in fairly detailed outline. Many bits and pieces of it are considered as all the prior steps are being planned. Yet, until they have been woven into an integrated plan, the bits and pieces can give no assurance that data collection will be possible. It is only as the relationship of each aspect of the data to the other is mapped out, as well as each individual's time, place, and activity in relation to the total scheme, that there can be certainty that "things will work as planned." And, of course, it is only with this planning that a time schedule for the data collection can be estimated. Essentially, without a detailed outline of the planning that composes Step 9, no plan for an investigation can be judged for its feasibility.

REFERENCES

1. Godfrey, A. E. A study of nursing care designed to assist hospitalized children and their parents in their separation. Nurs. Res., 4:52, 1955.
2. Abdellah, F. G., and Levine, E. Better Patient Care through Nursing Research. New York, The Macmillan Company, 1965.
3. Campbell, D. T., and Stanley, J. C. Experimental and Quasi-Experimental Designs for Research. Chicago, Rand McNally & Co., 1963.
4. The Nurse in Research: ANA Guidelines on Ethical Values. New York, American Nurses' Association, 1968.
5. Teranes, B. Patient Views on Nasogastric Tube Insertion. Unpublished masters thesis, Detroit, College of Nursing, Wayne State University, 1967.
6. Wandelt, M. A. Uninterrupted Patient Care and Nursing Requirements. Detroit, College of Nursing, Wayne State University, 1963, pp. 28-30.

STEP 10

ORGANIZATION OF DATA
Coding, Tabulation, Classifying

COMPLETING THE PROCESS CIRCLE

Beginning with organizing and classifying the data, the final four steps of the research process may be thought of as a whole new project. Indeed, some investigators consider that they have finished the planning stage when Step 9 is completed. They then move to the data collection phase and do not start planning for Steps 10 through 13 until they have collected their data. The process of research, however, can be thought of as a sequence of procedures, which begin with an irritation and move through a complete circle, with the final step completing the circle as the study findings are examined in relation to what they may contribute to alleviating the irritation. In this view of the research process, interrupting the planning at Step 9 would leave a great gap in the circle—a gap that might admit many errors that could prevent the circle from ever being closed.

Completion of planning for the closure of the circle, on the other hand, can reveal possible errors before they can be made. The type of error most likely to be revealed while Steps 10 through 13 are being planned relates to the data's potential for actually providing answers to questions under study. The planning can also reveal vagueness about the data's potential for lending themselves to organization and for supporting conclusions that the investigator expects to support with his findings. Of course, if the investigator doesn't do the detailed planning, he will not yet have committed any errors in these latter two areas; he won't have done anything! These generalizations will become clear as each of the subsequent steps is discussed.

Thinking Is Hard Work Wherever It Is Done

There are very practical reasons for careful planning of Steps 10 through 13 as a part of the research design. Among them are that errors may be avoided and that the investigator will not proceed through the costly data collection procedure only to find that the data gathered will not serve to answer his question. In addition, logic dictates that since these steps require much thinking (hard work) whenever and wherever they are done, they might just as well be done along with the other planning. Possibly some researchers avoid the knotty problems of planning Steps 10 through 13 on the basis of the delusion that they will be easier to do once the data are in hand. But the planning for these steps is just as difficult with the actual data as it is with hypothetical data. The big difference is that if the planning during the development of the design reveals flaws in the planned-for data, the investigator will be happy to have discovered them in time, whereas, if the flaws are not revealed until the actual data are in hand, the investigator must live with himself and wish. . . .

Results of Planning Usable in Doing

No labor is lost when Steps 10 through 13 are planned in advance, using hypothetical data. What is done in an early step does not have to be done at a later one. Plans for organizing and analyzing data that are made during the design stage will apply directly to the actual data handling steps. Admittedly, the actual data may fail to substantiate the hypothesis—a bitter truth no investigator will visualize in his anticipated data—but this will not change the manner in which any of the data are handled. Difference of actual data from hypothetical data may modify some of the conclusions and recommendations, but never all of them.

"Why Do the Study?"

Those who would delay the work of Steps 10 through 13 may argue that, if you already know what you are going to find, if you can propose realistic, albeit hypothetical, data, "Why do the study?" This question, rather than "Why collect the data?" implies that collecting the data is the same undertaking as "doing the study." The primary response, of course, is that no one *knows* what the findings will be until the data have been collected. Furthermore, unless the investigator has some idea about what his data are going to look like, he is not apt to find what he is looking for. No investigation will yield much that is useful unless the investigator has a fairly clear idea of what he expects to find. It is not that the researcher knows precisely what he will find; rather he knows the kinds of observations that will be needed to answer his questions. He does not know beforehand the frequency, variations, or distributions of the observations to be sought; rather he knows the nature of those he is seeking. An awareness of what he is looking for does not preclude the observer from noting other phenomena in the situation. Rather, it makes him sensitive to observing all phenomena in the situation, and it provides him with a base for judging the pertinence of each phenomenon observed. Feibleman has commented that it takes training for the researcher to see what is in front of him and not what he would customarily expect to be there.[1] The observer

Completing the Process Circle 241

who knows what he is seeking will not approach a situation with an attitude of noting only what he would customarily expect to see. He approaches with an attitude of attending to all he sees, and to sort from all phenomena those of pertinence to his concern. He will collect his data to determine whether the phenomena he seeks actually do exist as he suspects they do and the extent to which they exist. If the purpose of his investigation is to learn more about the existence of phenomena in a situation (descriptive study), then he must know something of what he expects to find. He may find something different, but it is through the guidance of his expectations that he knows where and how to look. Pasteur said, "In the field of observation, chance favors only the prepared minds." The researcher who has planned well will have identified, in Steps 5 and 8, the nature of the data he expects to collect. In Step 5, he first identified examples of each type of datum that he would seek. In Step 8, as he tested his tools by recording anticipated notations of hypothetical observations, he identified additional varieties of anticipated data.

In planning Step 10, the student might begin by envisioning the overwhelming feeling he may expect to experience if he collects his data without having first outlined plans for handling them. To do this, he must visualize all those individual observations, collected in various sizes and shapes of small "containers." They are all there in front of him, on and around his desk: each potentially identifiable as an individual datum. There may be a hashmark among 50 hashmarks on a single sheet of paper or among 30 sheets of paper. Or a single datum may be a brief paragraph on an index card in one of 50 stacks of index cards. There may be one sentence on a 3 by 5 index card, in one of five shoeboxes full of 3 by 5 index cards. He may envision an apple in one of five bushels of apples. Or his concern may be a nurse-patient interaction scene recorded on 43 inches of one of 20 500-foot rolls of video tape. He has anywhere from 20 to 10,000 or more individual items of data. He must so organize those data that he will be able to view large numbers of them at one glance. Where does one begin to arrange the brief sentences recorded on five shoeboxes full of index cards so that one can view large numbers of them at one glance? (Incidentally, this example is *not* hypothetical.) [2]

Quantity and Variety of Individual Data: 5 Shoeboxes Full

The first concern in planning organization patterns for the data will have been identified by the statement of purpose of the study. The investigator will think first of the data he will need to test his hypothesis, to answer his question, or to describe the many elements composing the situation he proposes to explore. He will attempt to visualize ways to arrange those data most closely pertaining to the primary purpose of his study. They must be so arranged as to serve as a basis for a generalization of what the data tell about the particular facet of the problem that he has chosen to study.

Statement of Purpose: Focus For Organization

For example, 1A wanted to know whether there was a relationship between the instructions received by patients preoperatively and the number of ambulatory activities performed during the early postoperative period; she was testing a hypothesis. She sought an answer to whether there was a difference in the number of ambulatory activities performed by all patients in her control group and the number performed by all patients in her experimental group. She had to develop a plan for how she would "move" the 185 hashmarks from the 40 "containers" for the control group and the 320 hashmarks from the 40 containers for the experimental group, so that she could see at a glance whether there was a difference. Looking at the hashmarks as they reposed in the two sets of 40 containers would not have enabled her to judge whether there was a difference. Certainly there was no way to arrange the 80 containers, or even the 40 for one group, so that the contents of all could be viewed at one glance. This example is a fairly simple one to illustrate the nature of the first organizational movement of the data when the purpose of the study is to test a hypothesis; it will be elaborated further in the discussion of tools for organization.

ORGANIZE DESCRIPTIVE DATA

Example: 10A

The second concern for planning patterns for organizing the data when the purpose is to test a hypothesis is comparable to the concern when the purpose is to describe. Again, the investigator will turn to the statement of purpose or to the definition of problem. For example, 10A's statement of purpose provided guidance for the preliminary organizational pattern for the data contained in the five shoeboxes full of index cards: "The purpose of the study was to identify responses of schizophrenic children, determine whether there are common behavioral patterns of these children, and report implications for nursing care based on knowledge of their behavior." The data were individual observations of single behaviors of five children. Her first organizational pattern would consist of categorizing the observations in terms of possible behavior patterns. She used behavior classifications developed along patterns implicit in combinations of findings from studies done earlier by others. In other words, she would have taken all observations that looked alike from the individual containers into which they had been gathered, and placed those that looked alike in a single container, labeled with one of the behavior categories. A process for doing this will be described in greater detail below.

When the purpose is to test a hypothesis, and the pattern is completed for organizing the data needed to meet that purpose, the researcher will address himself to eliciting descriptive findings from his data. The process is similar to that for organizing descriptive data. Since there will be no succinct statement of purpose to indicate the nature of the pattern, the researcher will turn to his definition of problem. There he will have identified various facets closely related to the one he chose to study. Descriptions of these facets will provide ideas about ways of looking at the data. Do his findings confirm those of others? To what extent are they in agreement? Disagreement? What is the nature of the differences? It may be expected that the data collected in relation to the facet of primary focus will cast light on the adjoining ones. These, in turn, can serve as guides to patterns for further organization and examination of various data and relationships among data.

BONUS FINDINGS

The third concern when planning organization of data will be the "bonus" findings. In any investigation, there will always be many more "findings" than can reasonably be reported. Some will be omitted because various potentially meaningful analyses of data will not be done; some, because they are minor compared to the many findings that are reported; and some, because they seem quite unrelated to the problem under study. All of these omissions are appropriate. On the other hand, there frequently are findings quite distantly related, or even unrelated, to the central theme or problem of the study, but which should not be left unreported. These findings have been identified by Dr. Rosemary Rich as bonus findings. They differ from the descriptive findings that should be reported from studies done to test hypotheses in that they are completely unexpected, unlooked-for findings. For example, 1A had findings in relation to the particular types of activities that were performed by each patient: she knew the age, sex, specific type of surgery, and complications of surgery for each patient. Findings related to these data were descriptive findings; they were facts about accounted-for variables. She had anticipated their having meaning in relation to her problem, she had planned to gather data related to them, and she had anticipated some of the analyses that would be done in relation to them. In contrast, bonus findings are not anticipated; no plan is developed for making the observations, and the analyses in relation to them are not outlined during the planning stages of the study. Rich might well have labeled her bonus findings as a matter of "serendipity."

Example: 10B

As an example, two investigators (10B) were testing the reliability of the Slater Nursing Competencies Rating Scale when they found that the frequency with which items were checked in the "not observed" column was in indirect proportion to the number of cues provided to guide the individual evaluating a nurse's performance of the activity identified in the items.[3] There had been no plan to examine data for this finding, yet it was extremely meaningful. Not all investigations will yield bonus findings, but the investigator should be sensitive to the possibility and should report them when they are discovered.

Essentially, then, there are three major types of concern when planning the organization of data:

1. Basis for generalization about the statement of purpose or focus of the investigation.

2. Generalizations about relationships of findings to facets in the problem that are closely related to the facet chosen for study.

3. Descriptions of bonus findings.

The next concern must be the tools for the organization: the "container" into which the data will be placed as they are taken from their original containers (the observation-recording tools) and sorted into like categories.

ORGANIZING TOOLS

Just as the planning for observation-recording tools must progress in relation to the nature of individual units to be recorded, to the setting in which the observer would be making the recordings, and to ideas gleaned from others, and just as this planning seems to require custom tailoring with repeated fittings, even more so do some of the forms for organizing the data require individual tailoring to fit. This is not true for all of them. For many it is possible to use a copy of the observation-recording tool or to modify that tool slightly to be used as the form for organizing the data. Exhibit 1 illustrates the simple modification that 1A made of her observation-recording tool (page 207) to provide a very usable organizing tool—one that lent itself well to various steps in the organization of the data.[4]

1. The first step was to convert the hashmarks to Arabic numeral totals for each type of activity for each day. The second step was to transfer the totals from four containers (Exhibit 2) for each patient to a single container (Exhibit 1) for each patient, and then to sum them for all four days combined (Exhibit 3). The third organizing move involved transfer of the numerical totals from the 10 containers (Exhibit 3) for the 10 patients in each group to a single container for each group (Exhibit 4). This was accomplished, not by writing the totals for each patient in the cells on a separate tool, but by summing the totals for the 10 patients for any one activity on any one day and entering that total into the appropriate cell on the total-group container (Exhibit 4). This final transfer was followed by calculating the total for all activities on each of the days and, finally, by summing the totals for the four days to determine the number of activities performed by the patients in the group. At this point, it was possible to see at a glance whether there was a difference in the number of activities performed by patients in the two groups. The organized forms also allowed ready identification of specific areas of similarity or difference.

It is theoretically possible to identify any individual hashmark in any one of the containers, even after the hashmark has been converted to the

EXHIBIT 1

OBSERVATION TALLY SHEET

Page _____ of _____ pages

Patient _____ Group _____

Post-Operative Day	Daily Total of Each Activity							Total Activities
	Coughing		Turning		Out of Bed			
	S	A	S	A	1	2	3	4	
First									
Second									
Third									
Fourth									
Totals									

composite of an Arabic numeral. Just as it is possible to attach radioactive tags or dyes to molecules or cells so that they may be traced when they become integrated into other substances, so it would be possible to label or tag a hashmark and trace its route from container to container. It could be traced from observation-recording tool, to organizing tools, to tables in Step 11, and even to the report of findings in Steps 12 and 13. This concept is particularly important as the student plans the handling of hypothetical data. Since planning for the processes through which the data will be put will not involve the quantities of recordings that will be repre-

Trace a Single Datum

EXHIBIT 2

OBSERVATION RECORD

Page _____ of _____ pages

Patient __E-1_____ Date __7/7/69__ Postoperative Day __1_____

Room_____ Type_____ Age _____ Sex _____ Marital Status _____

Date of Admission _____ Previous Major Surgery _____

Type of Surgery _____ Date _____

Complications _____

Time	Activity								Code
	Coughing		Turning		Out of Bed				
A.M.	S	A	S	A	1	2	3	4	
7:35				1					S = self
~~7:50~~									
8:05					1				A = assistance
8:15					1				
~~8:35~~									1 = sitting in chair
8:50				1					
~~9:10~~									2 = walking, back very bent
~~9:25~~									
9:45		1							
~~9:55~~									3 = walking, back slightly bent
~~10:10~~									
10:25						1			4 = walking, back straight
									— = no activity
TOTALS		1		3		2			

COMMENTS: Group __Experimental_____

Instructions __√__ Reinforcement __√__ Visual Aid __0__

EXHIBIT 3

OBSERVATION TALLY SHEET

Page _____ of _____ pages

Patient __E1__   Group __Experimental__

Post-Operative Day	Coughing S	Coughing A	Turning S	Turning A	Out of Bed 1	Out of Bed 2	Out of Bed 3	Out of Bed 4	Total Activities
First		1		3	2				6
Second			1	2	2	1			6
Third	1		2		2		2		7
Fourth			1	1	4			1	7
Totals	1	1	4	6	10	1	2	1	26

sented by the actual data, the student could conceivably "pull figures out of the air" to represent the figures in the organizing tool or in the tables.

For example, the figures that might have been used by 1A in her planning would have been hashmarks for one day for one hypothetical patient, on one copy of the observation record (Exhibit 2). She would have summed the hashmarks to derive the Arabic numerals for one day for each type of activity, then transferred those numbers to a copy of the organization form (Exhibit 3). Using these as a base for planning, she would then have written in hypothetical numerals for the other three days for the one

Deriving Hypothetical Data

Step 10: Organization of Data

EXHIBIT 4

OBSERVATION TALLY SHEET

Page _____ of _____ pages

Patient __All_____   Group __Experimental_____

Post-Operative Day	Daily Total of Each Activity									Total Activities	Control*
	Coughing		Turning		Out of Bed					
	S	A	S	A	1	2	3	4		
First		25		34	18				77	43
Second		32	6	10	20	10			78	49
Third	20	6	15	5	10	5	20		81	41
Fourth	8		10		40		18	8	84	52
Totals	28	63	31	49	88	15	38	8	320	185

*Figures for Control Group would be moved here to provide ready reference. The figures are such that this use of the tool will not lead to confusion or error.

patient and summed them. She would have written these sums in the totals row and total activities column on the organizing form (Exhibit 3) to represent the observations made for one patient. She planned to have ten patients in a group, so she would have done a rough multiplication of the sums for one patient by the number of patients and derived the hypothetical sums for all patients in one group for four days (Exhibit 4). Multiplying by 10 is simple, but the imaginative student would not have done an exact multiplication for each type of activity. For some activities there would be a few more than 10 times the hypothetical total for one patient, and for some, a few less. These hypothetical sums would be recorded in appropriate cells in the final organizing tool (Exhibit 4). The total for ten patients would in no instance be fewer than the total for one! Should the hypothetical data appear so (and that does happen when the beginning researcher picks figures out of the air rather than following a reasonable thought process for deriving the hypothetical data), the data are not realistic in terms of what may be anticipated in the actual study.

In Exhibits 2, 3, and 4, there are comparatively few cells, so hypothetical figures were written into each cell. Should a plan call for many more days of observations for each subject and many more types of observations, the hypothetical data could be placed in a block of cells measuring 8 to 10 cells on a side. From these, it would be possible to calculate roughly the totals to be expected for the rows and columns. This should be done for the rows and columns in which hypothetical data have been placed. From these, it is possible to calculate a realistic total for all columns and all rows. This figure should be written into its appropriate cell. *Partial Completion Adequate For Planning*

Such a pattern and process may seem to involve a great deal of busywork. It need not be overly time-consuming, however, since comparatively few figures must be handled. Comparatively few cells in the tools need to be filled, and the work will pay off many times: in planning later steps, in assurance of proceeding on a reasonably correct path, and in the value of the outcomes of the completed study.

Where the observation-recording tool will not serve, there are other prepared devices that can be helpful for organizing data. The student researcher would do well to examine detailed reports of studies that used data similar or analogous to his own. These reports will frequently describe the handling of the data and display the organizing forms that were used. Other sources of ideas and help can be an office supply store or the college bookstore, where there are varieties of graph and ruled forms from which useful ones may be selected. The statistics department of the school is another source of such help. The investigator should take a copy of each type of observation-recording tool with hypothetical data filled in as they may be expected to appear. A statistician can readily suggest a useful plan and will know where to secure needed forms. The 30 by 80 forms used some places for submitting data for key punching on IBM cards are useful where there is a large variety of data to be handled. *Existing Tools*

There are various mechanical devices for organizing data, such as IBM® punch cards, of International Business Machines, Incorporated, and the marginal punch cards and the Keydex® system of Royal.* Where there *Mechanical Organizers*

---

* Both International Business Machines and Royal have offices in all major cities.

are quantities of many varieties of data from a large number of subjects, the investigator should consider such devices. The relatively small amount of time required to develop the necessary coding of the data for use with these devices will save many hours of work during data analysis. In addition, there will be assurance that valuable analyses will not be omitted because of the time required to do them when data are less conveniently available for multiple rearrangements. The investigator thinking of using one of these mechanical devices should seek assistance from the computation center of a university or go directly to a local office of one of the companies that produce the machines and supplies. Sales representatives will assist with planning the organization of the data and the coding for transfer to the organizing "containers"—IBM® cards, marginal punch cards, or Keydex® cards.

"Mulling" While Organizing Data

Where many and varied interrelationships among a large variety of data are anticipated and the quantities of data are not prohibitively large, there is value in using a form where data are placed in the organizing "container" in paper-pencil form or in the marginal punch or Keydex® cards. This requires the investigator to handle the data repeatedly as he does multiple reorganizations of the data for various analyses. In so doing, he may pick up leads to other analyses that he has not previously thought of doing.

Some aspects of the reorganizing of the data can be tedious, but the multiple reorganizing tasks should not be considered a waste of time. Since the task at hand does not require a great deal of thinking, the investigator can be accomplishing the tedious aspects of the job and at the same time be thinking of various relationships among his data and of possible interpretations that may be made of them. As he mulls over his data, new ideas about relationships and interpretations will come to him. He will see meaning in his findings for facets of his problem other than the one he selected for study. The luxury of extensive handling of the data and the accompanying mulling cannot always be indulged but, when at all feasible, it can be rewarding.

Coding Narrative Data

Data recorded in the form of numbers have been used in the illustrations, but not all observations will be numerical ones. For example, Godfrey's data were narrative process recordings. She had to devise a plan for converting the data to numbers—to quantify the data—so that statistical analyses could be done. The processes devised for quantifying data are forms of coding; Godfrey's process was described in Step 5 (page 146). The planning for coding involves consideration of the nature of the data as recorded and the concrete observations they represent; it also involves the questions for which the data are expected to supply answers. Suggestions and descriptions of processes for coding data are described in various texts about survey research, and many reports of completed studies delineate the various processes used. Because the requirements for data for each study will be different, and because there are so many varied types of data handling requirements, no attempt will be made here to enumerate and describe samples. One exception will be to suggest a beginning step that can be helpful for organizing descriptive data.

The investigator will have developed details of each type of observation-recording tool. For each type of datum, he will have filled in hypothetical data representative of the recordings anticipated for one complete period of observation of one subject. This will be true whether the recordings are numerical readings from a scale, simple responses to a question, one-sentence reports of an observation, single paragraphs describing critical incidents, or lengthy process recordings. The investigator will decide the types of categories into which he expects his data to fall. He may have prepared detailed, operational definitions of each as he was planning for the data to be sought, or he may develop these categories and definitions as he prepares plans to organize his data. In some exploratory, descriptive studies, few categories may be identified and these may be only superficially defined before the actual data are in hand. Yet, even in such studies, some hypothetical data should be developed and some planning for their organization should be begun during design development. The investigator who neglects this planning on the excuse that he cannot know what he will find, cannot know what he is looking for. Since he can give no assurance that what study subjects contribute will benefit anyone, he has no justification for asking others to participate in his endeavor.

Hypothetical Descriptive Data

Once some categories have been identified and defined, the investigator may turn his planning attention to the process for moving the data from their original "containers" to containers labeled by category. The first phase may proceed in one of two directions: (1) each individual recording (datum) will be moved from the observation-recording tool to an organizing form, or (2) a code mark may be placed beside each datum on the collection tool to indicate the category or categories into which the datum is to be placed. The second process is usually indicated where categories are well defined and fairly complete, and where each datum to be placed in any single category is expected to be fairly similar in appearance and content to other data of the same category. An example may be drawn from 3N's study, in which the statement of purpose was:

Intercontainer Transfers of Descriptive Data

> The purpose of this investigation is to determine ways to facilitate gastric tube insertion for patients in terms of emotional preparation and support, and in terms of actual techniques of insertion.[5]

The data were recorded on seven pages of an interview schedule. The investigator was able to develop a set of categories into which all responses were expected to fit. She did a preliminary set as part of the plan for her design and completed it after she had all data in hand. After ascribing a code to each category of response, she then processed the interview schedules from several fictitious patients. She did not fill in hypothetical responses for several complete interviews, but did this for only a single major section of the several interviews, using the same section for each fictitious study subject. The hypothetical responses, of course, were recorded in relation to responses that might be anticipated, not in terms of the planned categories.

Before Taking Next Step

If hypothetical data are delineated, as above, at the time of tool construction, not only will the planning about the designs and format of the tool be more realistic, but the hypothetical data will be available for use in later steps. Also, the planner will hypothesize these data in terms of his concern for types of data needed and the design of the tool needed for efficient recording of the data as they are to be gathered. He will not be influenced by the requirements for organization. He will avoid an influence under which he might, inadvertently, propose data that fit the organizing plan, but that might be unrealistic in terms of the data he will record at the time observations are made. Here again is the reminder to write details while they are in mind, regardless of the step under consideration at the time. It will save time otherwise spent in deciding whether to write or not to write, and in most instances, it will mean having the materials when they are needed in later steps. "The longest way round is the sweetest (shortest) way home." Both variations of the adage are appropriate: details that are written as they are first needed will be the shortest way and will yield the sweetest results. For 3N, using several hypothetical responses to each of a limited set of questions provided assurance that responses would lend themselves to the categories. The process also provided hypothetical data to be used for planning later steps in the design. Once the responses have been coded, a tally sheet with the categories listed on it can be used to determine the number of responses in any one or all of the categories. There are a few other aspects of this planning, but they are similar to those pertinent to the first suggested means for categorizing descriptive data and will be described there (pages 253–256).

If data have been gathered by recording a single observation on a single tool—a critical incident or a single action recorded, each, on an individual form, for instance—the organizing may be somewhat simplied: these forms may be sorted into stacks, each stack representing a category. 10A was able to sort her five shoeboxes full of 3 by 5 index cards into nine stacks representing nine major categories and, in turn, into seven subcategories for each major category. Had she collected her data on running forms, such as 8½ by 11 typing paper, she would have had to transfer each datum to an individual form for organizing. Her plan for organizing the data alerted her to this, so she recorded each datum on an individual card at the time of the observation. This was a feasible plan, since she used a modified record analysis technique, and her data were taken from the clinical records of the subjects. 3N could not have done this, since her data were collected by interview, and it would have been most awkward to record each of some 75 responses on a separate card. The use of an individual form to record each datum is frequently appropriate for collecting critical incidents and is especially useful when the data gatherer is a participant observer. It is frequently more expedient to carry a small pack of cards for recordings than to carry a tool in the form of a sheet of paper or a sheaf of papers on a clipboard. Where it is not possible to record observations on individual forms and where data do not meet criteria to make coding feasible, the data must be transferred to other forms for organization.

Where descriptive data must be transferred and will be needed in descriptive form for later steps in the study, it will almost always save time to use, for the transfer forms, cards that can be readily sorted and re-sorted. For some types of data it may be best to transfer individual data to individual forms but, for many data, preliminary categorization can be initiated while accomplishing this step. The process is as follows: A 2- or 3-character code, identifying the subject of the record, should be written in one corner of the collection tool. As seen in Exhibit 5, 3B used only letters for the experimental subjects, and she added the suscript "c" for the control subjects.[6] The process is best envisioned by thinking of the sample questions noted in Exhibit 5 as being placed each on a separate 5 by 8 bibliography card. The number and letter of the question and subquestion would be placed in a corner of the card for ready reference. After cards have been prepared to accommodate responses to all subquestions, the data may be transferred from the data collection tool. The organizing cards will be stacked in numerical and letter sequence, beginning with subject A. From the appearance of the recording sequence in Exhibit 5, it may be presumed that 3B transferred her responses from her experimental group first. Each response will be transferred in complete or near complete form from the collection cards for subject A. Each datum will have the subject's identifying code letter placed before it. In addition, the category code will have been entered before it. 3B had but two categories, supported and nonsupported; in other studies, there may be several categories, or none. When all data have been transferred for subject A, the process will be repeated for subject B. Should the response to any one question be identical, in form or in intent, it will be necessary only to place the subject's identifying letter in front of the response already recorded on the organizing card. If B's response is different, his response will be written out and his letter, along with the category code, will be written in front of it. The illustrations in Exhibit 5 of handling responses (five subjects each from the ex-

Example: 3B Data Transfers

Step 10: Organization of Data

EXHIBIT 5

Codes: A through J, Identify Experimental Group Subjects
Ac through Jc, identify Control Group Subjects

(S) — Support   (NS) — Nonsupport

Question 2: What are your child's feelings in relation to his nurse?

<u>2a. What does he tell you about his nurse?</u>

Experiment / Control
        Groups

A	/	(S)	They come to visit often. They just sit and talk. Doesn't seem to hesitate to ask them questions. Says they always tell the truth, like when something is going to hurt.
B	/	(S)	Says his nurse never gets mad at him, even when he refuses to take his medicine or cries when he gets a shot.
C	/ Ac	(NS)	Tells me the nurses come to see him only when they have to give him medicine or a shot. Says they like to hurt people.
D	/	(S)	Calls her Terry. Is down in the dumps when she is not on duty. Says she likes sports too and that's what they talk about.
E	/ Dc	(NS)	Says never knows what's going to happen next. Never told anything, and no one answers questions.
	/ Bc	(S)	She introduces him to the new children. Plays games with them and helps them make decorations for parties they have. Brings him his favorite pop and tells him stories. Asks about his brothers, sisters, and school.
	/ Cc, Ec	(NS)	Never says anything about the nurses. Doesn't complain about anything, says you have to do what you are told, haven't any other choice.

<u>2b. Why does he think she is his favorite nurse?</u>

A,B	/	(S)	Says nurses "care," and always ask what he wants to do.
C	/ Ec	(NS)	Has to put his light on all the time. Never can find a nurse when he needs her. Never has anyone to talk to. Hates for me to leave.
D	/	(S)	She's fun to be with.
E	/ Cc	(NS)	Doesn't have a favorite nurse.
	/ Ac,Dc	(NS)	Says no one seems interested. Nurses are always hurrying to get out of the room.
	/ Bc	(S)	Always tells him where she'll be if he needs her.

<u>2c. How does she make him feel when she is with him?</u>

A,B	/	(S)	Seems confident. Nurses let him help them and do things for himself. Doesn't seem frightened or scared with the nurses.
C	/ Ec	(NS)	Seems frustrated and restless much of the time.
D	/	(S)	Seems to be kept occupied.
E	/ Cc	(NS)	Doesn't seem to trust anybody.
	/ Ac,Dc	(NS)	Is very demanding and irritable.
	/ Bc	(S)	Is content and relieved.

<u>2d. What does he depend on her for?</u>

A	/	(S)	Wants nurses to turn her. They move her gently.
B	/	(S)	Wants nurse to stay with him for a while after we leave.
C	/ Dc,Ec	(NS)	Doesn't seem to depend on any one of them.
D	/	(S)	Nurses help her with her meals.
E	/ Ac,Cc	(NS)	Wants me with him all the time. No one else will do.
	/ Bc	(S)	Asks to have nurses with him for treatments.

Organizing Tools

EXHIBIT 5a

Hypothetical Totals for Data Listed As Responses to Question 2 (10 subjects in each group)

	Supported	Non-Supported
Control	3	16
Experimental	10	8

perimental and control groups) to the four subquestions of question 2 from 3B's work make further describing of the process unnecessary. By placing the subject's identifying letter before the response, it is possible not only to count the frequency of any one response, but also to trace the sources of the response. The subjects giving any one response may be identified. Had 3B planned to have more than ten subjects in each group, she might well have planned individual cards for each question for each study group. Had the anticipated quantities of data warranted, she might even have had individual cards for each of the categories. Where the number of data is relatively small, there is advantage in using the plan devised by 3B, since it allows for ready comparisons of types of responses from the two groups of subjects.

The sequence for organizing the data in relation to category, and transfer to large container, may, in many instances, be arbitrary. In relation to 3B's data, it would seem advisable to have identified the categories, supportive and nonsupportive, by placing the appropriate code beside the response on the data collection tool. That way, the response could have been viewed in total and within the context of other responses, which would have provided a better base for judgments about the category.

Variety and Number of Containers Dependent on Variety and Number of Data

For this step in organizing the data, a plan that conceals the identity of the group on all collection tools is advisable; scrambling the tools is a good idea, too. Then categories can be assigned to all responses without the evaluator knowing the group to whom any set of responses belongs. An opaque cover may be placed over the identifying material on the face of the tool. Or identifying material may be placed on a separate sheet that may be detached from the rest of the tool. If the second device is used, identifying materials should be on the back of the forms, since it will be necessary to identify the group for subsequent analyses.

There are other means for eliminating or concealing group identification. The need to do it depends on the amount of potential subjectivity in the judgments and the importance of its influence on the outcomes of the study. The process requires varying amounts of planning and various devices for accomplishment, depending on the nature of the data and the identities of the individuals doing the categorizing. If categorizers are dis-

STEP 10: ORGANIZATION OF DATA

interested parties or if they do not know the hypothesis, eliminating individual subject identity would not be required. If the investigator is both data collector and categorizer, it is difficult to eliminate or preclude possibility of identification, but efforts should be made along lines suggested here.

Identifying Come-Alive Episodes

One further gimmick that may be useful in processing descriptive data is to plan a system of coding to identify particular observations that may be useful in reporting descriptions of episodes. Research writing is more interesting when it includes stories of living persons, not just stories of numbers of people. Particular observations or comments from subjects can illustrate points being made about numbers of people, and these illustrations can make the figures come alive. As the total responses for one subject are being categorized, while in context and before transfer from the collection tool, interesting episodes can be identified and coded. The code can be transferred at the time of the data transfer. It will then be simple, when it is wanted during the report writing, to return to the original record for a review of the episode in context. For example, 3B may have so coded the response of B_c to Question 2a (Exhibit 5). There may be an interesting story here about a child and nurse in the control group.

Once the preliminary transfer of descriptive data has been accomplished, plans can be developed for categorizing the various types of observations and for tallying frequencies of occurrences. These will be similar to the process described for handling data that have been recorded on individual recording forms. The planning of all these aspects of Step 10, it should be remembered, is being described in reference to hypothetical data.

Hypothetical Data For Sample Area of Exploration

Hypothetical descriptive data, like hypothetical numerical data, will be examples of descriptive data anticipated from only a section of the total number and variety of observations of any one fictitious subject. Complete planning will entail development of hypothetical data for the same section for only a few fictitious subjects. This is illustrated by 3B's use of responses to only four subquestions, from two groups each of five fictitious subjects. 3B's study indicated that there would be five areas of care needs: emotional, physical, psychological, social, and spiritual. In her design, she developed the hypothetical data displayed in Exhibit 5, and those for the subquestions under her question 8. Question 8 was designed to elicit information about physical care. The development of detailed anticipated data provided a basis for confidence in the nature of responses to be anticipated from other questions in other areas of concern.

The point is that the investigator should develop such hypothetical data as are necessary for a realistic plan about the nature of the data he may expect to have to handle. Sample data should be developed in sufficient number and variety that the investigator can plan how he may view a large number of them at a glance in order to make some general statements about them. These statements should be related to the purpose of his study and should be more definitive than, "Whew!" or some other mumblings of consternation at the amorphous character and the immensity of the quantities of data to be handled.

SUMMARY

In summary, Step 10 deals with the process needed to move from individual and specific facts to broad generalized facts. It is the step in research where a specific fact is drawn from among many facts known about a single subject and is placed alongside similar facts about many subjects. In this way, some general fact can be known about the sample group of subjects from whom the facts were derived. And this general fact, in turn, can be applied to the larger population of whom the study subjects were a sample. Put another way, a large variety and number of facts have been collected about each individual study subject. Each of these facts, as viewed in the observation-recording tools, tells us something about that individual subject, and each may be considered in terms of its relationship to other observations or facts about the subject. But as these facts are viewed on the recording tools, none of them can tell us anything about any of the other subjects in the group, nor can they be considered in terms of other types of facts recorded about other subjects. The purpose of Step 10 is to pull together sets of similar facts about all subjects. A set of facts will permit something to be said about one type of fact in relation to all, not just one, of the subjects in the group. In Step 10, the investigator moves facts from the individual recording tools on to one or more organizing forms, so that he can view at one glance the relationship of specific facts among a group of subjects. The object is to move the many facts from many tools to more compact situations on fewer tools. He places similar facts in similar "containers" (the organizing forms), rather than leaving them "scattered" among the many recording containers. In the recording container, the relationship of facts is to the individual subject from whom the facts were derived, rather than to each other or to the group from whom they were derived.

Movement From Individual to Group to Population

Organization of data can take many forms and will be unique for most investigations. Patterns for organization will depend on the nature of the data, the format of the recording tool, and the questions which the data are expected to answer. Organization forms must be developed and procedures planned. Several have been described as illustrative of types that may prove useful. There is perhaps a narrow line between Steps 10 and 11. The place at which data are sufficiently organized so that analyses may begin is not always readily recognizable. Essentially, the investigator should examine his organized data to determine that they meet a series of criteria. The data must be in such form that he can readily identify, from materials in a single container (organizing form) or a series of essentially identical containers, the experiences of all of his subjects in relation to a common fact. From this identification, he must be able to make a generalization about the subjects as a group. He must next be able, in similar fashion, to identify another experience common to all of his subjects and make a generalization about the relationship between these two types of experiences for the group. Finally, he must be able to do this in relation to many different common experiences. When he has his data organized to the point where he can do all of these things by referring to material on a single organizing form, then he is ready to begin analyzing his data: Step 11.

REFERENCES

1. Feibleman, J. K. The logical structure of the scientific method. Dialectica, 13:3/4: 209.
2. Bartociewicz, I. F. Behavior Patterns of Schizophrenic Children. Unpublished masters thesis, Detroit, College of Nursing, Wayne State University, 1964.
3. Jump, G. L., and Perkins, D. M. Reliability and Item Analysis of an Evaluation Tool. Unpublished masters thesis, Detroit, College of Nursing, Wayne State University, 1965.
4. Couture, N. A. Planned Pre-operative Teaching of Early Ambulation for Patients Having Major Abdominal Surgery. Unpublished masters thesis, Detroit, College of Nursing, Wayne State University, 1961.
5. Teranes, B. Patient Views of Nasogastric Tube Insertion. Unpublished masters thesis, Detroit, College of Nursing, Wayne State University, 1967.
6. Murphey, H. M. Greater Support for the Dying Child. Unpublished research design, Detroit, College of Nursing, Wayne State University, 1967.

STEP 11
ANALYSIS OF DATA

TERMS DEFINED

Analyze: Analyze means to separate or break up (any whole) into its parts so as to find out their nature, proportion, function, relationship, etc.; to examine the constituents or parts of; determine the nature or tendencies of.

Analysis: Analysis means a separating or breaking up of any whole into its parts so as to find out their nature, proportion, function, relationship, etc.; a statement of the results of this process.

CONCEPTS PERTINENT TO DEFINED TERMS

Although the term "analysis" is used with many connotations in research, this varied usage does not make for as much confusion as some of the terms previously discussed, such as "method," "technique," and "problem." The second dictionary definition of analysis, "a statement of the results of this process," is consistent with one use of the word in relation to the data in research. But it is difficult to understand why analysis is also defined as the process of so ordering the data that the statement of results can be made. Analysis, the dictionary says, is the separating or breaking up

Not Breaking Wholes Into Parts, Rearranging Parts Into Wholes

260   STEP 11: ANALYSIS OF DATA

of a whole into its parts. But the researcher, when working with his data, is working with nothing but many individual parts. He has no "whole" to separate into parts, unless all of the data collected are viewed as a single unit or a whole which, at best, can be viewed only as a conglomerate. There is nothing to hold similar individual units together in any kind of relationship until the process of "analysis" is begun. In other words, the researcher, as he analyzes his data, does not separate them into parts, but rather rearranges many individual parts into various integrated wholes.

It is true that, during the examination of the data, the individual items may be placed into relationship with other individual items to form one whole, and then these same items may be related to another set of individual items to form a quite different whole. This practice may possibly explain why the process of examining the data is identified as analysis: the separating parts from one whole to arrange them with different parts to construct a new whole. Yet this interpretation is not really logical, since the data used to construct any whole are not drawn from other constructed wholes, but rather from the original observation-recording tools and, more directly, from the organization forms.

The above "analysis" of "analysis," it is hoped, may help the student to recognize that the actual process of analyzing the data is exactly the opposite of what the term used to identify it seems to imply.

Essentially, the analysis of data consists of two distinct entities: (1) the rearranging of individual units of data into sets of like data to place them into various relationships with other sets of like data to form an integrated whole, "for the purpose of finding the nature, proportion, function, or relationship" of the various sets of units; and (2) statements of the results of the rearranging of the units of data (results here refers to the meaning gleaned from the examination of the rearranged data). Viewed in this way, the first step in the analysis of data is then the organization of the data: Step 10 of the research process.

Amorphous Mixture to Homogeneous Assortments to Planned Mixture

In Step 10, the individual units of data were taken from the amorphous mass of the collected data and arranged into piles of like units. In Steps 12 and 13, the statements of the meanings of various related sets of units of the data will be developed. Step 11 is intermediate between Step 10 and Steps 12 and 13. Analyzing the data is in many ways anologous to the steps involved in (1) converting materials (data) from an amorphous glacial morain into distinct and separate piles of sand, gravel, and stone, each composed of units of homogenous size and chemical composition (organizing the data, Step 10); to (2) mixture of measured quantities of units selected from various of the homogeneous piles (developing tables and graphic displays, Step 11); to (3) laying the concrete highway, plastering the wall, or building the stone fence (constructing interpretative statements of the meaning of the findings, Steps 12 and 13). Each of these steps is referred to as analysis of the data. When communicating about the process of research or about a particular investigation, the researcher has no way of knowing which of the steps is meant except by learning in some detail the context in which the term is being used.

Step 11, then, is the construction of integrated units composed of sets of homogeneous units of data. In the foregoing discussion of concepts of analysis, it was proposed that the process is the rearranging of units of data, with no reference to any original arranging. One is reminded of the small child who, when asked if he would like some molasses, protested: "How can I have molasses, I haven't had 'lasses, yet!" In terms of analysis of data it is the converse: there is no "arrangement" of data—there is only rearrangement. The original arranging of the data was accomplished as the observations were recorded on the data-recording tools. The student has been reminded, however, that some planning in relation to analysis actually should be done as plans are developed for making and recording the observations and as the observation-recording tools are designed. In light of this consideration, it could be said that analysis of data begins as early as Step 5, when the identities of the data are decided on. Here again is evidence of the interrelatedness of all the steps of the research process. If, however, research were thought of as the four-step process of planning the study, collecting the data, analyzing the data, and communicating the results, then analysis of data is an independent step. This view of independence, rather than interrelatedness, may lead to lack of planning for analysis until the data are in hand. Step 11 involves two distinct processes: (1) statistical analysis and (2) descriptive analysis. A thorough consideration of statistical analysis is beyond the scope of this text. There are many fine statistical references available to the student, and two or more of these should be in the personal library of every professional nurse, who should also own at least one introductory statistics text. The development of tables and graphs, of course, is basic to statistical analyses, and to this extent statistical analysis of data will be considered. Some brief comments about some interpretations of findings from statistical procedures will be presented in Steps 12 and 13.

Not Arranging But Rearranging

DEVELOPING TABLES

The general format of tables is described in any guide to writing research reports or manual of style; it need not be detailed here. There are, however, some pointers about various aspects of table presentation that may help the student to plan the tabular display of his data. Well-conceived tables are "worth a thousand words." Poorly conceived tables either fail to communicate or, worse still, confuse. Unfortunately, there are no simple

Uncluttered Tables

Example 11A: Data on Several Variables in One Table

guidelines for developing tables. The content and relationships to be shown will determine the general plan of the tables, and these will be different for every set of data reported and for every question to be answered. Nonetheless, some of the following suggestions may serve as cues and provide ideas for planning.

Tables should be uncluttered. It is better to display few data with few interrelationships in two or more tables, than to have too many data displayed in a single table. Where an excessive number and variety of data are displayed in a single table, the reader must work to determine the information he expects to find there. The investigator should think first of displaying the data that answer the primary question of his study, whether it be about a hypothesis or an area of exploration. For a report about the testing of a hypothesis, the table might consist of but two cells: one displaying a mean score for the control group and the other the mean score for the experimental group (presuming, of course, that the data are appropriate for calculating mean scores). For a report of an exploratory study, the table may run on to several pages. Neither of these extremes seems desirable, and seldom is either type displayed in a report, though either one may be developed during the planning for the report and its early writing stages.

To develop the table the investigator must turn to his statement of purpose and to his organized data. He must identify the data on which he may base a statement or statements about the purpose for his study. He must then plan the form in which the data can best be viewed to promote his own ready perception of them. They should be in such form that he can contemplate them without extraneous distractions as he thinks through the generalizations that he will make about them. Exhibit 1, a table taken from a masters thesis, illustrates several points in relation to tables.[1] Rather than limiting the table to the two cells with data needed to make the generalization about substantiation of the hypothesis, 11A arranged the data according to several pertinent variables, as well as according to the control and experimental groups. The information in the cells is readily viewed. This is a reasonable presentation, since it provides information about which several statements can be made. Actually, the table might have been improved, in relation to providing information about which comments could be made, if a column had been added in which the mean scores for all nurses in the control and experimental groups had been displayed. This would have provided the information about the hypothesis in the easily read table. Further, the horizontal row displaying mean scores for all nurses per tour of duty might have been omitted, since this information adds little to what can be readily grasped from the other two rows. Here is an instance where the investigator might just as reasonably have developed two or more tables, with fewer items in each, but where the more inclusive table serves equally well to display data for ready reference.

EXHIBIT 1

NURSES' MEAN SCORES FROM JOB SATISFACTION QUESTIONNAIRE
BY TOUR OF DUTY, BY HOSPITAL, AND BY ASSIGNMENT

Assignment	Mean Scores							
	Hospital A			Hospital B			Hospital C		
	Days	PM's	MN's	Days	PM's	MN's	Days	PM's	MN's
All Nurses per Tour of Duty	167.4 N-27	165.0 N-22	161.3 N-18	162.0 N-26	154.3 N-18	156.8 N-16	161.7 N-8	154.8 N-8	150.4 N-8
Nurses Assigned to One Floor	172.5 N-18	163.8 N-19	157.5 N-15	161.8 N-23	153.9 N-15	151.5 N-10	160.3 N-6	157.9 N-5	151.1 N-7
Relief Nurses	157.1 N-9	173.0 N-3	180.5 N-3	163.5 N-3	163.7 N-3	156.0 N-6	165.5 N-2	149.7 N-3	145.0 N-1

264   STEP 11: ANALYSIS OF DATA

Separate Displays For Data on Closely Related Variables

Exhibits 2 and 3 from the Uninterrupted Patient Care study are an example of moving in the opposite direction. The findings for both number of activities and amount of time spent in performing the activities might well have been plotted on a single graph. Originally, they were, but it was later decided that the findings could best be presented by first reporting the number of activities performed and discussing some interpretations of them, and then reporting and discussing the amount of time involved. If all the data had been displayed in a single graph, the reader would have had to turn back five to eight pages when he wished to view the data on the variable "time." Therefore, the data related to the two variables were displayed in two graphs, each placed near the discussion of the particular data.

Communicate With the Reader

A general rule-of-thumb is to develop tables that are not overly complex. Yet, an accompanying admonition might be: "Don't follow the rule over the cliff." To avoid either extreme, the investigator should consider the purpose of each table: how he expects it to facilitate his reader's ready understanding of the information displayed. The display that will best enhance his communication with his reader is the one that should be used. This often means that the investigator must remain flexible in relation to tables developed during the early stages of data analysis. That is, he may develop tables that will allow him to view his own data and generalize about them. Later, he may find it expedient, in order to improve and facilitate communication with the reader, to develop some modification of the table for the published report.

Cluttering" Permissible in Summarizing Table

Another exception to the rule about uncomplicated tables is the purpose that may be served by a summarizing table. Very frequently, data about many variables are closely interrelated, and there is value in displaying many in a single form so that examinations for interrelationships can readily be made. Again the prime consideration is the effectiveness of communication with the reader. Data about a limited number of variables —two, three, or four each—may be displayed in a sequence of tables throughout the report. For some purposes, it may serve to combine the data from all of these tables into one. Juxtaposing a variety of findings provides bases for broad generalizations to be made about larger, more complex, or multiple interrelationships—relationships that could not readily be visualized by viewing the data displayed in several tables. Obviously, the development of tables, from the preliminary analysis of data through the final draft of the report, will proceed on a somewhat play-it-by-ear basis, as will the decision about which tables to use in the report. The beginning researcher has already been reminded that research requires a great deal of imagination. Now he will recognize that the applications of imagination in the early planning stages were merely the warm-up for the final three steps of the process.

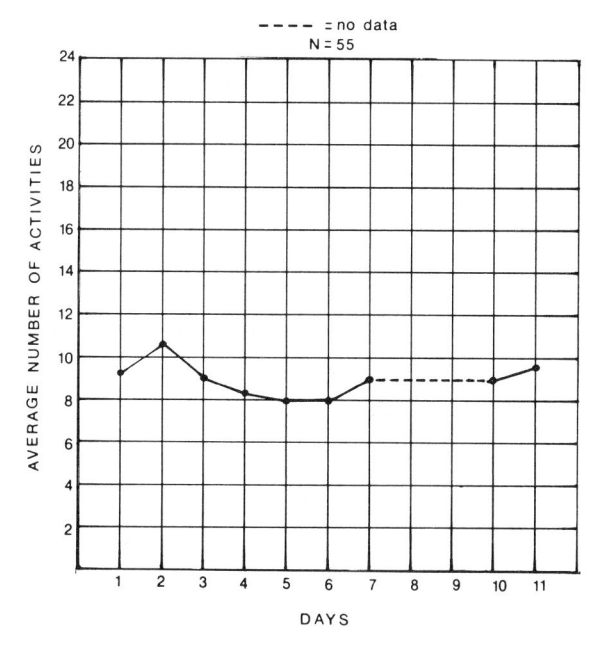

Exhibit 2. Average number of activities for the four hours immediately following experimental care 11 A.M. to 3 P.M. period.

Exhibit 4, a second table from 11A's thesis, exemplifies the display of varied data in a single table and also the combination of several tables into a single one. It also illustrates the utilization of accounted-for variables in the analysis of data, and the role they play in the rearranging of sets of data for the analyses. 11A's findings did not substantiate her hypothesis, which was a proposed relationship between type of assignment and job satisfaction of nurses. She had anticipated that other variables might relate to job satisfaction and had collected data in relation to a number of them. When the data were rearranged so that she might evaluate potential relationships between job satisfaction and various of the accounted-for variables, she found that each one examined made even less difference in job satisfaction scores than the independent variable, type of assignment. Nonetheless, since persons interested in her problem would undoubtedly wish to know about the influence of these variables, she displayed the findings in relation to those most frequently suggested (in the literature and by colleagues) as potentially related to job satisfaction. Since the differences were similar for each variable and since none was significant, there was little to be said about each separate examination. Therefore, rather than display the data for each examination in a separate table, she saved space, and more important, avoided redundancy, by combining the data from five tables into a single table. She then made a single and general statement

Combining Tables

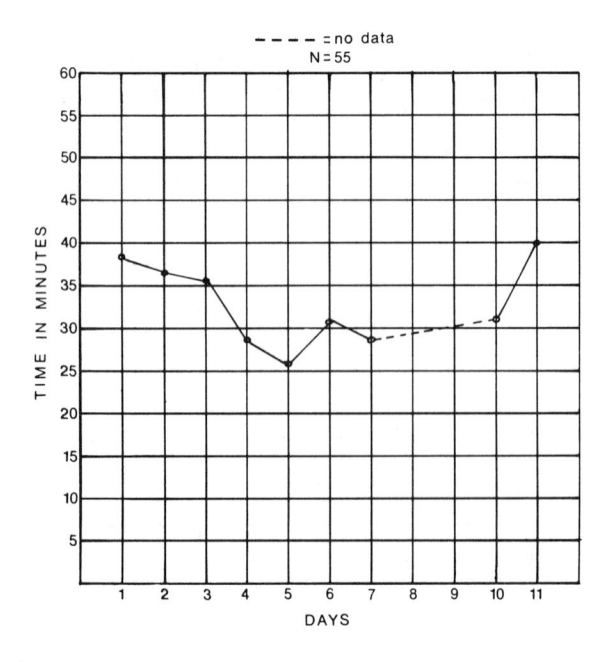

Exhibit 3. Average time in minutes for the four hours immediately following experimental care 11 A.M. to 3 P.M. period.

about the combined findings, rather than one general statement about each.

Combined tables should not be confused with summarizing tables. The former permits a single general statement applicable to findings related to each of several variables. The statement might be repeated as an individual statement about findings related to each variable. A summarizing table, on the other hand, permits several generalizations about interrelationships of findings related to several variables. Each generalization encompasses findings involving several variables.

Movement of a Datum Through a Series of Containers

The data displayed in Exhibits 5, 6, and 4, in that order, show the movement of data from the observation-recording tool (not exhibited),* to the data organizing form, to the various tables. If radiographic tagging were done on the job satisfaction score of one staff nurse who worked a regular assignment, full time, on day duty, and who was under 35, married, with one dependent, it would be possible to see the movement of that one score as it was moved from the data collection tool to the organizing tool, Exhibit 5. The code number for each subject would be listed along the left hand

---

* 11A used a multi-item questionnaire, which for purposes here can be envisioned (without need for display) as providing for calculation of a single score for each subject. In turn, single scores were processed through many rearrangements to provide for calculating a mean score for each of the various groupings of subjects.

EXHIBIT 4

MEAN SCORES OF JOB SATISFACTION OF NURSES IN GROUPINGS TO PLACE FOCUS ON SEVERAL POTENTIALLY INFLUENCING VARIABLES

Variable		Mean Score
Employment:		
Full-time	(N = 126)	160.9
Part-time	(N = 25)	160.0
Age:		
35 and under	(N = 91)	160.7
36 and over	(N = 60)	161.0
Tour of Duty:		
Days	(N = 36)	161.7
Evenings	(N = 37)	159.4
Nights	(N = 34)	159.8
Rotation	(N = 43)	162.0
No answer 1		
Marital Status:		
Single	(N = 42)	162.6
Married	(N = 94)	160.3
Separated, Divorced or Widowed	(N = 15)	160.0
Number of Dependents:		
None	(N = 114)	160.6
One	(N = 12)	160.4
Two or more	(N = 22)	161.6
No answer 3		

margin of the form and each of the variables about which data had been gathered would be listed across the top. In turn, the score (note in the exhibits the score for Nurse 1) could be traced to the various columns of figures that would be summed to determine the mean scores in relation to each of the several variables, Exhibit 6. There would be one column for all nurses working full-time, another that would be summed to determine the mean score for nurses under 35, still another for those who were married, and so forth. And it would be possible to identify the tagged score in each of the mean scores as they appear in the tables to the same extent that it would be possible to identify a radiographically tagged pebble from the Hudson Bay area of Canada, quarried from a glacial morain in southwestern Wisconsin, and currently composing a pavement of Interstate Highway 490 in northern Illinois.

EXHIBIT 5

11A's ORGANIZING TOOL #1
(Incomplete, there were many more columns, and as indicated, 151 rows. Adequate for design)

Nurse #	Mean Score	Assignment Reg.	Assignment Relief	Age	Shift Day	Shift PM	Shift Nights	Marital Status	# Dependents 0	# Dependents 1	# Dependents 2-3	# Dependents >3
1	182	✓		26	✓			M		✓		
2	179		✓	42		✓		M			✓	
3	138	✓		54			✓	S	✓			
150	139		✓	34	✓			M				✓
151	168		✓	41		✓		W	✓			

EXHIBIT 6

11A's ORGANIZING "TOOL" #2
(Incomplete, Adequate for design)
Nurses on Regular Assignment (Experimental Group)
MEAN SCORES ACCORDING TO ACCOUNTED-FOR VARIABLES

Fulltime Nurse #	Fulltime Score	Parttime Nurse #	Parttime Score	Under 35 Nurse #	Under 35 Score	Over 35 Nurse #	Over 35 Score	Married Nurse #	Married Score
1	182			1	182			1	182
6	171			4	139			2	179
21	153			9	173			12	143
22	160			11	166			62	138
26	157								
149	177			147	152			150	139
Total Score	20273			14624				15168	
Number	126			91				94	
Mean Score	160.9			160.7				160.3	

DESCRIPTIVE DATA IN TABLES

Exhibit 7, from 1A's thesis, represents a detailed display of descriptive data.[2] Had the sample size been larger, these data would have been grouped into various category levels for each variable, and the number of subjects in each category would have been indicated. With small samples, it is more meaningful to display the data as shown here (there is a comparable table for the experimental group) and to make the few generalizations permissible in the narrative. For example, two generalizations were: (1) The two groups were comparable in age, with ranges being 33 to 65 for the control group and 30 to 64 for the experimental group, with medians of 48.5 and 48.0 respectively, (2) The patients in each group were divided about equally between six-bed wards and semiprivate rooms.

LABELS FOR TABLES

The matter of how tables should be titled is a controversial subject. Some advocate the-briefer-the-better, and others believe that the title should describe the content of the table with all major variables or qualities of variables identified in the title. There seem to be good reasons for suggesting that the title really identify the content of the table. A primary reason is that it facilitates communication, providing the reader with readily grasped information for an overview examination. A useful procedure is to read the stated purpose, read the titles of tables and skim their content, and finish by scanning the summary, conclusions, and recommendations. The stated purpose, along with the summary, conclusions, and recommendations, give some notion of the aim and results of the study. But these materials alone, since they provide only gross facts and declarations of the investigator, do not allow the reader to make judgments about the value of the study to him. If the tables are well done and have clear, informative titles, however, the reader has access to extensive factual information. He can readily identify the population, the sample size, the explicit nature and quantity of data, and other pertinent factors. He can then make judgments about the meaning of the study for him, both in terms of the scope and soundness of the study and in terms of the information about specific population and facts.

Descriptive titles for tables also clarify for the investigator himself the precise nature of the data displayed in his tables. It may seem impossible that an investigator could construct a table from his own data and not know the identity of the data displayed. Nevertheless, there have been

EXHIBIT 7

TABLE 1.—INFORMATION CONCERNING PATIENTS IN THE CONTROL GROUP

Patient	Age	Sex	Marital Status	Number of Days in Hospital Before Surgery	Surgery	Complications	Room*
A	33	F	M	1	Abdominal Hysterectomy	None	W
B	46	F	M	3	Abdominal Hysterectomy	Foley catheter Steam inhalations	W
C	53	M	M	7	Hiatal Hernia	Levine Tube IV's	SP
D	65	M	M	7	Gastrectomy	Levine Tube IV's	SP
J	52	M	M	1	Cholecystectomy	T-Tube IV's	W

*SP = Semi-private
W = Ward (6-beds)

actual instances where the figures in the cells represented numbers of individuals, but the title stated that they were mean scores. The narrative about content in such a table moves freely back and forth between number of subjects and scores, and the delineation of findings portrays complete confusion of thought. Where a table displays data related to several variables, the development of a title that identifies each of the major variables can be a considerable task. Without a pattern, there is repeated casting and recasting of the sequence of phrases, and there seems never to be an entirely satisfying title. Yet there is a simple pattern for developing the title that can ease considerably the problem of sequence and yield a satisfactory title. The pattern, as illustrated by 11A's table in Exhibit 1, page 263, has two keys. First, the title should start by identifying precisely the data displayed in the lower right hand cell of the table: what observations are represented by the figure in the cell. This is followed by identification of the variables to which the figure in the cell is related and which identify the exact subcategory to which the figure belongs or which it represents. The procedure entails using the second key: The label is developed in logical sequence, by moving diagonally upward and to the left across the table, and listing, as part of the title, each variable as it appears in the headings of the columns and rows. 11A identified the figure in THE LOWER right-hand cell as: "Nurses' Mean Scores from the Job Satisfaction Questionnaire." She then identified the subcategory represented by the score in that cell by moving upward and listing the first variable encountered: "by tour of duty," followed by the second variable: "by hospital." She then moved to the left and identified the variable in the rows: "by assignment." The resultant title described the data displayed in each cell of the table. It may be proposed that the sequence could have been changed so that the movement went first to the left and then upward. Or that the same planning could be done by describing the data in the cell in the upper left-hand corner of the table. These observations are true —for this relatively noncomplex table. But when data in any single cell of a table represent a subcategory identified by a large number of variables, the only pattern that allows for smooth sequential flow is the one proposed: (1) identify precisely the nature of the data in the lower right-hand cell and then (2) identify the subcategory to which the data belong by moving diagonally upward and to the left, listing the variables indicated in the column and row headings.

Precise Identification of Content in Tables: Two Keys to the Pattern

The title of Exhibit 8 illustrates not only the efficacy of the procedure just described, but also some exceptions to the rule. It will be noted that the two cells of number and percent are treated as a single cell after the exact nature of the data are identified and in relation to the precise subcategory which they represent. It will be further noted that the pattern is modified somewhat, when the sequence lists first the "four ranges," which

Exceptions Preclude Extremes

EXHIBIT 8

TABLE SII 2. NUMBER AND PERCENT OF STUDENTS IN FOUR RANGES OF BEGINNING AND FINAL SCORES FOR THE SOCIAL INTERACTION INVENTORY BY QUARTER AND BY HOME SCHOOL

Home School	Quarter	N	4 – 9 Begin #	4 – 9 Begin %	4 – 9 Final #	4 – 9 Final %	10 – 15 Begin #	10 – 15 Begin %	10 – 15 Final #	10 – 15 Final %	16 – 21 Begin #	16 – 21 Begin %	16 – 21 Final #	16 – 21 Final %	>21 Begin #	>21 Begin %	>21 Final #	>21 Final %
	2	46	16	35.	10	22.	22	48.	8	18.	8	18.	20	44.	—	—	8	18.
Totals	3	162	52	32.	22	14.	76	47.	54	33.	21	13.	47	29.	8	5.	37	25.
	4	105	32	30.	10	9.	49	47.	30	29.	20	19.	36	35.	2	2.	29	27.

272

Group	Quarter	N															
1	2	—	1	33.	1	33.	1	33.	—	1	33.	—	—	—	—	2	66.
1	3	50	12	24.	3	6.	29	58.	15	7	14.	21	42.	2	4.	11	22.
1	4	92	92	31.	8	9.	45	49.	26	16	17.	32	34.	2	2.	26	28.
2	2																
3	3																
4	2	8	4	50.	2	25.	4	50.	1	—	—	5	—	—	—	—	—
4	3	41	15	36.	4	10.	19	46.	13	4	10.	12	30.	1	2.	12	29.
4	4	0	0	—	—	—	—	—	—	—	—	—	—	—	—	—	—

Note 1: Quarter in Basic Educational Program during which students began clinical experience in Psychiatric nursing.
Note 2: Note small N's in some cells.
Note 3: Per cents have been rounded to nearest full percentage; where per cents have been omitted, they have not been calculated because of small N.

273

actually are encountered second in the upward movement. Also, the variables, "beginning and final scores," are encountered first, but listed second in the sequence. This was done to eliminate repetition. Rigidly following the pattern would have necessitated: "Number and Percent of Students with Beginning and Final *Scores* for the Social Interaction Inventory in Four Ranges of *Scores*. . . ." Further, in this illustration, beginning by describing the data in the cell in the upper left-hand corner would not have served to identify the data in other cells of the table. In other words, it is unnecessary to "follow the rule over the cliff" by attempting to include in the label the identity of the data in the cells containing the summarizing data, the totals. In planning labels for tables, two of the criteria of a good hypothesis suggested by Feibleman may be pertinent: (1) as complex as necessary and (2) as simple as possible.

Advantages of Repeating Phrases

Another "helpful hint" is to follow, in the title of each table, the exact sequence for phrases that are common to a number of tables. For example, in the study from which Exhibit 8 was taken, many tables were needed. The labels of two additional ones illustrate the point just made: (1) "Number and Percent of Students in Three Ranges of NLN Achievement Scores, by Age, by Home School," and "Number and Percent of Students in Four Ranges of State Board Test Scores, by Group, by Length of Experience." It may be argued that such repetition indicates lack of imagination and that some variety should be introduced. On the other hand, anyone who reads a report, especially one with many tables that require lengthy titles, will quickly recognize the value of the repetition of the phrases in sequence. With this device, as soon as the sequence is identified, the reader needs only to seek the phrases that vary in any one table to learn the identity of the data and the subcategories to which data in various cells belong. He can move quickly from table to table without having to read carefully the full title of each table and yet not overlook pertinent detail. When the sequence and terms identifying each variable are changed from table to table, it is necessary to read carefully the entire title of each table, and also to adjust thinking to identify each precise variable that is denoted.

Try Several Constructions

The two suggestions, (1) presenting common elements from the tables in the same sequence in titles of successive tables and (2) following the pattern of moving diagonally from lower right to upper left, can serve numerous useful purposes. They facilitate both the development of the titles for the tables and the reading of the tables. In addition, once the first few tables have been developed, these two suggestions can facilitate the development of later tables. Note that the suggestions will aid after the "first few tables," not after the *first* table, have been developed. This is proposed for two reasons: (1) It is unlikely, during the early phases of working with the data, that the investigator will recognize anywhere near all the commonalities in the various data to be analyzed. (2) The investigator undoubtedly will cast various types of data into various formats. For example, when working with the set of data displayed in Exhibit 8, the investigator may have developed a table with rows indicating identity of the scores and the scores ranges, and the columns indicating the Quarter and Home School. Then, when working with the data to be displayed in the table titled, "Number and Percent of Students in Three Ranges of NLN Achievement Scores, by Age, and by Home School," he may have used the format of Exhibit 8. After developing three or four such tables and thinking through the definitive titles and some of the statements to be made about the information in each, he would recognize the commonalities and proceed to use a common format for displaying all analogous data.

The recognition of commonalities and the identification of the "best" format can facilitate analyses of data in two ways: (1) saving time in relation to the mechanics of developing the format of the table and (2) permitting establishment of a pattern for ways of approaching each new set of data and of thinking about statements to be made about them. In turn, repetition of effort and reporting can be limited. For example, the patterned procedure used by 11A as she analyzed the data in relation to the various accounted-for variables in Exhibit 4 (page 267) enabled her to recognize the possibility of combining five similar tables into a single table and to make a general statement applicable to the findings about each of the accounted-for variables. The single table and one general statement could be used rather than displaying five tables with five titles and narrating essentially the same statement in discussion of each table. Each investigator must develop the general format of the tables in relation to the unique characteristics of his purpose and data. Once he has identified a useful format, he is able, by following the suggestions for developing labels for tables, to follow the pattern for displaying his data in many varied relationships.

Commonalities in Format Facilitate Analysis

Exhibit 9 is an example of what can happen when the investigator uses as brief a title as possible. The reader could not possibly know what the figures in the cells of the table represent. The alternative title given below the table is not overly lengthy, yet it informs the reader about the nature of the data displayed in the cells. It will also be noted that the figures in the cells represent neither time nor number of toys, despite the table's title. The investigator was so close to his data and knew so well what the figures represented that he forgot to inform his reader. He also failed to provide another important kind of information: the number of subjects from whom the observations were derived. The omission of the "N's" in the headings of the group rows forces the reader himself to add the 1's and 2's in each row, whereas the "N" entered in each heading would have permitted this information to be grasped at a glance.

Title as Brief as Possible

EXHIBIT 9

TIME AND NUMBER OF TOYS PLAYED WITH*

	Number of Toys	Time Spent Playing in Minutes			
		10-15	16-20	21-25	26-30
Control Group	.25	2	2	1	
	.50		2	2	1
	.75	1	2	1	
	1.00				1
Experimental Group	.25	1	1		
	.50		1		1
	.75		2	1	1
	1.00	2	1	1	2

*Suggested title: Number of children playing with varying percentages of toys by periods of time spent playing.

Identify All Column and Row Subcategories

There are further reminders to be gleaned from the table (fictionally adapted) in Exhibit 9. The title of the column identifying the variables related to the data displayed in the rows is omitted. The label of each row, of course, is explicit in this instance but the investigator would do well to identify the variable to be subcategorized in the labels of all rows and columns and to report its identity in the heading of the column. In this instance, the heading should have contained the identification, "Group," and the labels for the rows could then have been "Control" and "Experimental." The proposed alternative title for the table, it will be noted, does not move all the way to the left: it does not include the phrase, "by Group," nor "by Experimental and Control Groups." This is another example where simplicity may be served. It is not necessary in a table as simple as this to include the identity of the group variable in the title of the table; it would add nothing to facilitate quick reading and grasp of the table contents. In general, it is usually unnecessary to include the identity of experimental and control group in the title of the table. If, however, there are several experimental groups, it may be well to identify them in the title or at least to indicate that there are several. Judgment about communication with the reader should be the basis for including or omitting the identity of group in the title.

Yet Another Easily Avoided Neglect of the Reader

Only by reading the narrative of the report accompanying the table in Exhibit 9 could the reader know that the labels of the rows related to the variable, "number of toys," refer to the percent of toys played with, from a particular 100 percent provided. On the other hand, and on the basis of the data presented, it is almost impossible to improve the presentation, since one does not know whether the figures in any one cell represent the number of children playing for a particular number of minutes who played with a particular number of toys during the entire study period, or for one play period, or for one day. It may be presumed, from certain elements in the table, that the investigator intended the data displayed to serve as bases for statements comparing the control and experimental groups. Possibly the data were meant to support a generalization about the hypothesis of the investigation. If indeed such was the intent, the student will readily grasp the import of the limitations in the data presented in Exhibit 9.

From this example, the student may see the effect of failure to identify precisely the nature of the facts represented by the figure placed in one individual cell in a table. Conversely, he may recognize the degree to which precise identification of the figure in an individual cell clarifies understanding of the facts displayed. The extent to which the precise identification contributes to thinking about generalizations that may be made about the data is also obvious. In Exhibit 9, the failure to identify precisely what the figure in one single cell represents, in terms of the nature of the data and of the subcategory to which the data belong, resulted in failure to display data that have any meaning and about which general statements might be made. Even reading the narrative discussing the data displayed in the table could not reveal the precise nature of these data, since it hardly seems possible that a generalization about similarities or differences in groups could be reconciled with the figures displayed in the various subcategories identified by the labels of rows and columns in the table.

Raw Data Versus Averages, Percentages, and Ratios

There are no general rules as to when and when not to convert raw scores into averages or rates; the investigator must be guided by a sensitivity to communication with his reader. Where there are large numbers of subjects, and particularly where there are many subjects in varying numbers of subcategories, there is little problem. Under those circumstances, the only way to make meaningful comparisons is through conversions to averages or rates. When the number of subjects is small, say fewer than 100 in the total sample, it frequently is best to retain the raw numbers when making various comparisons among groups. For example, Godfrey studied 23 children in her control group and 27 in her experimental group. Here, the unequal distribution of three-year-olds within the two groups is made clearer to the reader by using numbers rather than percentages: i.e., 4 three-year-olds in the control group and 10 in the experimental group, rather than 17 percent and 37 percent, respectively. Stating that 29 percent of the three-year-olds were in the control group and 71 percent in the experimental group would not have been very meaningful, either. Neither of these extremes—very large numbers or very small numbers of subjects—can alone be a guide to the decision about conversion of raw scores, but it is one factor to be taken into consideration.

Number of Subjects Entered in Column or Row Headings

Regardless of the number of subjects, all displays of data about them should include the number of subjects from whom each particular item of data derives. The full meaning of providing the reader with the information about the number of subjects from whom any set of data was obtained is illustrated in 11A's table, Exhibit 4 (page 267). For example, the relief nurses on midnight tour of duty in Hospital A (N-3) have the highest mean score for job satisfaction, and those (N-1!) on the same assignment in Hospital C have the lowest mean score. The mean scores alone might lead to many speculations about these subcategories of nurses. But when consideration is given to the relatively small number of subjects represented in these categories in relation to the number of subjects represented in some of the other categories, it is readily realized that these scores permit no generalizations about nurses in these subcategories. Nor do they permit comparisons of them with those of nurses in other categories.

Wherever data are presented in calculated combination form, such as mean scores or percents, it is important to provide the information about the number of subjects represented. This is illustrated in Exhibit 8 (page 272). For students from Hospital I who had their psychiatric nursing experience during the second quarter of their educational program, 33 percent had final scores in the range below 10, and 66 percent had scores in the over-21 range. For students who had the experience in the fourth quarter, only 9 percent were in the below-10 range and only 28 percent were in the over-21 range. But in the second quarter the percentages derive from only 3 subjects and therefore have little meaning. No generalizations could be made about second quarter students in relation to students in other quarters from the same school or in relation to students in the same quarter from other schools. These are extremes, but they are, nonetheless, meaningful and pertinent for reporting all data.

Using raw numerical data where the number of subjects is small will eliminate much stilting and repetition otherwise needed for clarity in the discussion of the findings. For example, where conversion is used unnecessarily, there may be such comments as "three patients or 33 percent in the control group failed to respond, while only one patient or 25 percent failed to respond in the experimental group." This statement must then be followed by an explanation that, though the percentages are large, the small number of subjects does not permit a generalization to a larger population. If analyses were to be done in relation to 20 or more variables, it is easy to imagine the repetition and boredom that would characterize the report.

Graphic Displays: Forced or Natural

Many beginning researchers assume that displaying data in graphic form is an essential part of "research" and that certainly their data must be cast into some sort of graphic form. But they may not be able to visualize a form suited to the data and to what they expect to say about them. Rather than being concerned about a suitable graphic form in which to display data, the researcher should concentrate on reporting his findings to his reader and thinking about how he can best display his data in relation to what he wants to tell his reader about them. Once he knows exactly what his data represent and what he wants to communicate to his reader, the graphic forms will suggest themselves to him. There is little point in forcing data into graphic forms when tables or narrative would tell the story better. On the other hand, as the researcher is trying to tell his reader about his findings, he sometimes almost unconsciously begins to visualize them in some graphic form. He will suddenly realize that he is describing his findings and his thoughts about them as though he were discussing a graphic display. When this happens, he should try a rough sketch of the graph or pictorial display. If he then finds that his discussion is clearer, he should plan to include the graph in his report.

A small section of a graphic display from the Uninterrupted Patient Care study, Exhibit 10, can add to the discussion and make an additional point.[4] In this instance, the reverse of the process described above occurred. In the early analyses of these data, the investigators moved them through various steps: (1) From the 363 observation records, (2) to 33 sheets of the first organization form, (3) to a second organization form, 12 cells long by 44 cells wide, (4) to a form 12 cells long by 32 cells wide, and finally, (5) to 3 hystograms, one of which is displayed in Exhibit 10. This seemed the best way to display these data, but the problem of communication to the reader was not yet solved. The narrative that reported the findings and their interpretations of them was developed in reference to the 3 hystograms. The many relationships displayed were of great complexity, and all attempts to describe the relationships among the subjects resulted in lengthy explanations about the display. In fact, the explanations about the display tended to be lengthier than the discussions of the relationships displayed. Yet the explanations still did not seem sufficiently clear to ensure reader comprehension, let alone ready grasp. After three or four tries from different approaches, the decision was made to omit the hystograms from the report and to report the findings in narrative only. This is not to say that the development of the hystograms was a waste of time and effort. Quite the contrary: the report could not have been written without the visual form provided by the hystograms in which the relationships could be viewed.

Narrative Describing Graph Instead of Telling Story of Findings

The experience with the hystograms illustrates one way in which graphic displays are developed, how they may be used, and decisions that must be made about them. For almost all numerical data that describe relationships among groups of subjects, it is possible to develop forms for graphic display. One or two forms should probably be tried out in the process of analyzing the data from any study. Nonetheless, the researcher should discriminate among those graphic displays that enhance his communication, those that serve no real purpose, and those that may even confuse and interfere with communication.

Graphic Display and Honesty in Reporting

Honesty in reporting is another consideration. Whether the form be a bar-graph, a histogram, a pie-graph, or any other "picture," the portion of the figure shaded to represent a particular set of the data should be in the same proportion as the quantity of data in the set is to the other sets of data or to the total set of data. For example, if 33 patients failed to improve and 66 patients showed improvement, one third of a pie-graph would be shaded to represent the 33 patients; the remaining two thirds would remain unshaded. One-sixth of the surface would not be shaded to represent the 33 patients, in the hope that such a graph would better support the contention that "the treatment seemed 'relatively' effective and would be recommended for use with similar patients." Occasionally, but not very often, this ruse is used.

Another, also infrequent, flaw that may be encountered in graphic displays of data is illustrated by Exhibits 10 and 11. In Exhibit 11, when the histogram was being developed, the number of observations of each subject for each activity was plotted at the appropriate height in each column. This plotting yielded the beginning of a running graph, needing only the drawing of the lines to connect the various plottings across the 32 columns of the graph. The original work was done in color, with a color for each subject, and the result was a very pretty picture. But then came the realization that a mark in one column had no relationship whatsoever to a mark in any other column. The activities might have been placed in any sequence along the graph without changing the information contained in the observations being depicted. The relationships to be visualized in the plottings were the differences between the four subjects on any one activity. In other words, the marks plotting the observations for any one subject could not be connected by lines running between any two columns. The histogram, on the other hand, with the solid columns in different colors, permitted ready visualization of differences in frequencies of observations on any one activity made by the various subjects. They do not depict a relationship of fluctuation between frequencies of observations from one activity to another. Warning against this may seem superfluous, but the error does occur and research reports have been published with data so displayed. How investigators can write about the data so displayed, without discovering the lack of relationship between observations that they have erroneously connected with lines simulating a running graph, is an enigma!

The student can avoid this error by asking himself one simple question. After he has plotted the data at the appropriate columns-and-rows intersections and as he is about to draw the connecting lines, he should ask himself: "Just what is the relationship between the number plotted in

EXHIBIT 10

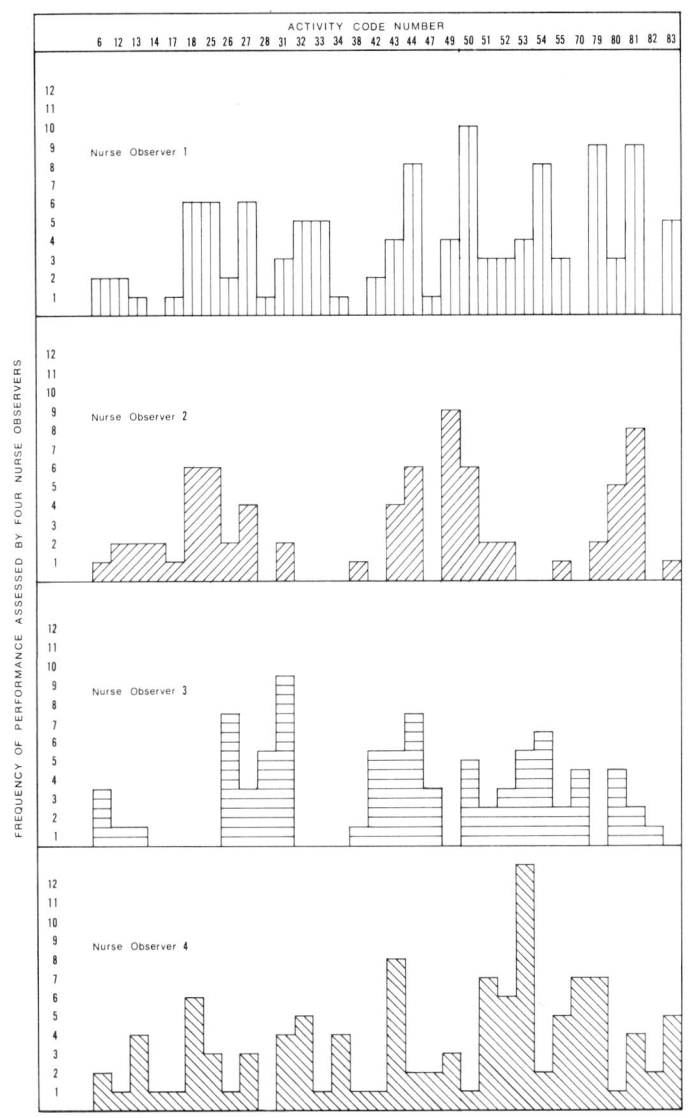

[Exhibit 10: Four histograms showing Frequency of Performance Assessed by Four Nurse Observers (y-axis, 1–12) against Activity Code Number (6, 12, 13, 14, 17, 18, 25, 26, 27, 28, 31, 32, 33, 34, 38, 42, 43, 44, 47, 49, 50, 51, 52, 53, 54, 55, 70, 79, 80, 81, 82, 83) for Nurse Observer 1, Nurse Observer 2, Nurse Observer 3, and Nurse Observer 4.]

one column and that plotted in the next?" A further test, and perhaps a simpler question to answer, is the question: "What difference would it make if the columns were arranged in another sequence?" Or: "What dictated the sequence in which the columns are arranged?" Sometimes the columns are arranged in terms of the variables having been arbitrarily labeled, in numerical or alphabetic sequence, at some point during the data collection procedure. When data related to them are analyzed, though

Answer Simple Questions to Avoid Major Error

EXHIBIT 11

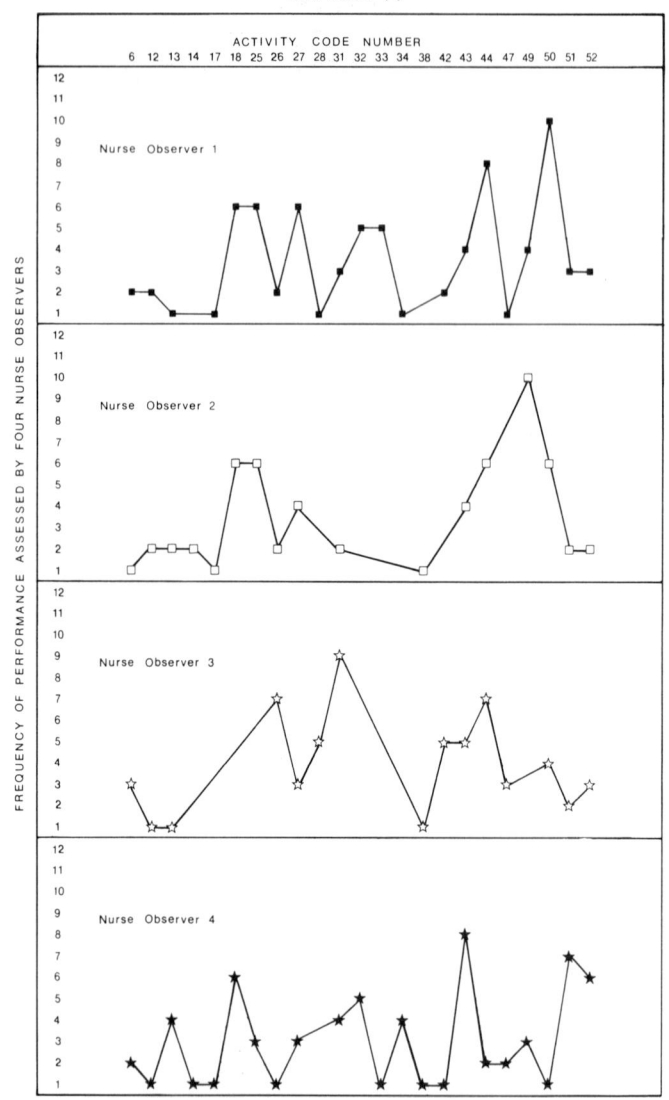

there is no inherent sequential relationship among the variables, the identification is retained. This is what happened in the arrangement of columns in Exhibits 10 and 11. The need to elaborate precisely the nature of the facts represented by any figure in an individual cell of a table applies equally to the need to understand precisely the nature of the facts represented by any individual plotting in a graphic display.

Labels for Tables

Essentially, most data that will be displayed in tabular form will be numerical data, either in the form of scaled measurements or frequencies. Occasionally, however, descriptive data will also lend themselves to a tabular format. For example, if the purpose of the study is to identify facts and principles from a particular basic science that are pertinent for nursing patients with a particular illness, the data might be displayed in a form wherein (1) the symptoms and needs common to these patients would be listed in one column; (2) the outcomes desired from nursing intervention in response to the symptoms and needs, in an adjacent column; (3) the facts and principles that could serve as bases for planning the appropriate nurse actions, in the third column; and (4) in the fourth column, the nurse actions proposed in the light of the materials listed in the first three columns. A display of such data would include no numbers, yet a quasi-tabular format such as described would be useful for reporting the findings from the study.

The investigator preparing a display of descriptive data will follow a procedure similar to that used for numerical data. That is, in the process of accomplishing Step 10, he will have placed like data from various subjects into common organizing forms. He will then decide about the generalizations that he expects to be able to make about his findings. The first generalization will relate to accomplishment of the purpose for which he collected his data. When the purpose is to test a hypothesis, this generalization can be made in about two sentences: (1) "The hypothesis seems to be supported by the data displayed in Table 1," followed by (2) a succinct statement about the specific data and the rationale justifying the proposal that they so relate to the variable as to substantiate the hypotheses. (See examples of typical statements in discussions of Steps 12 and 13.) When the purpose is exploration, the generalizations about accomplishment of the purpose may be quite lengthy as they identify many elements inherent in the situation explored. There will be narrative reporting the observations made in relation to various elements and describing the relationship of each to the other and to the total situation.

Although the generalizations about achievement of purpose may thus vary, depending on whether a hypothesis was tested or an exploratory study done, preparing the data for display is no more detailed or time-consuming for one than for the other. The planning of format for presentation of data in the exploratory study, however, may sometimes seem more difficult, since the precise forms of data can not be anticipated with the same degree of specificity as when data are in the forms of scaled measurements or of frequencies. Even where the general nature of the data can be visualized, descriptive data are not apt to fit into nice neat boxes, all

Tabular Display of Nonnumerical Data

Planning For Nonnumerical Data, Thinking and Procedure Same As For Numerical Data

of similar size and shape. As in the example on page 283, the amount of data to be fitted into each of the separate columns may vary. For instance, the notation about a particular nursing need may require two lines; the desired outcomes, six lines; the pertinent facts and principles, 20 lines; and the nurse actions, 40 lines. Such requirements do not lend themselves to tidy formats. For such planning the student will want to seek ideas about presentation in reports of studies that have had analogous or similar type data. Pages 148–149 provide an illustration by analogy.

After examining several studies and gleaning some ideas, the researcher should use as the primary guide, in determining his own presentation, his aim to communicate with his reader. He needs to decide who his primary audience is and gauge his writing to ensure understanding and interest by that audience. The student researcher might do well to think in terms of communication with a fellow student who is as knowledgeable, but no more so, about research as himself. He should envision helping this student to understand what he, the researcher, has in mind and having him become as interested in the problem and the process of its investigation as he is himself.

Specific Audience to Enhance Communication

The student researcher should *not* aim at communication with his teacher: such a guide can only lead to stilted writing through over-consciousness of need to display erudition. And it frequently leads to omission of pertinent details on the assumption that the teacher knows what he means. The latter can only result in trouble all around: (1) The teacher does not always know what the student means. (2) The teacher has no way of knowing that the student knows what he means. And (3) the student may fail to reveal to himself that he is not sure what he means. Still another reason for addressing other than the teacher is that, if the communication is clear to a peer, the teacher, too, may be expected to understand it.

In planning the display of descriptive data, the investigator should try out a plan early in his considerations. He should put something on paper, not just sit and stare at volumes of data. Such early action will preclude his entertaining the thought that there is no logical form for presentation. Once something is on paper, there is a concrete base from which to proceed, and other ideas will follow.

Ingredients of Research Are Facts— Not Figures

Facts are observable phenomena; figures are merely symbols representing facts. A frequent barrier to planning for descriptive data is a mind-set about numbers being a part of research. Students often struggle to make something meaningful out of the frequencies with which various observations occurred. But in many instances, frequency is of very little import to the concern of the particular study. One means of handling this is illustrated in Lesser and Keane's descriptive study, *Nurse-Patient Relationships in a Hospital Maternity Service*.[5] The only figures appearing in the report were the number of subjects and the fact that each subject was interviewed two times. The investigators' reason for not reporting any frequencies was that their purpose was to describe. They wanted to give no impression that the various facts fell into any reported hierarchy of importance. Studied avoidance of numbers seems a very wise way of handling the problem of over-concern for frequencies in descriptive studies. Analyzing data and proposing generalizations are hard work at best. Granted, it is easier to think in terms of frequencies, since these are more concrete and since this is "what is expected in research." Yet, where the purpose of the study is to explore and describe, the investigator should concentrate on reporting the findings and delineating descriptions of relationships discovered. When he has exhausted all possible meaningful ways to describe the situation in terms of his findings, he might then consider frequencies that could be potentially meaningful.

NUMBER OF TABLES FOR PLANNING

As part of the planning of the design for a study, the investigator, of course, does not develop all tables that he anticipates will be needed to report his findings. He does only those needed to complete his planning. The purposes to be served by developing two or more tables displaying hypothetical data are the same as those served by precise planning for previous steps. A primary purpose is to ensure that the data will lend themselves to organization into forms that can be used as bases for generalizations about their relationship to the stated purpose of the study and to the problem. The planning for this step is, indeed, the final test of whether all will move as envisioned. When tables are developed with realistic hypothetical data and are logical facsimiles, in form and content, to the real tables to be developed, the investigator may be assured that the observations he plans to make are the right ones. Tables developed with hypothetical data will also test the usability of the data-recording form. Part of the process of developing tabular and pictorial displays of data will be doing the appropriate statistical tests and indicating the outcomes of the tests, either as part of a display or as a footnote to it. Detailed planning for Step 11 will include application of the planned statistical test to the hypothetical data displayed in one of the planning tables. The most useful trial test would be one using the hypothetical data from the display intended to be the basis for the generalization about the hypothesis. Such a planning exercise will reveal the fitness of the form of the data to the planned statistical testing. Developing illustrative displays of grouped data will ensure that the data can be organized into forms that will reveal facts about the particular facet of the problem being studied and about other facets of the problem.

Therefore, the investigator should plan to develop at least two tables with hypothetical data: the first, to display data relating to the generalizations to be made regarding achievement of the purpose of the study; and the second, to display data dissimilar to those in the first table. They may be descriptive data; they may be data analyzed in relation to one of the accounted-for variables; or they may be data that seem to the investigator to represent new knowledge of importance second only to that directly related to the stated purpose of the study. Some findings not directly related to the purpose of the study may be of even greater import to the problem than those directly related to the purpose. Such import, however, is not likely to be anticipated nor recognized until all data are in hand or even until analyses are well along.

Save Some Energy For Final Steps

The suggestion that the investigator develop the two tables is to ensure broad thinking about the nature of the observations to be made during this crucial final planning about the "shape" of the data. It does not imply that only two tables should be planned; rather, it is that at least two be done. On the other hand, the student researcher should remember that there is still one final step that must be planned—one that will require considerable thinking. He should not put this off by developing more and more tables. If he does so, he will lack both time and energy for his final and most important step: planning interpretation and write up of his findings. When planning for the tables with hypothetical data, the investigator is essentially planning displays that are illustrative of what he expects to do when the data have been collected. Construction of tables with hypothetical data tests the goodness of his planning to this stage and provides a pattern for what he will do when the data are in hand. Displays developed prior to collecting the data provide assurance about the validity of expectations about outcomes of the study.

Detail Sufficient For Planning, But Short of Busy-Work

For the development of tables with hypothetical data, the same common sense guide should be used as in earlier steps in planning: if the tables require a large number of cells to accommodate a variety of data, not all of the cells have to be filled. A table should be completed in sufficient detail for it to serve as a test for feasibility of so arranging the data that generalizations may be made about them. For example, in the planning stages, the table in Exhibit 8 would have had only the cells of the top six rows and of the first three columns filled, along with all of the labels of rows and columns and the N's for each school. These hypothetical data would have been sufficient for determining the feasibility of the arrangement and the applicability of the planned statistical analyses, and for providing a basis for planning the generalizations to be made.

TABLE FORMAT AND STATISTICAL ANALYSES

Another part of Step 11 is planning for the statistical analyses that will be done. Actually, this should have preliminary consideration at the time that the data are being identified and during the planning for the observation-recording tools. The statistical tests to be used will have been decided during the earlier steps, but the arrangement of data into tables will be influenced by the statistics to be done. The planning, as well as the work with the actual data, may move in either of two directions: (1) the arrangement of the data in the tables may be planned to facilitate the drawing of the data from the tables for performing the statistical analyses; or (2) the statistical analyses may be completed first, and the tabular arrangements then done in terms of the results of the analyses. Actually, the arranging of the data for the computation of a statistical test is a process similar to arranging data for tabular display. There is a fine line between what may be classed as an organizing form utilized in the work ascribed to Step 10 and what would be classed as a table to be developed as part of the work of Step 11. Exhibits 5 and 8 illustrate this point. Both require all of the format features of a table; yet neither would be likely to be displayed in the published report of the study. They provide more information than the majority of readers would be interested in and, particularly in the case of Exhibit 8, are far too cluttered to be helpful to a reader. These arrrangements and displays of the data might be called "worktables." This type of arrangement of data can be thought of as a bridge between the steps of organization and analysis.

WORKTABLES INTERMEDIARY BETWEEN ORGANIZATION AND ANALYSIS

One reason for proposing that planning development of worktables is more appropriate to Step 11 than to Step 10 is that the task of Step 10 is to organize units of data so that all data on one variable can be placed in a single container or set of similarly categorized containers. This permits all data on one variable to be seen at a glance. In Step 11, on the other hand, the task is to so arrange data that sets of data from *two* or *more* variables are placed in a single container, the purpose being to show the relationships among data from two or more variables. Thus, Exhibits 5 and 8 display the data from several variables, so arranged as to portray relationships among them.

Another reason for planning development of the worktables in Step 11 rather than Step 10 is that they are so intimately tied to the planning for statistical testing and development of analytical statements. The detailed worktables will be developed where there are few data and the statistical tests will be done without the aid of a computer. Since the computer will perform many organizing tasks, as well as computations of test results, there is frequently no need to develop the detailed worktables. In these instances, the investigator may develop only the more compact tables for display of summarized data in the report. Essentially, then, the investigator must consider statistical analyses at three points in his planning; their consideration in Step 11 ensures that what he plans to do is feasible and may be expected to yield meaningful results.

NARRATIVE REPORT OF FINDINGS

As a final aspect of planning for Step 11, the investigator will delineate a portion of the narrative that he expects to use to explain the data in his tables. This may seem an unnecessary detail, but it can provide the base for planning interpretations and implications of the findings. The most plaguing factor here is drawing the line between adequate and excessive detail. Of all the portions of a report of research, it is perhaps this one that most clearly reveals the personality traits of the investigator. One individual will describe the content of a table in one or two sentences. Another may report in narrative the content of every cell and repeat the figures from each, followed by pointing out comparisons between groups with repetition of the figures from the appropriate cells. Such a report of the findings displayed in Exhibit 8 would be horrible to comtemplate. This does not mean, however, that figures from cells of tables should not be repeated in the narrative report of findings. Indeed, there are times when they must be repeated; unfortunately, those times cannot be identified in a "rule of procedure." The investigator must rely on his sensitivity to the needs of the reader and to the degrees of emphasis he wishes to place on various findings. Repetition may be a powerful force in communication, working either to its enhancement or as a complete barrier to it. Delineating, during planning, a few paragraphs of the narrative expected to accompany a table serves as still one more test of the nature of the data and the character of the arrangements that may be expected.

The value of executing a minimum illustration of the hypothetical narrative presentation of the data has been described in the discussions of Exhibits 9 and 11. If even one paragraph had been developed to narrate the nature of the findings displayed in Exhibit 9, the investigator would have realized that what he wanted to tell his reader was not really displayed in the table. The mere contemplation of the narrative about Exhibit 11, before a word was put on paper, would reveal that the display did not represent the relationships the investigator had thought were being portrayed. As well as serving as a test for the precise nature of the data being displayed, the narrative about the data in the tables will provide the introduction to planning the final steps in the study.

SUMMARY

Analysis denotes a dual concept. An analysis is the breaking of a whole into its parts, so as to examine the nature and function of the parts. An analysis is a statement of the results of that examination. It is proposed that, in relation to analyzing data obtained in a scientific investigation, the first denotation of the dual concept does not apply. There is no whole to be broken into parts. The data obtained for an investigation are parts; the only whole is any single observation or piece of data. When data are "analyzed," no whole is separated into parts. Rather, many individual units of data are repeatedly rearranged into a variety of multifarious "wholes." In data analysis, the units placed in the various rearrangement patterns are usually figure or narrative generalizations derived from combining many like parts which, in Step 10, had been arranged so that like parts were grouped into a single container or several similar containers. The purpose for rearranging units or sets of data into various wholes is to display relationships among the data from two or more variables. The process of the multiple rearrangings of the data is referred to as constructing the tables and graphs to display the data about which generalizations will be made. The generalizations, of course, represent the second element of the dual concept of analysis, statements of results of the examination. In Step 11, there are suggestions for guides to determining tables that appropriately should be constructed, and for facilitating their construction. Included are precautions that can preclude errors. There is note of the place of statistical analyses in the scheme of data analysis. The rationale is presented for detailed planning for data analysis during the planning of the design, rather than delaying until the data are in hand. Planning Step 11 can serve as one further test of the potential goodness of the planning in all the preliminary steps of the design. The test is effected through explicit and precise planning, using hypothetical data, for illustrative analyses that may be anticipated for the actual data. The planning will test most specifically the extent to which the planned data will relate to the statement of purpose and to closely allied facets of the problem. Specifics delineated in the planning will also provide bases for planning the final two steps of the design.

REFERENCES

1. Sangala, J. M. Satisfaction of Regularly Assigned and Relief Staff Nurses in General Hospitals. Unpublished masters thesis, Detroit, College of Nursing, Wayne State University, 1960.
2. Couture, N. A. Planned Pre-operative Teaching of Early Ambulation for Patients Having Major Abdominal Surgery. Unpublished masters thesis, Detroit, College of Nursing, Wayne State University, 1961.
3. Wandelt, M. A. Outcomes of Basis Education in Psychiatric Nursing. Detroit, College of Nursing, Wayne State University, 1966.
4. ——— Uninterrupted Patient Care and Nursing Requirements. Detroit, College of Nursing, Wayne State University, 1963.
5. Lesser, M. S., and Keane, V. R. Nurse-Patient Relationships in a Hospital Maternity Service. St. Louis, Mo., The C. V. Mosby Co., 1956.

STEPS 12 & 13
OUTCOMES

From the title of this section, it would appear that it will treat but one step in the research process: the step concerned with reporting outcomes of the study. Indeed, the discussion is of outcomes, but the process of identifying and communicating the outcomes is composed of two very distinct entities. Each entity may be identified by the title used by most researchers: the first, Step 12, may be titled "Findings, Interpretations, and Implications"; the second, Step 13, titled, "Summary, Conclusions, and Recommendations." The two steps are distinct, one from the other, yet they are composed of congruous elements, which may be identified in the vernacular as, "Facts, Meanings, and Suggested Actions." Each title identifies the same three concepts, with the terms that denote any one concept placed in the same sequential position in each title. As the researcher plans for or works through the final two steps of the process of his investigation, to determine and report the outcomes of his investigation, he will address himself to three conceptual areas for each step. He will plan for reporting: (1) the facts collected, (2) some of the meanings of the facts, and (3) some actions that might be suggested on the basis of the proposed meanings of the facts. Although there are similarities and it is expedient to consider the two steps in a single discussion, yet it is necessary to recognize the essential independence in sequence and process of the two steps.

STEPS 12 AND 13 DISTINCT IN DETAIL

The proposal that the two steps are independent of each other relates to the process of accomplishing each; it does not mean that the factual and ideational content of one is independent from that of the other. Perhaps the simplest distinction is the matter of detail. Step 12 is the process of (1) reporting all of the findings, (2) describing all of the analyses to which the findings were submitted, (3) proposing all of the potential meanings of the facts, and (4) suggesting actions that might be warranted on the basis of the many facts and meanings. Step 13 is the process of summarizing the detailed facts to point up those judged as most meaningful in relation to the purpose of the study and to the problem of concern. Step 13 is drawing conclusions—proposing the most pertinent meanings—that might be inferred from the summarized, generalized facts. It is recommending actions that seem warranted by the proposed meanings of the generalized facts. In other words, Step 12 is the report and discussion of the detailed findings, and Step 13 is the report of the highlights of the study. The student will, of course, recognize the sections of the report of an investigation represented by the two steps, with Step 12 resulting in the "Findings" and "Discussion" sections of a journal report and the chapter titled, "Findings" in the full report. And (remarkably!) Step 13 yields the section or chapter titled, "Summary, Conclusions, and Recommendations."

Facts, Findings

Much of the thinking in relation to planning Step 12 will have begun in the development of the plan for Step 11. Decisions about the facts to be reported and the forms in which they will be displayed required anticipating what might be said about them. Essentially, planning the report of the findings involves planning the sequence in which the tables, graphs, and results of statistical tests will be presented and developing the narrative to make explicit the nature of the materials presented. The findings are the facts—the observable phenomena—from the study. They may be reported in the form of raw data (recordings of individual observations) or in the forms of categorized data, where similar individual observations have been combined and are represented by a symbol in a cell in a table. The symbol (figure in the cell) may be a frequency number, one indicating a conversion to a rate, or one identifying the results of a statistical test. The facts represent objective observations of phenomena. What is a fact to one person considering the collected data will be a fact to another considering those same data.

The investigator is obligated to accept the facts as he found them and to report them in full. This can sometimes be painful, as when the beautiful hypothesis is slain by the ugly fact. Nevertheless, the detailed report of the findings is the display of the facts revealed in the study and the narrative describing the precise nature of the facts as they were observed and are displayed. When planning the design for the study, the investigator will refer to the tables and graphic forms he has developed and in which he has displayed hypothetical data. He will delineate the narrative that will illustrate what he expects to say about his data and the manner in which he plans to say it. (See later portion, Step 11.)

Accept the Facts

FORMATS: CLASSIC AND OTHERS

As the investigator delineates the narrative description of his data, his thinking will frequently move on to the interpretation of his facts. Indeed, thinking tends to move rather freely back and forth between these two elements, and the reporting itself often blurs their common boundary. The classic format for reporting findings and interpretations is that of reporting all of the facts, followed by discussion in which possible meanings of the facts are delineated. The two units are presented in two specifically identified, separate sections of the report. The use of the classic format might be expected to eliminate fuzziness of thinking and blurring in reporting. Yet, even when the classic format is followed, the problem is not always avoided. Where there are extensive data of great variety, the investigator may choose to report the data in small segments with interpretations accompanying each segment. This format makes it unnecessary to repeat the identification of many data during the proposals about interpretations. This moving back and forth between facts and interpretations does not reflect confusion and uncertainty in the investigator's thinking. In other words, there is nothing wrong in forsaking the classic format, and juxtaposing the report of the facts and the delineations of their interpretations, so long as the investigator reveals clarity of thinking and does not report interpretations as though they were facts.

Fact or Interpretation

Whether a statement delineates a fact or an interpretation may be judged by using two tests and determining (1) whether the content alludes to observable phenomena or to the meaning ascribed to observed phenomena and (2) whether the statement would be accepted as being true by all persons, regardless of individual interest or discipline. A fact is a fact and is so recognized by all persons considering it. On the other hand, a fact may *mean* one thing to one person and quite a different thing to another person. Furthermore, a single fact may have several meanings for a single individual.

IMPLICATIONS FROM INTERPRETATIONS

The facts are immutable; they are readily recognized and accepted as facts by all considering them, regardless of personal bias or interest. In contrast, interpretations, or the meanings of the facts, will relate to the interests and concerns of the individual viewing the facts. Consequently, they may be different for different individuals. In turn, the implications, suggestions for actions to be taken in light of the findings of the study, will depend on the interpretations the individual makes of the facts, and on his interests and discipline. It follows that implications, too, will vary according to the individuals suggesting them. Essentially, the implications are not based directly on the facts. Rather, they are based on the meaning ascribed to the facts and on the interests and concerns of the individual suggesting the actions. In consequence, from a single fact may stem multiple interpretations (meanings) and, from a single interpretation, there may stem several suggestions for varied actions. The student may want to think through his own example that will clarify these concepts for him.

Dennie Stole a Dime

The homely example proposed here is simple and concrete. The fact (the observable phenomenon) is that 7-year-old Dennie stole a dime.

INTERPRETATIONS (meanings)	IMPLICATIONS (suggested actions)
For Grandmother: Poor Dennie, all the other children had dimes.	*Grandmother:* I'll give Dennie a dime each week.
For Mother: Dennie did wrong.	*Mother:* Dennie must understand his error, and a plan must be made for him to have an allowance and guidance for planning its use.
For Father: No son of mine is going to be a thief!	*Father:* (Off with his belt) "It's to the woodsh . . . — garage — with you, young man!"

The fact was the same for each, but the meaning for each was quite different. The suggested actions, each consistent with the meaning of the fact to the individual, stemmed directly from the interpretations and could not be related to the fact without the link of the meanings. It is quite obvious that other interpretations might have been inferred from the fact. For example, what might the meaning have been for Dennie?—before discovery?—after Father learned of the fact? And there are many other possible implications—implications in relation to Dennie and generalizable to all 7-year-olds, or to other acts of transgression by 7-year-olds.

That interpretations of facts are markedly influenced by understanding and interest of the individual proposing the meanings is illustrated repeatedly in the literature of "nursing" research. There are, for instance, so-called nursing studies that are really psychological or sociological studies, and not studies of nursing problems. In reports of such studies, usually carried out by psychologists or sociologists, many of the facts are interpreted in terms of meanings for the psychologist or sociologist, rather than in terms of meanings for nurses and nursing. This is not to say that such studies were not good studies and worthwhile or that they had no meaning for nurses. But they were not studies of nursing problems, per se, and since interpretations were not made by persons knowledgeable about nursing, the suggestions for actions were not particularly pertinent to concerns of nurses.

Interpretations and the Interest of the Investigator

In order for facts to be meaningfully related to concerns of nurses and to lead to suggestions for actions expected to improve nursing practice, they must be interpreted by nurses. This distinction between what is nursing research and what is not nursing research introduces a topic for endless discussion. The discussion here is sufficient to indicate the writer's intent: nursing research is that which concerns itself with problems of direct concern to nurses and for which the special knowledge possessed by nurses is required for meaningful interpretation of the facts.

Nurses Investigate Nursing Problems

It would seem that research described as being of or belonging to a particular discipline or another should mean that the study is concerned with the basic problems that are concerns of that discipline. In light of this concept, studies to be considered as nursing research might be measured against Henderson's definition of nursing. If the attention is addressed to improving the practice of nursing and the care delivered by nurses, the research may be described as nursing research. This proposal permits a wide latitude, and these is no need for a fine line to be drawn between studies to be classified as nursing research and not nursing research. The words "nursing research" and "not nursing research" are frequently used. It is suggested here that a simple distinction might be applied to the two concepts. What is considered to be nursing research may encompass a wide variety of studies and involve cooperative effort and interest with many science disciplines. Discussions should not become diverted from meaningful focuses to oratory about what is and what is not nursing research.

Interpretations of the facts do not derive from a vacuum. When the investigator moves from describing the facts that he proposes are those that allow generalizations about his hypothesis, he proposes a meaning for

Interpretations and the Statement of Purpose

his facts. For example, 11A reported that the mean scores of her control and experimental groups were 162.2 and 160.5, respectively (facts), and that the statistical test for significance was: $t = 0.54$ ($p. > .05$) (a fact). She interpreted the results of the t test to mean that the observed difference between the mean scores of the two groups of nurses could have occurred by chance, and that the two groups of nurses did not differ in relation to the dependent variable, job satisfaction. From this she moved on to the meaning of the facts in relation to her hypothesis: that is, she proposed that the facts did not support her hypothesis, that type of assignment does not make a difference in job satisfaction of the nurse. Her statistical test did not tell her that type of assignment did not make a difference; the observed result of the t test told her that the two groups did not differ in relation to the scores that were statistically analyzed, which happened to be scores of job satisfaction. But other data told her that the two groups *did* differ in relation to type of assignment. Since they did not differ in relation to job satisfaction, however, she proposed that the meaning of these two sets of facts was that the two phenomena, type of assignment and job satisfaction, were not related to each other. The first meaning that the investigator will seek from his facts will be their meaning in terms of the primary purpose of his study.

The sequence for considering interpretations to be reported is the same as for considering the report of findings. There will be movement from statements related to the primary purpose of the study, to facts closely related to the statement of purpose. (11A's second consideration would have been related to the accounted-for variables.) Next considered will be facts judged to be of major importance in relation to the problem, followed by descriptive facts and their potential relationship to proposed meanings of other facts. Finally, there will be consideration of "bonus findings." Frequently, the investigator will proceed with the interpretations of his data as he contemplates them in his tables and graphic displays. He relies on his knowledge and awareness of the various facets of the problem to provide him with ideas about interpretations; and this is entirely correct.

Interpretations and Definition of Problem

Before the investigator considers his task completed, however, he should reread his definition of problem, where he will undoubtedly discover many suggestions for additional meanings in his data. The rereading of the definition of problem as an aspect of analyzing the data accomplishes two things. (1) It moves the process of the research full circle—it begins and ends with consideration of the problem and its many components. (2) It enhances the probability of the investigator's relating his findings to those of other researchers—to previously known knowledge. The latter contribution is not merely additive. It casts new light on earlier findings and permits new and extended interpretations of all findings: those from

Implications from Interpretations

the current study and those from past studies. The process of relating findings from the current study to those of earlier studies is one of reporting agreement-nonagreement with earlier findings and of new meanings that can be attached to all. The step of tying the findings to those from earlier studies is frequently neglected in the process of analyzing and reporting findings from studies. There seem to be two primary reasons for this neglect. (1) The investigator wishes to move the report to publication as quickly as possible, so he omits this important facet of Steps 12 and 13. (2) The problem has not been defined in detail, so there are no suggestions in the definition of problem to stimulate the investigator to propose relationships with findings of earlier studies.

One of the purposes served by a detailed definition of problem is to provide a framework on which to hang findings. This is the point at which that framework should be put to use. This aspect of the study is of particular importance to nurses who express concern about development of a "body of nursing knowledge." It is as each nurse researcher fully defines the problem to be studied and analyzes her data in detail, examining from every possible angle the relationship of findings of the current research to reveal relationships to findings from earlier studies, that the body of nursing knowledge will develop. It will not be developed in a single project, nor will it result from one great attempt to weave all the bits and pieces from many studies into a single body. Rather, it will develop as each nurse researcher defines problems and delineates interpretations of findings by integrating ever more detailed findings from wider and wider ranges of scientific investigations.

Hang Findings on Framework in Step 1

This phase of the report of findings may be thought of as a repetition of components 5, 6, and 7 of the definition of problem, where the researcher delineated the facts that he judged relevant to his problem. He used findings and thinking of others as bases for his thinking and as supports for his proposals. In component 7, he identified his personal view of the problem and the perspective from which he was viewing it. In the culminating discussion of his report of findings, he will report the extent to which his findings agree or disagree with those of others. He will propose new meanings of facts in the light of his findings. He will revise his frame of reference about the problem and various facets of it.

An illustration of analyzing data in terms of elements identified in the definition of problem is found in 11A's study. Her findings did not support her hypothesis. She had hypothesized that nurses on regular assignment (continuous assignment on one nursing unit) would have higher job satisfaction scores than nurses on relief assignment ("float" nurses, assigned each day to a nursing unit where there was need for them). She did, however, find significant differences between the two groups from one hospital in relation to tour of duty, Exhibit 1. For regularly assigned nurses,

EXHIBIT 1

RESULTS OF STATISTICAL ANALYSES OF JOB-SATISFACTION SCORES OF REGULARLY ASSIGNED AND RELIEF NURSES FROM ALL TOURS OF DUTY AT HOSPITAL A

Assignment	Days Mean Score	Days Standard Deviation	Evenings-Nights Mean Score	Evenings-Nights Standard Deviation
Regular	172.5 N=18	12.0	161.0 N=6	20.9
Relief	157.1 N=9	10.5	176.8 N=6	19.5

VARIABLE: Days		VARIABLE: Regularly Assigned	
Regular:	172.5	Days:	172.5
Relief:	157.1	PM's-MN's:	161.0
t = 3.42*		t = 2.51*	

VARIABLE: Relief		VARIABLE: PM's-MN's	
Days:	157.1	Regular:	161.0
PM's-MN's:	176.8	Relief:	176.8
t = 2.66*		t = 2.13*	

*Significant at .01

the mean score was higher for those on day duty than for those on the evening and night tours. For relief nurses, the mean score was higher for those on evening and night tours than for those on day duty. When scores were compared in terms of tour of duty, for day tour the regular nurses had a higher mean score than the relief nurses; while for the evening and night tours of duty, the relief nurses had the higher score. As 11A was preparing the definition of her problem, she noted that supervision can greatly influence worker job satisfaction. One factor in supervision that has been found to make a difference is the matter of change of supervisors. That is, job satisfaction is usually higher among workers who receive supervision from one person over a period of time, in contrast to workers who have frequent changes of supervisors. Nurses on regular assignment on day tour of duty usually have the same head nurse and the same supervisor. Relief nurses on day duty have a different head nurse with each change of nursing unit assignment (which may be each day) and, very frequently, they will have a different supervisor. Relief nurses on the evening and night tours of duty, even though they may be assigned to a different nursing unit each tour of duty, are apt to have the same supervisor over a prolonged period of time. This does not completely explain the findings, of course, since the nurses on regular assignment on evening and night tours of duty would also have had the same supervisors for a prolonged time, yet they had a lower mean score than the regularly assigned nurses on day tour. Nonetheless, there is at least a hint of corroboration of consistency of supervision, in the form of having the same person as a supervisor, tending to favorably influence worker job satisfaction. These analyses and interpretations of the facts not only serve to relate facts from a current study to those found in earlier studies, but also serve as a basis for suggesting further investigation of the influence of supervision on job satisfaction of nurses. They suggest also the need for scrutiny of the possible interacting influence of tour of duty.

Freedom to Interject Self

The researcher has a responsibility to report the facts as he has found them. The only latitude for allowing his own personality and imagination to enter into the reporting of the facts is the skill, imagination, and originality that he may introduce in relation to the display of his data. Yet even in this he must be straightforward and honest, allowing no nuances that might mislead the reader. In interpreting the facts, however, the investigator is not so restricted. He may allow his interests and biases to show; he may use his imagination; indeed, he may even propose seemingly wild ideas. Not only may he do this, he should be encouraged to do so.

Excuses! Excuses!

On the basis that each individual will interpret facts as having different meanings and that each will propose different actions as warranted by the interpretations, some researchers do not write interpretations or implications as a part of the report of their investigations. Their job is to "reveal the facts," they say; "let others place on them whatever interpretations they wish." This posture may reflect one or more of several conditions. (1) The investigator is too lazy to think through the various possible interpretations of the facts. (2) He is too insecure about his own grasp of the total problem to attempt to find meanings in the facts. (3) He is afraid to stick his neck out and express his ideas about the meanings of facts, lest others disagree with him. (4) The problem has not been well defined and there is little base for proposing meanings in the facts. (5) The facts do not relate to the problem as it was defined nor to the stated purpose of the study, and the investigator does not wish to say so in so many words. There may be still other reasons for an investigator to refuse to delineate interpretations and implications from his study, but none, it seems, can be considered a valid reason for neglecting or avoiding this important step in the study.

Excuses Invalid

Perhaps the primary reason the investigator should propose interpretations and suggest implications is that he has done more thinking about the entire problem and about "his" facts in relation to it than has any other person. As he thought through these matters during the planning of the study and the collection and organization of data, he could not help but have thought of some possible meanings of the facts as they relate to the problem. Therefore, the writing of at least a few interpretations will involve only the work of putting on paper thoughts he has already formulated as he accomplished other steps of the investigation. Anyone else attempting to identify possible meanings of the facts would have to undertake extensive study of the problem and the facts in order to make even a beginning at proposing interpretations.

Furthermore, as another interested person considers the report of the investigation and moves from the facts revealed by the study to the interpretations proposed by the investigator, his own thinking will be stimulated, and he will more readily identify interpretations of his own. That is, interpretations proposed by the investigator will kindle thoughts of an interested reader. No investigator should withhold delineation of his interpretations for fear of disagreement from others. Disagreement in interpretations is the very essence of interpretation. Not that each person considering the facts will disagree with every other person considering the facts. Rather, it is only as there is disagreement—be it friendly or antagonistic, positive or negative, enhancing the ideas of the investigator or knocking them down—that the full worth of the facts will be extracted. It would be ridiculous for an interested person to infer another meaning from the facts and then not to express it, simply because two or more interpretations have already been proposed. Indeed, the investigator who has qualms about others disagreeing with him should realize that, as he proposes more than one meaning for any one of his facts, he is, in effect and to some degree, disagreeing with himself. Disagreement by others does not negate the validity of his interpretations. Furthermore, proposal of more than one interpretation is not tantamount to disagreement; frequently, additional interpretations are extensions of meanings and may even support earlier interpretations. Each individual has a right and an obligation to interpret the facts as he sees them, to bring to them knowledge from his own field of expertise. By the same token, each individual has the right to agree or disagree with interpretations made by others.

The event of the facts not relating to the problem or to the stated purpose of the study may lead to one of two courses of action, neither of which is particularly helpful or scholarly. The one course may be that mentioned above: the investigator omits reporting his interpretations of the findings. The second course, too frequently taken, is overanalysis of the data, in vain attempts to make something meaningful of them. This second course can result in many words, but it will not yield any more meaning than the first. The middle course is for the investigator to make explicit the relationship, or lack thereof, of the data to the problem and specified purpose of the study. He should then identify where the study got off the track and, if possible, describe what would have been a more fruitful line of procedure. This latter is a scholarly approach, which may be

Implications from Interpretations 301

expected to contribute to future work in the field. In this instance, again, the investigator has been thinking about the matter and, while he has all elements of the situation in mind, it will take him relatively little time to write interpretations of the facts and the lack of their relationship to the problem. He may serve by delineating "what might have been," and how his new awareness may be used in future studies.

The findings should be "squeezed" to extract all possible good from them. This general rule is another that should not be followed over the brink of the cliff. In writing the first draft of his report of findings, the investigator should not worry about going too far in proposing interpretations. It is frequently easier to elaborate all ideas that come to mind, and later to eliminate some, than to decide which considerations should or should not be pursued in the early analysis stages of the work. *"Squeeze" the Data*

It has been pointed out earlier, however, that this going too far can go too far. That is, when the investigator finds that he is pursuing lines of analysis to avoid getting on with analysis of the next set of data, he is going too far. What happens is that the investigator has considered a particular set of data in relation to several variables. For example, 11A considered mean scores on a job satisfaction test for nurses in relation to her independent variable, type of assignment. She then analyzed them in relation to tour of duty, hospital, educational background, marital status, age, number of dependents, and many more potentially related, accounted-for variables. Fairly soon, she had developed a neat pattern for pursuing each new analysis. How comfortable it might have been to continue through a series of 50 or more potentially related variables! Days or weeks could have been spent rearranging data into new tables, doing repeated significance tests, and writing the narratives to describe the procedures and outcomes. On the other hand, it is possible, after a certain number of similar analyses, to examine grossly a set of data and determine with reasonable certainty the results to be obtained by completing the analysis of the set. Indeed, investigators have commented, as they examined reams of plotted data, that they could have come nearer to the value of the correlation by guessing rather than by performing the mathematical calculations. This does not mean that extensive numbers of analyses should never be done in relation to many variables, but it warns against doing analyses because a comfortable pattern has been established and the next analysis *just might* show something meaningful. It suggests moving to the next set of analyses or the next step in the process, both of which will require greater thinking than continuing in the established pattern. Squeeze the data for all their possible good is worthy advice—but it should be followed by advice to leave the rind and pulp unprocessed. *A Comfortable Rut*

The situation of how detailed to be when elaborating the interpretations is similar to that encountered when defining the problem: when an idea occurs, it usually takes less time to write it than it does to make a decision about whether or not to write it. Once it has been written, it can be handled as 11A did the work she reported in relation to the table in Exhibit 4. Indeed, she had still other analyses that she did not mention in her report, except to say that other analyses had been done but had yielded no meaningful information and therefore were not individually identified in the report. The researcher must, within reason, exhaust the potentials of his data in the work of analyzing them. He must also be aware of the interest and needs of his audience and limit his report to the most meaningful findings—those adequate to support proposed interpretations. He should avoid overshadowing the relatively few findings of major interest and meaning with the many findings of limited import. There are no firm guides to determination of what specifically identifies the important and the less important. This is a matter of judgment. The investigator should be aware that he must make judgments and that the report of a limited number of important findings is more likely to be helpful than one of an *exhausting* number of minor findings. He may find the rut comfortable; his reader is not apt to.

Concepts Apply, Whether Real Data or Hypothetical

The concepts delineated in relation to interpretations of data in hand apply equally well to planning for this step as a part of developing the design. The difference is that, in the planning stage, the investigator will use hypothetical data and will limit interpretations to the three or four that he expects he will make about his data. To get on to the work of planning for thorough analysis, the investigator should probably propose three or more possible meanings for a single fact or set of facts, rather than one interpretation each, for several sets of facts. A useful procedure is to continue work with the hypothetical data displayed in the sample tables, and to think through several interpretations for data of two or more types. This should be followed by indicating the particular types of data for which similar processes of analysis may be expected to be used during the study.

INTERPRETATIONS OF DESCRIPTIVE DATA

Where the facts will be those needed in an exploratory, descriptive study, the approach and process will be similar to those described for facts used to test a hypothesis. The investigator will consider the broad generalization describing the meaning of his findings in relation to the stated purpose of the study. He will then select a particular, well-defined set of facts and propose possible meanings of the facts in relation to the stated purpose. An example may be seen in the study identified in Example 3N: The purpose of this investigation is to determine ways to facilitate gastric tube

Interpretations of Descriptive Data 303

insertion for patients in terms of emotional support, and in terms of actual techniques of insertion. 3N anticipated that patients might vary in relation to wanting to know ahead of time about an uncomfortable treatment, that some might worry if they knew a long period ahead of time, and that most would want to know at least far enough ahead so that they might learn what they would experience and what would be expected of them. Among the potential interpretations that she proposed for these hypothetical facts were: (1) Patients wish to know, so that they may have some control of the situation and can plan for their own actions. (2) A single "routine" will not serve to provide information for all patients who are to experience the same treatment. (3) Patients would rather know the truth about what they will experience, than be told, "It won't hurt." (4) Patients will experience less emotional and possibly less physical trauma during treatment, if they have been told what to expect with detail and explicitness. For planning in relation to a broad general statement about the stated purpose of the study, 3N might have anticipated that her findings could be interpreted to mean that there are several types of emotional support that can be provided for patients and that will result in facilitating the insertion of the gastric tube. She might have suggested that the facilitations would be in terms of both less emotional tension and physical discomfort for the patient and less time needed for the treatment. In her planning, she would have delineated several additional broad statements and indicated that they were illustrative of statements she expected to make about meanings of the facts she expected to find.

Particularly where hypothetical data are used, the investigator should elaborate planning to the extent that he has a clear, written description of what the counterpart processes will be and materials will look like when the actual data are analyzed and reported. The delineation should clarify for him exactly what he will be doing and the appearance of the results. It should be such that another knowledgeable reader would have no difficulty understanding the plan. One characteristic that distinguishes research from other types of studies is the complete design that permits others to replicate the study. Some believe that detailed explicitness of design can wait for the writing of the report of the study. Most, however, believe that the design should be such that another researcher might complete the study, whether or not the designer ever does so. Again, since all may interpret findings according to individual bias and interest, it may be argued that planning potential interpretations is moving beyond that needed as a part of the design. However, it is no more difficult to do it as part of the planning of the design than to delay it until data are in hand. Still more important is that thinking through these details, and putting some on paper, can serve one additional test of the goodness of the

Sufficient Elaboration to Provide Usable Pattern

plan. It can serve to justify asking others to give of their time to contribute to the study.

Differences Should Be Encouraged

Just as interpretations of the facts may reflect the interest and bias of the individual making the interpretations, so implications, suggested in the light of the interpretations, will reflect the interest of the individual making the implications. There may be many suggestions for actions stemming from a single interpretation. There may be seemingly unlimited numbers of suggested actions stemming, indirectly through the interpretations, from a single fact or set of facts. According to the individuals making them, there will be differences in suggested meanings of facts. Similarly, there will be differences in suggestions about actions to be taken. Researchers should be encouraged to suggest as many and varied actions as are warranted by the interpretations of the facts.

Limitations Imposed on Execution of Suggested Actions

The same freedom that prevails in relation to interpretations and suggested actions does not, however, apply to executing actions. That is, an individual may place any interpretations on the meaning of a fact. Within reason, he may make suggestions for any type of actions he wishes. But these privileges of interpretation and implication do not extend to the execution of the actions. The matter of executing the suggested actions need not be of great concern to the investigator, except that consideration of the potential for executing the actions may limit the number of suggestions that reasonably should be made. On the other hand, the investigator should not too greatly limit his suggestions for actions on the basis of obstacles to execution. What is impossible today may well be not only possible but entirely feasible tomorrow.

Audiences: For Step 12, Worker, For Step 13, Management

The identification of the content of implications and recommendations may be clarified by thinking of another means for distinguishing between Steps 12 and 13. As mentioned above, the two steps are made up of three congruent sets of concepts: (1) the detailed facts (findings) and summarized facts; (2) the meanings of each detailed fact (interpretations) and meanings of each summarized set or each major fact (conclusions); and (3) suggestions for detailed actions (implications) and suggestions for broad-reaching, major actions (recommendations). But the distinction between the two steps may also be viewed in relation to the audience toward which the communication about each is addressed. Materials in Step 12 may be thought of as being addressed to the persons on the production line. The materials elaborated in Step 13 will be addressed to management, to persons who provide the materials and programs through which those on the production line are able to apply knowledge to improve the product. This distinction between the two steps applies most directly to the third element: suggested actions. Yet it is not exclusively applicable to any, since management will be interested in details of the findings as well as in summarized findings and recommendations for programs of action.

Interpretations of Descriptive Data

Discussion of materials from a fictional study can illustrate the points being made. This fictitious epidemiological study was done in relation to falls from bed by hospitalized patients. Some of the fictitious findings were reported in terms of frequency of falls per 10,000 patient hospital days associated with each variable listed:

Illustration: 12A

VARIABLES	NUMBER OF FALLS
Bed with short siderails in place	20
Bed with long siderails in place	44
Patient instructed about siderails	14
Patient not instructed about siderails	50
Short siderail, and instructed	4
Short siderail, not instructed	16
Long siderail and instructed	10
Long siderail, not instructed	34

The facts are the same for all persons viewing them. The interpretations might be: (1) For the staff nurses who provide care (production line worker): there apparently are relationships (a) between falls from bed and type (length) of siderails used, and (b) between falls and instructions provided patients about the use of the siderails. (2) The supervisor would ascribe the same meanings but, in addition, she would infer that staff nurses are allowing something to interfere with their providing a very important element of care to patients. (3) The hospital administrator would concur with those interpretations, but he might add the interpretation that the number of falls from bed could be drastic in terms of additional hospital days (should the falls result in bodily injury) and of law suits claiming negligent care (whether or not there was bodily injury). (4) There may be additional interpretations cited for other concerned persons (patient, family, physicians), but for purposes of illustration discussion will be limited to concerns of the two nursing groups and hospital administrators.

Interpretation and Individual Interests

The fictitious facts may be interpreted to mean that, should a patient attempt to get out of bed, if he has been instructed about the use and purpose for short siderails, he will use the siderail to help steady himself and thereby avoid a serious fall. Whereas, with the long siderail, should he try to get out of bed, it means that he must climb over the rail and, though he may be holding onto the rail, he cannot reach the floor with his feet and therefore falls from a height. Another interpretation may be that, when patients receive instructions about siderails, they do not attempt to get out of bed as frequently as when they have not received instructions.

General Interests

Short siderails may have a different meaning for nurses as well as for patients. As nurses instruct the patient about short siderails, they would identify for the patient the purpose the rails are meant to serve and those for which they are not intended. The short siderail is meant primarily to prevent the patient from rolling out of bed. Where a patient wishes to get out of bed, it may serve the additional purpose of providing a firm handle to hold onto for support. The short siderail never holds the connotation, for either the patient or the nurse, of confinement. It is not thought of as a means to *prevent* the patient from getting out of bed. It holds only the connotation appropriate for siderails: a safety device to prevent accidental falls, never a restricting device to confine the patient to the bed.

Staff Nurses Interests

The interpretations in relation to staff nurses might lead to several suggestions for actions (implications). (1) Nurses would consider effective instructions for patients who have siderails placed on their beds. (2) Nurses would provide instructions about siderails whenever they are used, and they might think in terms of reinforcing the instructions several times during the first few days of their use. (3) Staff nurses would use short siderails whenever they had a choice. (4) Staff nurses would be even more careful in their instructions of patients and would be more vigilant where long siderails are in use.

Supervisors Interests

The interpretations would lead, naturally, to implications for actions by the supervisor. (1) The supervisor would check each patient with siderails and confer with the nurse to determine that the patient had been instructed. (2) The supervisor would determine that all of her staff understood the type of instructions needed by patients and that they understood that short siderails were to be used whenever available. (3) The supervisor would assist in planning differences in instructions in relation to long and short siderails. (4) The supervisor would requisition short siderails to replace long ones. (5) The supervisor would plan with her staff to attempt to determine whether differences in patient orientation to time and place and degree of alertness to surroundings make differences in relation to the effectiveness of short or long siderails in preventing falls from bed.

Hospital Administrators Interests

The interpretations for hospital administrators might lead to suggestions for some of the following actions. (1) Review current and pending budget to plan replacement of long siderails with short ones as expeditiously as possible. (2) Seek legal counsel concerning liability and planning for types of reports of such accidents. (3) Establish an accident review committee, consisting of members of several services, including medicine, nursing, pharmacy, engineering, and administration. (4) Check with nursing director to determine policy and planning for promoting staff nurse understanding and alertness to special needs of patients for whom siderails are used.

Conclusions (Abbreviated)

Conclusions to be drawn from these findings are essentially the same as the meanings proposed as interpretations addressed to the staff nurses.

Interpretations of Descriptive Data

There are relationships between falls and length of siderail, with the short siderail being associated with fewer falls than long siderails. There are relationships between falls and instructions of patients about the use and purposes of siderails, with fewer falls associated with instruction than with omission or limited instruction. The most favorable condition is associated with the combination of the two variables: short siderails and instruction of the patients, a condition in which only 4 out of 64 falls occurred.

The recommendations that might be proposed on the basis of the conclusions are: (1) Nursing services should review their supervisory practices to determine means used to ensure that persons providing direct care to patients understand the needs of patients for instructions when bedrails are used. (2) Nurses should identify the content of instructions needed by patients and, through inservice education programs, ensure that all nursing personnel know these and understand how to provide the instructions so that they are meaningful for each individual patient. (3) Hospitals should provide only short siderails. (4) Hospital administration groups might propose to manufacturers that production be limited to types of short siderails. (5) Hospital associations might direct convention discussions to problems and programs of patient safety, with particular concentration on factors associated with falls from bed.

Recommendations (Abbreviated)

Other interpretations and implications may be proposed and, as the interpretations are considered, many questions come to mind about other potentially related facts. For example, what medications patients may have had; what were their ages, what was the lighting situation, how long had siderails been in use at the time of the accident, and others. Other conclusions and recommendations might have been proposed. However, the purpose here was only to delineate sufficient detail to illustrate distinctions between the various processes and outcomes of the analyses of data, which result in the elements of research commonly labeled "findings," "interpretations," "implications," and "summary," "conclusions," "recommendations."

Points Made By Illustration

The illustration makes obvious that the elements of Step 12 are not neatly distinct from those of Step 13. Quite obviously, the investigator will make a generalized statement about the accomplishment of the stated purpose of the study, in the section on detailed report of the findings. He will make a similar, if not the identical, statement in the section devoted to summary, conclusions, and recommendations. Similarly, statements about other major findings will be reported in the detailed report of findings and repeated in the summary section. Nonetheless, the concept of addressing the communication about detailed findings to the persons on the action line can serve as a guide for making the report understandable to all who may be expected to have an interest in one or more aspects of the findings of the study. Addressing the summary, conclusions, and recommendations to management helps the investigator to think in terms of more encompassing facts, of meanings pertinent to persons with extended responsibility, and of actions to be undertaken by persons who provide the means by which persons on the scene of action can effect changes indicated by the findings. The concept of addressing recommendations to management can help remind the investigator of a prerequisite to a study's being considered research: the findings must be generalizable to a population larger than the one from which the findings were obtained. This, in turn, will lead to applicability in settings other than the one in which the findings were obtained.

The proposal that the detailed report of findings, interpretations, and implications be addressed to the worker and that the summary, conclusions, and recommendations be addressed to management is not a necessary procedure in thinking about and reporting research findings. It is really only a gimmick to help the student identify some distinction between these two important sections of a research report. It can also serve as a guide for organizing materials and for decisions about what content to include in what section. But even when the student does use this concept to organize his thinking, he should not allow it to preclude discussion of particular materials in one section or to force discussion of particular materials in another. The suggestion is not meant to be another Procrustean bed.

IDEAS AND RECOMMENDATIONS WITH NO BASIS IN FINDINGS

An additional area to be considered in relation to reporting the outcomes of the study is that of including comments that have no direct base in the findings of the study. This matter is of more concern in developing the report of the study; it seldom needs consideration during the design planning. Nonetheless, materials having no direct base in findings of the study are sometimes included in the report, and students frequently are faced with questions about inclusion of such materials in their own work.

There are actually two distinct types of reporting that may be classified as reporting beyond the basis in the findings. (1) The first type is seen most frequently in enumerations of recommendations that have no basis in the findings. The situation may arise either where the data-gathering plan and process failed to secure anticipated data, or where the design did not include a plan for securing data that would support the recommendations. (2) The second type of reporting beyond the basis in findings occurs when, through the extensive thinking and reading involved in the execution of the study, the researcher has hit upon some ideas that are particularly pertinent to the problem. These ideas evolved after the design was completed and data gathering had begun. There will be no basis for the ideas in the findings of the study, yet anyone interested in the problem of the study would be served by information about the new ideas.

Several factors may influence the first type of recommendations that go beyond the data. (1) The design may have been superficially executed and the data planned for and gathered not relevant to the stated purpose of the study. (2) Through no fault in the design planning, but for various other reasons, data secured were inadequate to support recommendations. For example, the rat sat down in the maze, or the disoriented patients slept the whole night through—there were no "behaviors" to be observed. (3) The researcher had established a mind-set on preconceived ideas and, regardless of the findings, listed the recommendations he had previously thought should be made.

It might seem that this latter influence could be a result of the detailed definition of problem. (Aha! An excuse for limiting that exacting task! Not so.) The researcher who lists recommendations unrelated to his findings and without basis in them usually approached his study with the preconceived ideas that were established even before defining his problem. His motive for undertaking the study was that he might expound his ideas and give weight to his declarations. Such motivation is not necessarily faulty, but it is a detriment to scientific inquiry if it causes blind spots in thinking. Actually, there is merit in approaching a study with preconceived ideas. It is when the preconceived ideas are expressed in the recommendations in the study and have no basis in the findings reported that the reporting is faulty. Where a design has been thoroughly planned and the data identified as being needed are examined in the processes suggested in Steps 10 and 11, there should be no need for the researcher to resort to recommendations that derive directly from preconceived ideas and have no basis in the findings.

Preconceived Ideas

Sometimes factors beyond the investigator's control result in failure to secure needed data. Even then there is no need to list recommendations that have no basis in the findings. The investigator, in such circumstances, should report what actually happened. He should report the data he did secure and the interpretations and recommendations that are warranted by those data. Yet he may believe that others would want to know about recommendations that he believes would have been warranted had he secured his planned-for data. He may be entirely right and he may well include these in his report, but he will identify them for what they are. He will not list them under the major heading, "Recommendations," which, by implication, contains statements based on actual findings. Instead, he will add a section following his listed recommendations, introducing it with an explanation of the nature of the comments in that section.

The Plan Failed

Quasi-Appendages

Similarly, the researcher who has developed some meaningful ideas during the course of his work with the data may very well report the ideas in a separate section. He will do this even though no data have been obtained to serve as bases for comment. The section should be introduced with an explanation of the nature of the comments and the rationale for including them. The researcher will *not* use this device, however, as a catch-all for trivia. These quasi-appendages to the report will report only ideas of major import and with marked pertinence for others who may be interested in the problem, or who may engage in future studies of it.

RECOMMENDATIONS FOR FURTHER STUDY

Recommendations from studies almost always include proposal that further research be done. The less imaginative investigator enlarges this section of his report with recommendations for repetitions or extensions of various facets of his own project. These include suggestions for repetition with a larger sample; with different, but analogous settings; for further testing of the tools, again with larger samples and with different populations; and others. The more imaginative investigator handles suggestions for replications and further testings in a single broad statement. Should a related specific recommendation be indicated, he delineates the rationale for it and describes the specific purpose that may be expected to be served by the repetition or extensions. The imaginative investigator develops recommendations for actions that may be taken on the basis of knowledge revealed in his study to improve various aspects of the problem in various settings. In addition, recommendations developed by the imaginative researcher will include hypotheses to be tested in future studies. When this point is reached in the design, it should be said, the investigator has moved full circle in his planning. If he is developing the report of his investigation, he will have moved full circle in executing his study.

The investigation is begun with the definition of the problem. The problem-defined will include many theories that serve to explain why things are as they are and to provide ideas for actions. From it will derive the statement of purpose for the investigation. Both the statement of purpose and the definition of problem will provide bases for developing hypotheses for future testing. One good hypothesis generates another. The purpose for doing exploratory research is to learn enough about the problem to be able to propose hypotheses. Whether a study's purpose (focus) was to test a hypothesis or to explore an area of concern, what is learned from it should lead to development of hypotheses. When planning Step 13, the researcher will not delineate in detail hypotheses that he expects may be developed in recommendations. He will have intimated some of them in his definition of problem. He will delineate some of the phenomena that may possibly suggest interrelationships and that will be given consideration in the light of new knowledge anticipated from his investigation. He will have begun the thinking that, months or years later, during terminal writing of the report, will result in proposing hypotheses for future testing.

THE COMPLETED STUDY

The goal of research is to reveal new knowledge, and its ultimate goal is to discover relationships among phenomena. The relationships will be described in generalizations that are validated theories and principles. The investigator starts with a specific irritation about which he thinks something should be done and about which he seeks new knowledge. Through his research, he is able to propose a general statement pertinent to his irritation—a generalization that helps to explain the existence of the irritation, to suggest actions that may modify the existence of the irritation, and to indicate the nature of the modification potentially extending from the actions. His generalization may, in turn, serve others as they use it in their specific situations to effect modifications of their specific irritations.

The researcher will have "completed" a study. He will have experienced and acknowledged an awareness of a specific irritation. He will have thought about it, learned about it, and proposed a generalization about irritations similar to and including his own. He will have carefully examined extensive observations of phenomena intimately related to his irritation and to others like it. He will have determined the fitness and validity of his generalization in relation to many specific and individual similar irritations. He will have reported his concern and his observations and consequent thinking about it. He will have provided a generalization supported by facts, to be used to explain specific observations, to guide actions in specific situations, and to predict outcomes of those actions.

In completing his study, the researcher will have revealed new knowledge about the goal he had established in his statement of purpose. Though he may not have reached his goal, he will have served his own purpose by moving toward it. And he will have served others by revealing new knowledge about one facet of an area of concern to many—ultimately, to all.

Glossary

Analysis: Analysis means a separating or breaking up of any whole into its parts so as to find out their nature, proportion, function, relationship, etc.; a statement of the results of this process.

Analyze: Analyze means to separate or break up (any whole) into its parts so as to find out their nature, proportion, function, relationship, etc.; to examine the constituents or parts of; determine the nature or tendencies of.

Assumption: An assumption is a statement describing a fact or condition that is accepted as being true on the basis of logic and reason. The reason for accepting the conditions on this basis is so that the investigator may get on with the study he wishes to do without having to stop to demonstrate that the stated conditions are indeed as logic or reason would lead knowledgeable people to believe them to be.

Component: A component is any of the simple or compound parts of some complex thing or concept.

Component of a Problem-Defined: A component of a problem-defined may be thought of as being composed of many elements and possessing many facets. (See problem-defined, below).

Concept: A concept is a complex of ideas so united as to portray a large general idea. A concept may be essentially ideational, as the concept of liberty, or it may encompass concrete elements, as the concept of table; both of which involve a complex of ideas in contrast to a single idea (if such a thing as a single idea is possible).

Conception: A conception is the complex of ideas that portray a general idea for an individual. One person's conception of liberty may differ in some ways from that of another person, yet both would be examples of the concept of liberty.

Criterion Measure: A criterion measure is a quality, attribute, or characteristic of a variable that may be measured to provide scores by which subjects or things of the same class may be compared with respect to the variable. (The term is most frequently used in relation to a dependent variable, but the concept applies to any variable for which measurements are to be sought or about which observations will be made for the purpose of comparisons among subjects or things.)

Crux: Crux is a crucial point; the essential or most important point; a critical moment.

Crux of the Problem: The crux of the problem is the focal point around which the problem will be defined. It is the "irritation" identified and selected by the researcher as the one about which he thinks something should be done. It is the manifestation of the problem about which he proposes to seek new and extended knowledge, with the view to contributing to alleviation of the problem.

Data: Data is the plural of datum.

Datum: A datum is a fact: a single observable or potentially observable phenomenon. (See phenomenon, below.)

Definition: A definition is an arbitrarily imposed description that allows common understanding.

Definition of Terms (Variables): A definition of a term (any term that designates a variable) is an arbitrarily imposed description that allows common understanding and is composed of three parts or phases:

1. A dictionary or general definition; a generalization that fits all "cases."
2. A pertinent general definition; a generalization that fits only specific cases: those pertinent to the concerns of the study for which the term is being defined.
3. A for-instance definition; an identification or description of a single entity or phenomenon representative of an attribute of the variable being defined. A for-instance is a single case illustrative of the cases identified in the pertinent general, which in turn, are illustrative of the cases described in the general definition. For example: A rose is illustrative of a flower is illustrative of an object of natural beauty.

Criterion measures of the variable are identified in the pertinent general phase of the definition. Single measurements or observations of an attribute of the variable are identified (described) in the for-instance phase of the definition of the term (variable).

Element: An element is a basic, irreducible part or principle of anything, concrete or abstract.

Entity: An entity is a being or existence; a thing that has real and individual existence, in reality or in the mind; anything real in itself. (See phenomenon, below.)

Facet: A facet, literally or figuratively, applies to any of the faces of a many-sided object (facets of a diamond, personality, etc.).

Fact: A fact is an observable phenomenon. (See entity, above, and phenomenon, below.)

Hypothesis: A hypothesis is the delineation of a relationship believed to exist between two phenomena; when substantiated by research, the statement moves to the realm of theory or principle.

Method: Method is "a way of doing anything; mode; process; especially, a regular, orderly, definitive procedure or way of teaching, investigating, etc."

Method of Study: Method of study is the general pattern (the blueprint) for organizing the procedures for gathering all the data for the investigation.

Operational Definition: An operational definition is a definition that uses observable processes, actions, or structural analogues (or explicit and detailed word descriptions of them) to describe concepts represented by the term being defined; an operational definition is an explicit description of a single entity or phenomenon considered to be a concrete referent of the term being defined, whether the referent be an object, a process, or an action; it specifically identifies a single entity or phenomenon to be measured to provide one component of a score of the variable or characteristic being measured and evaluated. Put more succinctly, an operational definition is a description or actual display of a process, action, or object suggested as an analogue or single representative example of what is meant by the term being defined. It is the for-instance portion of a three-phase definition of a term.

Phenomenon: A phenomenon is any fact, circumstance, or experience that is apparent to the senses and that can be scientifically described or appraised: as bereavement is a psychological phenomenon; the appearance or observed features of something experienced as distinguished from reality of the thing itself. The concept of phenomenon encompasses the concept of entity. That is, phenomenon is a more encompassing concept than entity. An oversimplification, for the sake of distinguishing the two, is to view an entity (a being or existence) as a "thing," and a phenomenon as a "thing" *or* a "process." From this, all entities may be classed as phenomena, but not all phenomena are limited to the category of "static" entity. For example, the fact or observation of a leaf on a tree may be identified as either an entity or a phenomenon. The fact or observation of a leaf falling from a tree would be classed as a phenomenon; it would not be classed as an entity.

Population: Population is the general group or category of entities under study; individual entities in the population may be animate or inanimate; animal, vegetable, or mineral. The population is represented in the study by selected subjects from whom the facts needed as data derive.

Problem: The problem may most simply be thought of as an "irritation": the irritation that stimulates interest and prompts investigation.

Problem-Defined: The problem-defined must be thought of as a complex entity, and it may be viewed as being made up of seven components:

1. The irritation or crux of the problem;
2. Elements in the situation; factors supporting, causing, impinging upon the problem;
3. The problem in its largest universe; what others have experienced, learned, and thought about the problem;
4. The ideal situation: no problem exists;
5. Suggestions for moving toward the ideal;
6. Potential results of each suggestion in Component 5;
7. Investigator's frame of reference.

Technique: Technique is "the method of procedure (with reference to practical and formal details) in rendering an artistic work or carrying out a scientific or mechanical operation."

Technique of Data Gathering: Technique of data gathering is the process of making individual observations of phenomena or entities. A technique is a process by which data are collected, one datum at a time. All accumulated observations will compose *the data* for the investigation.

Theory, Principle, Law: A theory, principle, or law is the delineation of a relationship between two facts that may be used to explain phenomena, guide actions, and predict results of actions.

Tools for Obtaining Facts: A tool for obtaining facts (an observation-making tool) is a tool or instrument that is used to assist in the process of securing observations that are to compose the data for the study;

GLOSSARY

examples are a thermometer, a yardstick, an electrocardiograph, a rating scale, a true-false test, an interview schedule, and many, many others.

Tools for Recording Facts: A tool for recording facts (an observation-recording tool) is a form on which observations are recorded; examples are a temperature graph sheet, an electrocardiogram tape, a video tape, a checklist, a bibliography card, a diary, and many, many others.

Type of Research: Type of research refers to the general purpose for doing a particular investigation, such as pursuing a study for the purpose of describing, demonstrating, applying, testing. For example, as a type of research, descriptive research is done for the purpose of revealing new knowledge by describing situations or conditions. Applied research is done for the purpose of learning how to utilize knowledge. General purpose is not to be confused with the definitive statement of purpose, which makes specific the focus of the study.

Setting for Study: Setting for study is the general locale in which the sources of the data are expected to be located and in which the data collection procedures will be carried out.

Source of Data: Source of data is an entity from which facts needed for study are obtained by the investigator. A source may be the study subject from which the facts are obtained by direct observation. A source may, also, be an object or person from which the needed facts, as observed and recorded or reported by others, are obtained. By way of example, the datum, age, may be available to the investigator from various sources. One source may be the study subject: the investigator may ask the patient his age. Another source may be a person who knows the patient: the investigator may ask the patient's relative, his nurse, or his physician. Still another source may be a record: the investigator may obtain the datum, age, from the patient's clinical record. Essentially then, the study subject is the ultimate source from which the facts needed for study derive, and from which the facts needed for study may be directly or indirectly obtained. The study subject may be thought of as a direct or indirect source of the data, but not all direct sources are study subjects. The study subject is the entity which possesses and manifests the observable phenomena of concern (the data sought). The data may be obtained either directly, by observation of the study subject as the source, or indirectly, from other sources, by excerpting or eliciting observations recorded or reported about the study subject.

Study Subject: Study subject is an entity from which the facts needed for study derive: the object of study that manifests the qualities and actions to be observed. (See source of data, above.)

VARIABLES

Variables: A variable is a measurable or potentially measurable component of an object or event that may fluctuate in quantity or quality, or that may be different in quantity or quality from one individual object or event to another individual object or event of the same general class.

Independent and Dependent Variables: The independent and dependent variables are the two variables about which a relationship is delineated in a hypothesis.

Independent Variable: The independent variable is that phenomenon in the hypothesis that, in the experimental study to test the hypothesis, is manipulated by the investigator.

Dependent Variable: The dependent variable is that phenomenon in the hypothesis that, in the experimental study to test the hypothesis, is not manipulated, but is accepted as it occurs.

Extraneous Variables: Extraneous variables are all variables in a hypothesis-testing investigation that are not the independent variable, the dependent variable, or criterion measures of the dependent variable.

Accounted-for Variables: Accounted-for variables are those variables about which observations are gathered during the study for the sake of additional information they will provide, but which actually are not needed in relation to testing the hypothesis.

Controlled-for Variables: Controlled-for variables are those extraneous variables that are apt to affect the dependent variable in a manner similar to the affect of the independent variable. It is to be noted that the designation is controlled-*for*, which should not be confused with controlled, one of the common terms used to refer to the independent variable. These extraneous variables will be controlled for, they will not be controlled or manipulated, per se. The reason for controlling for them is to eliminate the influence of potentially confounding variables.

Confounding Variables: Confounding variables are extraneous variables that influence the dependent variable in the same way the independent variable influences it. There are those who would class confounding variables as those of prime concern, after the independent and dependent variables. It will be noted, however, that, if variables that are apt to confound the findings are controlled for, there will be no confounding variables. Their confounding influence will have been precluded from occurring.

Index

Analysis of data, 259-290
   "rearranging" data, 260-261
   statement of results, 259-260, 288
Assumptions, 127-132
   those made explicit, 128, 130-131
   validity, 129-130

Bias of investigator, 59-60, 84, 294, 299, 304

Cause-effect relationships, 69-70
Component of problem-defined, 1-24
   Component 1, 7-10
   Component 2, 11-13
   Component 3, 13-17
   Component 4, 17-19
   Component 5, 19-23
   Component 6, 19-23
   Component 7, 23
   definition, 2
   seven components, 1, 7-24
Conclusions, 291-292, 306-308
Co-relational relationships, 69-70
Criterion measures, 101, 111-113, 122, 150-154
   relevance, 152-154
   validity, 152-154
Crux of problem, 2, 34, 36
   influence on definition of problem, 39
   natural, 34, 37
   selected, 34, 37-40, 57-59

Data, 133-159
   analysis, 259-290

Data (continued)
   from definition of problem, 136, 139-140, 141, 147-148
   in definition of terms, 119-120, 122, 122-124, 136, 141-143, 147-148
   descriptive, 144-149, 155-158, 206-211, 215-219, 242, 250, 253-257, 269, 283-285
   display, 261-288
   ground-ham-on-rye, 137-139
   hypothetical, 214, 247-249, 251-257, 302, 303
   kinds needed, 134-135, 136, 149, 155-158
   number needed, 223-224
   one-at-a-time, 134, 144, 147, 181, 183-184, 205-206, 244, 252, 267-268
   qualitative, 144-149
   quantification, 145-147
   quantitative, 144-149
   raw versus calculated, 277-278
   sources, 162, 167-173
Datum, 133, 135
   tracing a single datum, 244-249, 267-268
Data collection, 223-238
   "actual study," misnomer, 223
   what, 225-234
   when, 235
   where, 235-236
   who, 224-238
   with whom, 226-229, 233
   informing participants, 226-229
Definition of problem, 1-62
   components, 1-24
   purposes served, 53-54, 61, 296-299

Index

Definitions of terms, 101-126
   from definition of problem, 116-117
   investigator's right, 116
   terms defined by others, 117-119
   terms that must be defined, 119-123
   three phases, 102-104, 122-124, 125-126, 141
Display of data, 261-288
   calculated data, 277-278
   descriptive data, 283-285
   graphics, 278-282
   tables, 261-288

Fact, 2, 63, 64-65, 74-76, 135, 136, 292-293
   observable phenomena, 2, 284-285
   and principle, 73-76
   raw materials of research, 135, 136
   use, 74-76
Findings, 292-310
Focus of study, 63, 83-93
   statement of purpose, 63-100

Geodesic dome, 24-48
   analogue to problem-defined, 24, 31-48
Ground-ham-on-rye, 137-139

Hypothesis, 63-93
   attributes, 65, 71-76, 80-82
   descriptive proposition, 76-80
   focus of study, 83-93
   statement of purpose, 83-93
Hypothetical data, 214, 247-249, 251-257, 302, 303

Implications, 291-308
   from interpretations, 291, 294-296, 299-300, 304-308
Interpretations of data, 291-308
   interest of investigator, 295, 299, 305
   responsibility of investigator, 296, 299-300
   tie to definition of problem, 297-299
   tie to statement of purpose, 295-296

Labels for Tables, 260-277
   content, 269
   process of development, 269-277

Method, 161-180
   analogue of diagnosis, 164-167
   confusion with technique, 162-167
   experimental, 174, 176
   four methods, 173-176
   historical, 173, 175
   philosophical, 173, 174
   and sources of data, 167-172
   survey, 174, 175-176

Nurses study nursing problems, 195-196, 295
Nursing diagnosis, 165

Operational definition, 70, 102, 113-115
Organizing data, 239-258
   bonus findings, 243
   descriptive data, 242, 250, 253-257
   fundamentals of process, 249, 251
   manual organizing—advantages, 250
   mechanical organizers, 249-250, 252
   questions as guides, 241-243
   statement of purpose as focus, 241-242
   tools, 244-256
   tracing a single datum, 244-249
   using observation-recording tool, 244-249
Outcomes, 291-311
   conclusions, 291-292, 306-308
   findings, 292-310
   implications, 291-308
   interpretations, 293, 295, 299, 305
   recommendations, 291-292, 307-308, 310

Precision
   of definition, 111-114
   identity of facts, 277
   of statement, 85, 92, 104, 133

Principle, 63-83
  attributes, 65, 72-76, 80-82
  law, 62
  theory, 63-70
  use, 73-76
Problem, 1
  definition of, 1-62
  versus purpose, 3-4
Problem-defined, 1
  analogy in geodesic dome, 24-48
  components, 1, 7-24
Purpose, 2-4, 63-100

Questions:
  in definition of problem, 45-46
  as guides to organization of data, 241-243
  in questionnaire-interview schedule, 215-220
  as statement of purpose, 83, 98-99

Recommendations, 291-292, 307-309, 310
Relevance, 150-152
Review of literature, 15-16, 49-52, 99
  annotated bibliography, 50

Sources of data, 162, 167-173, 224
  existing records, 171
  influence of cost and time, 170
  permission to use sources, 225-226
  relation to method, 167-172
Statement of purpose, 2-4, 63-100
  declarative sentence, 83-85, 94-98
  focus of study, 83-98
  hypothesis, 83-93
  interpreting findings, 295-296
  organizing data, 241-242
  question, 83, 98-99
Statistics:
  analysis of covariance, 110
  numbers and relations to facts, 157-158, 250
  planning data analysis, 286
  planning numbers of data, 223-224
  representatives of facts, 157-158, 250

Study subject, 162, 168-170, 224, 227-229, 230-233
  consent, 228-229
  representative of population, 233
  rights of human subjects, 232

Tables, 261-288
  calculated data, 277-278
  communicate with reader, 264, 277, 284
  descriptive data, 283-285
  labels for tables, 296-277
  raw data, 277-278
  uncluttered tables, 286-287
  work tables, 286-287
Technique, 161-167, 181-200
  adopt, adapt, combine, 184
  analogue to prescribed treatment, 166
  one-datum-at-a-time, 181, 183-184
  using concept rather than process, 185, 191
Techniques, 186-198
  activity analysis, 195
  content analysis, 190-193
  critical incident, 191, 193-194
  diary, 194
  interview, 190
  nonparticipant observation, 187-188
  nursing audit, 192
  participant observation, 186-187
  process recording, 193-194
  projective techniques, 197
  Q-sort, 198
  questionnaire, 188-190
  record analysis, 192-193
  time sampling, 195-197
  time study, 196
  work sampling, 195
Theoretical framework, 16, 52-54, 297-299
Theory, 62, 63-83
  law, 63-70
  principle, 63-70
Tools, 201-222
  adopt, adapt, combine, 203-205
  data-observing, 201-203

Tools (continued)
   data-organizing, 244, 249-250
   data-recording, 201-203
   develop from scratch, 205-214
   one-datum-at-a-time, 205-211
   pretest, 188-190, 205-206, 214
   questionnaire/interview schedule, 215-220
   written instructions for use, 208-211

Variables, 101
   dependent, 101, 105, 120
   extraneous, 101, 105-111
   independent, 101, 105, 120
   introduction of independent, 224, 230-237
Variables, extraneous, 105-110
   accounted-for, 106-108
   confounding, 105-108
   controlled-for, 105, 109-110